A HISTORY OF EDUCATION IN PUBLIC HEALTH

HEALTH THAT MOCKS THE DOCTORS' RULES

A HISTORY
OF EDUCATION IN
PUBLIC HEALTH

HEALTH THAT MOCKS THE
DOCTORS' RULES

EDITORS

ELIZABETH FEE

AND

ROY M. ACHESON

'Health that mocks the doctor's rules
Knowledge never learned of schools'
JOHN GREENLEAF WHITTIER

1991

OXFORD UNIVERSITY PRESS

OXFORD   NEW YORK

Oxford University Press, Walton Street, Oxford OX2 6DP

Oxford New York Toronto
Delhi Bombay Calcutta Madras Karachi
Petaling Jaya Singapore Hong Kong Tokyo
Nairobi Dar es Salaam Cape Town
Melbourne Auckland

and associated companies in
Berlin Ibadan

Oxford is a trade mark of Oxford University Press

Published in the United States
by Oxford University Press, New York

British Library Cataloguing in Publication Data
A history of education in public health: health that mocks the doctors' rules.
1. Public health, history
I. Fee, Elizabeth II. Acheson, Roy M. (Roy Malcolm) 1921–363.09
ISBN 0–19–261757–5

Library of Congress Cataloging in Publication Data
Data applied for

Typeset by Promenade Graphics
and Printed in Great Britain by
St Edmundsbury Press,
Bury St Edmunds, Suffolk

ARTHUR VISELTEAR

A RESPECTED SCHOLAR AND

A WISE FRIEND

CONTENTS

CONTRIBUTORS

ROY ACHESON, MD, SCD, FRCP, FFPHM, FFOM
*Professor Emeritus of Community Medicine, University of Cambridge
and Fellow of Churchill College*

★

ELIZABETH FEE, MA, PHD
*Associate Professor of Health Policy, Johns Hopkins School of Hygiene
and Public Health, Baltimore, Maryland*

★

MARGOT JEFFERYS, BSC(ECON)
Professor Emeritus of Sociology, University of London

★

JOYCE LASHOF, MD
*Dean, School of Public Health, University of California,
Berkeley, California*

★

JANE LEWIS, PHD
*Reader in Social Administration, London School of Economics,
London*

★

DOROTHY PORTER, PHD
*Assistant Professor, Department of the History of Science,
Harvard University, Cambridge, Massachusetts*

★

BARBARA GUTMANN ROSENKRANTZ, PHD
*Professor of the History of Science, Harvard University,
Cambridge, Massachusetts*

★

ARTHUR VISELTEAR, PHD, MPH
*Associate Professor of the History of Medicine and Public Health,
Yale University School of Medicine, New Haven, Connecticut*

ACKNOWLEDGEMENTS

The editors have received generous assistance from the Rockefeller Foundation of New York and the Wellcome Trust of London. Their contributions towards the costs of library and archive research, travel, and general support have made the preparation of this book possible. They enabled all the authors to spend a week together to discuss plans for the book in the Rockefeller Foundation's Study and Conference Center in Bellagio in August 1987. The editors are grateful for the opportunity to write and edit as Scholars in Residence in Bellagio in the spring of 1989.

The editors also thank Bill Bynum, Gordon Smith, Penelope Poole, and Ann Smith for their support and advice, and Corelli Barnett for his wise and detailed criticisms of parts of the text.

Introduction

ROY ACHESON AND ELIZABETH FEE

1. Preamble

This book examines the historical development of education and training in public health in Britain and the United States. Although the two countries share many of the same political, scientific, and medical cultures and traditions, there are important differences between them in the organization of public health, many of which stem from the different relation of public health to the medical profession.

In Britain, as public health developed, it became a medical specialty; in the United States, where the boundaries of public health have always been more permeable, those entering the field may come from a range of disciplines and professions, including medicine, law, engineering, nursing, administration, mathematics, biochemistry, sociology, and economics. The differences between the relations of public health to medicine in Britain and the United States have in turn been a result of the different conditions in each country during the period when their systems for public health education were first developed. Britain took its first steps towards the organization of public health training in the mid-nineteenth century; the United States did not do so until 50 years later.

2. The origins of public health in Britain and the United States

The development of public health in Britain and the United States began in the context of industrialization. The disastrous social consequences of the industrial revolution for the working class, who were crowded into insanitary housing and subject to periodic outbreaks of cholera and other epidemic and endemic diseases, aroused Edwin Chadwick's concern for the 'sanitary conditions of the labouring classes in Great Britain'.[1] Chadwick himself had stressed the importance of sanitary engineering

---

[1] Chadwick, E. *General report on the sanitary conditions of the labouring classes of Great Britain, 1842*, edited and reprinted by M. W. Flinn, 1965. Edinburgh University Press.

but the issue was soon taken up in broader terms by the medical profession who supported a demand for 'state medicine', with medical officers of health, paid by local governments, responsible for the public health services. A postgraduate certificate in state medicine was first introduced in 1871; it was awarded by examination to medically qualified persons and provided in effect a licence to practice public health on a full-time basis. The General Medical Council laid down the rules and regulations governing the qualification, thus providing a form of central control for the profession of public health as a medical specialty. Then and for some decades to come, there was an abundance of medical practitioners who had great difficulty in eking out a living by providing patient care on a fee-for-service basis. Some of these undertook public health work part-time for extra income, and some were only too glad to do the extra study necessary to obtain what was to be called a Diploma in Public Health (DPH) in return for a full-time job with a steady local government salary. In Britain, there is only one school specifically devoted to public health, the London School of Hygiene and Tropical Medicine, which was founded with support from the Rockefeller Foundation in 1924. While the London School would play an important role in research and in training both national and foreign specialists, it had a considerable degree of independence within the University of London. Its principal activity on the domestic side was to provide courses in preparation for the statutory DPH examination. It rapidly became the most important centre in the country in this respect. In the early 1970s, the DPH was discontinued and a University of London master's degree in social medicine took its place.

In the United States, similarly wretched social conditions in the industrial cities and the rural areas of the southern states stimulated progressive voluntary movements, physicians, and other concerned citizens to campaign for increased attention to public health. A weak central government left public health organization to the individual states, with the result that the development of public health varied widely across the country. In several cities, most notably Boston and Philadelphia, universities and colleges began courses and programmes to train public health officers. The United States Public Health Service, the United States Army, the Rockefeller Foundation, and the American Public Health Association were the main organizations concerned with public health on a national and international level. In 1914, the officers of the Rockefeller Foundation decided to create a national system of education for public health to train national and international public health officers. By this time, however, the medical profession had already become well organized. The system of medical education had already been reformed along scientific lines, the numbers entering medicine had already been strictly controlled, and the profession was jealously guarding its autonomy and the basis of its new-found economic success. State salaries in public health proved unattractive to physicians when contrasted with the high incomes to be made in clinical practice. Choosing a career in public health administration meant that a physician would have to sacrifice at least half, and often far more, of his potential earning power. Hermann Biggs, for example, one of the great pioneers of public health administration, was in a position to take up the banner for public health and devote himself to community well-being because he had first become wealthy through a successful medical practice.

As a result of the economic differential between clinical medicine and public health in the United States, careers in public health have never attracted large numbers of physicians. In the early decades of the twentieth century, schools of public health were established in the United States. These were usually separate institutions, sometimes departments of medical schools, but always connected to universities. Four of the first eight universities to have accredited schools of public health were private: Johns Hopkins, Harvard, Columbia, and Yale. The other four were public: Michigan, Minnesota, North Carolina, and California at Berkeley. When schools of public health were built, they were open to physicians and other professional groups: engineers, nurses, statisticians, bacteriologists, chemists, administrators, sociologists, and economists. The contributions of these professions to public health research and practice have broadened the scope and perspectives of public health; in the United States, public health has thus never been simply a medical specialty. Now, there are a total of 25 schools of public health in the United States. Graduates of these schools enter a large variety of roles in the health system, in federal and state government, academia, private organizations, and foundations.

Britain and the United States also have quite different forms of organization of their curative health services. In Britain, the organization of the National Health Service provides an opportunity for planning to be based on epidemiological knowledge of community needs; it also allows for considerable attention to be paid to preventive medicine, both through public health and general practitioner services. This potential is not always realized in practice. In the United States, the dominance of fee-for-service medicine, the plethora of private and governmental reimbursement mechanisms, and the large population of the uninsured and the under-insured, all mitigate against rational planning of health services based on need. In the former context, a reasonable distribution of resources between public health, preventive services, curative care, and long-term care is possible, at least in principle; in the latter context, public health services are left to provide all the services rejected by the private medical care system as unprofitable. While the medical care system absorbs the lion's share of the resources, the public health service may be placed on a semi-starvation diet. The major problems of public health in the United States are thus political and economic, as indeed, they also are in Britain.

3. New schools of public health

The British and United States' models of public health and medical care have been influential in many other parts of the world. Interest in public health is again growing rapidly and many countries are now anxious to establish new schools or institutes of public health, or to reopen, modify, or update the ones they already have. We therefore believe that it is both appropriate and necessary to examine, in some detail, the problems and issues that have emerged in the history of education for public health in Britain and the United States. The purpose of such an analysis is not to propose answers to the questions of contemporary training and education in public health; rather, it is to provide information and perspectives which we hope will be of value to those facing similar issues now and in the future.

Basic questions about the form of education for public health have endured and will continue to be debated. Who should receive specialized education for public health? What should be taught and who should do the teaching? How should such education be financed and organized? What is the appropriate mix of disciplines that the public health practitioner needs to know—basic biological sciences; social and behavioural sciences; laboratory and field research; management and administrative methods; epidemiology and biostatistics; the history and philosophy of public health? What is the appropriate balance between theoretical knowledge and practical experience in the training of future practitioners? How should the educational structure relate to professional practice in terms of the specific credentials appropriate for particular roles in the health system? How can practical training best be provided to prepare public health workers for their future responsibilities? What is the proper role of physicians, nurses, engineers, statisticians, sociologists, economists, etc., and how should these different professional groups relate to each other within the larger endeavour of public health? These questions, and more, are all of considerable contemporary interest and the experiences of the United States and United Kingdom during the last century can provide instructive examples—for themselves and for others.

4. Public health: theory and practice

Charles-Edward Amory Winslow called public health the Great Crusade, and those who have chosen to enter this field have usually combined a commitment to social reform with a concern for scientific analysis and understanding. The particular issues dominant in public health and the methods chosen to confront problems have, however, changed radically over time. In the mid-nineteenth century, public health relied on epidemiological methods and chemical analyses to identify polluted water supplies. With the discovery of bacteria, laboratory identification and study of specific micro-organisms overshadowed interest in general environmental reform. When the limits of bacteriological knowledge became evident, great emphasis was placed on public health nursing and popular health education as a means of changing people's behaviour. Epidemiology and biostatistics became the most important tools for analysing the causes and distribution of disease. After the Second World War, with increasing concern about chronic illness, mental illness, and the problems of ageing populations, the social and behavioural sciences received more attention—although the potential applications of these sciences to public health have still not been sufficiently realized. Issues newly defined as social and health problems in the 1960s, 1970s, and 1980s have in turn shaped and reshaped the boundaries of public health: the field has expanded to include such major issues as population control, international health, environmental health, occupational hazards, medical care organization, health economics, alcoholism, drug abuse, and AIDS. With the emergence of new health problems on to the national and international stage, new forms of knowledge and analysis have been needed, and the mix of sciences, professions, and disciplines in public health have altered in response to the new needs.

Public health has therefore always been a multidisciplinary field, in which the mix of contributing disciplines changes constantly.[2] This means that training in public health will always be subject to revision to ensure that the knowledge and insights from all relevant fields are being put to the best possible use. In the past, there has been a tendency to

[2] Acheson, Roy M. (1980). Community medicine: discipline or topic? profession or endeavour? *Community Medicine*, **2**, 2–6.

favour the methods and approaches of the biological and laboratory sciences and this still needs to be balanced by an equivalent emphasis on social analysis: public health problems are both social and biological. Similarly, the emphasis on the production of new knowledge by research needs to be balanced by an equivalent emphasis on the application of that knowledge in practice. The application of knowledge may involve a large range of methods and techniques: management and administration, mass communications, legislation and lobbying, and the ability to organize diverse communities towards specific goals. These techniques must be taught and public health practitioners must be capable of choosing the most appropriate techniques for dealing with specific problems.

It means also that there will be a wide range of variation, within each of the component disciplines, in the material taught and the perspectives of the teachers. An issue such as drug addiction will be dealt with from the point of view of sociological, psychological, biochemical, and economic theory as well as in terms of practical field work and programme administration. The current system of rewards within the university takes account of research and scientific publications, and gives little credit for the practical application of knowledge. But public health without practical application is a theoretical exercise of scant worth. If schools of public health want to provide their students with practical training of a high quality, better methods will have to be found for recruiting, evaluating, and rewarding those responsible for the practical training component of the curriculum.

Schools of public health are part of a university structure and, like schools of law or medicine, their orientation is professional and practical. Many of the disciplines contributing to public health have nevertheless their own established corpus of knowledge and identity in universities. Statistics, economics, history, sociology, microbiology, and other subjects which compose the public health of today often have generic departments in the university. There is frequently a problem when the career development of teachers responsible for applied work in public health is judged by their academic peers in the basic disciplines because again, theoretical work is generally more highly valued in the academy than are its practical applications. On the other hand, many institutions of higher education are having to reconsider their objectives in the light of increasing demands from employers for individuals capable of exercising leadership while also possessing expert knowledge in specific technical areas. This problem of finding the proper balance between theoretical and practical knowledge is fundamental to education and training in public health.

5. Range of needs for education and training

Another dimension of complexity in the education and training of people for careers in public health is the variety of different positions for which people in public health may be prepared, and the philosophy and content of the education and training appropriate for different levels of responsibility and expertise. Some will be accountable for the management and administration of large bureaucratic organizations; some will be developing statistical or microbiological methods for seeking the source of a disease outbreak; some will do routine testing of the water supplies and some will conduct the population surveys necessary for health planning. How are all these to be given appropriate levels of education and training?

In the paper Wickliffe Rose presented to a small, but important Conference at the Rockefeller Foundation offices in New York in 1914, he suggested that there should be three grades of public health workers: the leaders, responsible for planning, organization, and administration; the specialists, who would be experts in specific disciplines of public health; and the 'foot soldiers' or field-workers who would do most of the practical tasks. This division was accepted by those at the conference, and is compatible with much that has happened since. In this form of organization, the first two groups, the leaders and the specialists, have advanced university degrees in medicine or the sciences and specialized training in public health; the third group, the 'foot soldiers' are likely to have had short practical training programmes. Such an organization, however, is hierarchical and rather rigid; ideally, there should be mechanisms for leadership to develop from the base, for lower level workers to be involved in planning and organization, opportunities for continuing professional education, and the organizational flexibility to make the best use of whatever talents are available. Too often, public health agencies have suffered from a bureaucratic stuffiness that stifles initiative and creativity.

We have already stated that some look upon public health as a profession in its own right; to others, it is a specialty of medicine. In some countries medical people have an important role to play in the administration and control of public health services at all levels of government. But developing countries may well ask whether physicians should have the dominant role either in the administration of the public health services or in the training and education of those who are to work there. Should, for instance, Third World countries which have inherited the British colonial system of administration continue to adhere to it, or should they encourage a new cadre of public health professionals? The

British tradition which has dispersed medically trained health officers throughout developing countries in much of the world is not now necessarily an appropriate one for countries with a low per capita income. Economic realities help determine the balance between public health workers who are medically trained and those who are not. The economic and professional issues are complex and will vary according to place and time, but they cannot be ignored by planners or educators.

6. A multiplicity of names

The continuing struggle over the relationship of public health to medicine explains why so many terms have been used in the field, either to define public health or to indicate the specific contributions of the medical profession. Chadwick, the English pioneer, used the expression 'public health' and called the Parliamentary Act of 1848, of which he was the chief architect, the first Public Health Act. 'Public health' clearly referred to the health of the public in broad terms and had no necessary connection to medical practice. The terms 'sanitary reform', 'sanitary engineering', and 'sanitary science', were popular at that time, and were all associated with the movement to clean up the industrial environment and city streets, to provide clean water, air, milk, and food, and to remove and dispose of wastes safely. None of these activities had a connection with the medical profession *per se*. They were associated with voluntary reform movements, and with the contributions of engineers, chemists, biologists, and bacteriologists (Chapter 1). The older French term *hygiène* was also used in the sense of maintaining and promoting health; Edmund Parkes, who was the first Professor of Hygiene in the Royal Army Medical Corps School of Medicine at Netley, used it for his remarkable textbook, *A manual of practical hygiene*, which dominated the field for a couple of decades towards the end of the nineteenth century.[3] In his introduction, Parkes defined hygiene as 'the art of preserving health' and he laid no more emphasis on 'disease' or 'medicine' in his concept of hygiene than had Chadwick in his view of public health.[4]

In contrast with the terms: public health; sanitary reform; sanitary engineering; sanitary science; and hygiene, others were specifically coined to stress the medical contribution to public health: state medi-

[3] Parkes, Edmund A. (1864). *A manual of practical hygiene* (1st ed). Churchill, London.
[4] To add further confusion, William Henry Welch would later introduce the term 'hygiene' into the American context in a different sense: he used it to refer to the German research tradition in 'physiological hygiene' as exemplified by Max von Pettenkofer's Institute of Hygiene in Munich—the rallying standard for his own campaign to strengthen the medical and scientific contribution to public health in the United States.

cine; public health medicine; preventive medicine; social medicine; community medicine; and even clinical epidemiology, to which we shall return. State medicine and public medicine (or public health medicine), originated in the nineteenth century with Henry Rumsey and William Farr respectively. Although neither their origins nor their early usage are clear, social medicine dates back for over 100 years and preventive medicine probably for longer.[5] Community medicine is a concept of the twentieth century and one which in Britain at least appears to have fulfilled its purpose (see Chapter 6).

William Farr used the expressions 'public medicine' or 'public health medicine' to emphasize that public health had a medical component and that medicine had a responsibility for the public health. He was an active member of the British Medical Association and believed that the state should accept responsibility for surveillance and promotion of the public health. His special interest was the development of nosology and the classification of death certificates by cause of death and by social circumstances of the decedent. Accurate and sound statistical information, he said, was essential to monitor the public health and learn about the epidemiology of disease. The data necessary to do this could neither be collected nor analysed without the active participation of the medical profession.

It was Henry Rumsey who coined the expression 'state medicine' in England. He and his supporters, among whom Farr was very active, asserted that medical contributions were essential to public health and that there should be a cadre of properly trained 'medical men' working full time. Full-time work meant full-time pay, and this was quite incompatible with depending for a living on providing care to fee-paying patients. The patient of the state physician was the population, so the population in the form of the State should reimburse him. Rumsey and the British Medical Association directly confronted the government with this argument and won their case (Chapter 2). Not only was state medicine a specialty of medicine, but it was one with its own state-controlled training programme. The term had fallen out of favour in Britain by the turn of the century. By then, the term 'public health' had been reinstated and had, in the interim, absorbed the associations and responsibilities of 'state medicine'.

The term 'social medicine' has been associated through the years with

---

[5] Rosen, George (1947). What is social medicine? *Bulletin of the History of Medicine*, **21**, 674–733; Porter, Dorothy and Porter, Roy (1988). What was social medicine? An historiographical essay, *Journal of Historical Sociology*, **1**, 90–106; Leavitt, Judith W. (1980). Public health and preventive medicine. In *The education of American physicians* (ed. Ronald L. Numbers), pp. 250–72. University of California Press, Berkeley and Los Angeles.

writers such as Jules Guérin, René Sands, and Henry Sigerist. Their interest lay in the larger social determinants of health and illness—a perspective not limited to the effects of disease on an individual's body or mind, but encompassing the total influence of the physical and social environment on human well-being and disease. In Britain, from the late 1930s, the term acquired a sense very much its own, because it was adopted by members of an important movement in academic medicine and population research (Chapters 6 and 8). In Britain, Ireland, and some of the Commonwealth countries, the term 'community medicine' subsequently came in vogue for 15 years and was used to replace both public health and social medicine. It described a new medical specialty which attempted to reunite service and academic public health at a time when the British National Health Service was undergoing its first major reorganization in the 1970s. The term 'community medicine' has different meanings in different contexts. In the United States, the term is often applied to medical institutions or departments concerned with the community context of health and medical care, and in Britain it has now been replaced by 'public health medicine'.

'Preventive medicine' is an old expression and the idea that medicine might prevent disease as well as ameliorate, if not cure it, dates back for centuries. Medical officers of health in Britain in the late nineteenth century used the term 'preventive medicine' to express a contrast with curative medicine and to claim an equal importance for it, and therefore for themselves; preventive medicine was often used by them as a synonym for public health (Chapter 3). In the twentieth century, preventive medicine has come to acquire the more restricted connotation of clinical preventive medicine: the endeavour on the part of doctors to prevent disease in individual patients.[6] This contrasts with the interest of public health in preventing disease on a population basis. The two are not mutually exclusive, however. Immunization, for example, can be used in either setting: when a doctor immunizes one child, it is preventive medicine; when he or she plans an immunization campaign for a whole population, it is public health. During the 1960s in the United States, medical school departments of preventive medicine became involved in demonstration health programmes for under-served populations and many changed their names to 'community medicine', or added this to their title. Departments that continue to be concerned with the broader community aspects of health and health care delivery usually call themselves departments of community medicine, or more complexly,

---

[6] Leavitt, Judith W. (1980). Public health and preventive medicine. In *The education of American physicians* (ed. Ronald L. Numbers), pp. 250–72. University of California Press, Berkeley and Los Angeles.

departments of community medicine and/or preventive medicine and/or family medicine.

Since its establishment in 1913, the Rockefeller Foundation has been concerned to forge a productive link between public health and clinical medicine. The first, and perhaps the most important of all the steps it has taken in this direction was to create the Johns Hopkins School of Hygiene and Public Health on the same campus in Baltimore as the Johns Hopkins School of Medicine, which it had taken as the model of modern science-based medical education (Chapter 5).[7] This move had the dual purpose of enabling scientific public health to develop alongside scientific clinical medicine, and more fundamentally, to forge a link between medical science and public health in the United States.

The Rockefeller Foundation also surveyed all the medical schools in the United States to determine the extent to which preventive medicine was a regular part of the curriculum, as a move towards ensuring that it would become a fundamental component of medical education. More or less simultaneously in Britain, Sir George Newman, the first Chief Medical Officer to the Ministry of Health, conducted a similar survey and, through the authority of the General Medical Council, introduced preventive medicine as a compulsory subject in the national curriculum. These were the first of many renewed efforts to promote the teaching of preventive medicine in medical schools. But despite these repeated efforts, preventive medicine teaching has rarely thrived in medical schools, either in the United States or in Britain. Those responsible for teaching the subject sometimes forget the strength of the emotional concern among students to learn how to heal. This together with pressures toward concentrating time, attention, and resources on curative medicine overwhelm virtually all efforts to establish an effective and balanced curriculum.

The potential benefit to be derived from a close partnership between clinical medicine and public health is still great, yet attempts to realize it have been disappointing. Throughout the world clinical medicine has tended to concentrate its efforts and resources narrowly—albeit successfully—to the detriment of the real health problems of the times. The Rockefeller Foundation in attempting to overcome this problem has developed a programme which draws the attention of clinicians to the importance of epidemiology in the practice of clinical medicine by providing a perspective that sets the work of the hospital and the doctor's

---

[7] Fee, Elizabeth (1987). *Disease and discovery: a history of the Johns Hopkins School of Hygiene and Public Health, 1916–1939*. The Johns Hopkins University Press, Baltimore, Maryland.

office against the health needs of the total population.[8] Following John Paul and others, Kerr White used the term 'clinical epidemiology' to suggest that the medical profession must learn how to make its resources available equitably by taking into account the true health needs of the population, rather than confining its attention to expressed demand.[9] Implementation of such a programme would require the close co-operation between an epidemiologically informed medical profession and health planners with the political will and economic ability to distribute resources according to need. Although some countries have made considerable progress in this direction, it remains an ideal for the future. The problems of rational resource allocation between various public health, preventive services, curative care, and long-term care, are still to be solved.

7. Organization of the book

In this book we present a series of co-ordinated essays which are concerned with how—and how differently—two prosperous countries with different methods of government, but sharing a common language and many of the same cultural and political values, have tackled the establishment of a training system in public health. We believe that it will be the first publication to bring together the contributions of historians, from both sides of the Atlantic, who have been engaged in extended his-

[8] Evans, John R. (1982). Measurement and management in medicine and health services: training needs and opportunities. In *Health and populations* (ed. M. Lipkin and H. Lybrand), pp. 3–43. Praeger, New York.

[9] The introduction of the term 'clinical epidemiology' is attributed to John Rodman Paul, Professor of Preventive Medicine at Yale University. He in turn attributes the concepts upon which he drew to William H. Welch and W.H. Frost, both of Johns Hopkins University. Paul stated that whereas epidemiologists deal with large groups of people, the clinical epidemiologist dealt with small groups, a family or small community. The clinical epidemiologist, said Paul in 1938, started:

. . . with a sick individual and cautiously branches out into the setting where the patient became sick . . . He is anxious to analyze the intimate details under which his patient became ill. He is also anxious to search for other members of the patient's family, or community groups who are actually, or potentially ill. It is his aim to thus place his patient in the pattern in which he belongs, rather than to regard him as a lone sick man who has suddenly popped out of a health setting; and it is also his aim to bring his judgment to bear upon the situation, as well as on the patient.

See Paul, John R. (1958). Definitions and attitudes. In *Clinical Epidemiology*, pp. 7–8. University of Chicago Press, Chicago, Illinois; Paul, John R. (1971). A clinician's place in academic preventive medicine: my favourite hobby. *Bulletin of the New York Academy of Medicine*, **47**, 1263; Viseltear, Arthur J. (1982). John R. Paul and the definition of preventive medicine. *Yale Journal of Biology and Medicine*, **55**, 167–72.

torical research on aspects of the development of education and training in public health.[10] Our aim is to make our work accessible to those who can make practical use of the book's insights and conclusions as well as to lay the foundations for a new field of historical study. The chapters discuss various issues and problems in education and training for public health which have recurred over the decades, and which we can confidently predict will continue to recur. The reader will note some differences of interpretation between our authors; we have not tried to impose a single editorial view but have welcomed the expression of a variety of perspectives. In some instances, the same events will be discussed by several authors in different contexts; we believe that the resulting overlap between the chapters is in the best interest of our readers.

In the first chapter, Elizabeth Fee and Dorothy Porter provide an historical introduction to what follows by explaining the development of public health in Britain and the United States in the nineteenth century. They discuss the different responses of the medical profession, and the relative importance of sanitary engineering, bacteriology, and social reform in shaping responses to the health problems produced by industrialization. They show why education and training patterns were to develop in such strikingly different ways in the two countries. In Chapter 2, Roy Acheson traces the development of the Diploma in Public Health in Britain and its practical and academic requirements through the nineteenth century. He describes the roles played by the British Medical Association, the universities, the Royal Medical Colleges and the General Medical Council in the creation of standards, rules, and regulations governing a state controlled specialist qualification. Dorothy Porter, in Chapter 3, then describes how the new Medical Officers of Health in Britain had to struggle to achieve a professional identity. She delineates the ways in which the specialty was stratified along social and educational lines, leading to a division of interests between full-time and part-time practitioners. In Chapter 4, Arthur Viseltear writes about the early development of education in public health in the United States, and describes the important role played by bacteriologists and engineers in these pioneering programmes. He places them in the larger social

---

[10] For brevity we sometimes use the expression 'public health education'. By this we mean professional or graduate level education to prepare people for careers in the field of public health. Occasionally we refer to popular health education—often known simply as 'health education'—which, although it is an activity of public health professionals, is peripheral to the main theme of this book. Education in public health, like education in any other profession, strives to provide a realistic theoretical basis for the practices and structure of that profession, and seeks to indicate how such knowledge can be advanced. It contrasts with training which is concerned primarily with the teaching of practical expertise and the application of knowledge.

context of the movement to develop specialized scientific and technical educational institutions. The fifth chapter, by Elizabeth Fee, continues the story by explaining how the Rockefeller Foundation became involved in professional public health education. She describes the alternative proposals considered in the early twentieth century for creating a national system for education and training, the decisions made at that time, and some consequences of those decisions. Jane Lewis in Chapter 6 traces the complex development of public health in Britain in the twentieth century, and considers the tensions between public health, preventive medicine, and curative medicine. She also shows the relationship between the changing contours of public health, the social medicine movement, and community medicine. In a parallel chapter, Chapter 7, Elizabeth Fee and Barbara Rosenkrantz examine the troubled relations between public health and clinical medicine in the United States in the context of a political system which favours fee-for-service medicine and underfunds public health services. They explore the contributions of schools of public health, state and federal health services, and philanthropic foundations in attempting to educate public health professionals and reduce the gap between preventive and curative services. In Chapter 8, Roy Acheson follows the fate of the British Diploma in Public Health from its success and relative popularity in the early twentieth century to its end in 1974. He describes and analyses many of the factors leading to the demise of the Diploma in Public Health and its transformation into what is now the Membership of the Faculty of Public Health Medicine. Finally, in Chapter 9, Margot Jefferys and Joyce Lashof reflect on the current condition of education and training for public health, consider the lessons of the historical experiences discussed in the previous chapters, and suggest the directions that education and training in public health may take in the future.

1

Public health, preventive medicine, and professionalization: Britain and the United States in the nineteenth century

ELIZABETH FEE AND DOROTHY PORTER

1. Introduction

Public health in both Britain and the United States began as a response to the social and health problems of rapid industrialization. In both countries the public health movement had initially been created by social reformers and included, but was not led by, the medical profession. As public health became professionalized, physicians came to play a more dominant role. Medicine began to dominate public health in Britain from the mid-Victorian period. In the United States, public health would retain a considerable independence from medicine; as the medical profession remained wedded to fee-for-service practice and displayed little interest in salaried public health positions, public health evolved as a somewhat separate professional specialty, staffed by biologists, statisticians, engineers, and others with specialized training. In both Britian and the United States, however, the professionalization of public health involved a certain distancing from the original social reform impulses which had given it birth. Scientific methods tempered, when they did not replace, the initial commitment to improving the lives and living standards of the poor.

The origins of public health in social reform may be traced to France and Germany in the mid-nineteenth century. In Europe, 1848 was a year of revolution. Social, economic, and political crises in France and Germany were matched by the material and health crises of urbanism in the industrializing nations of the continent. Growing epidemic diseases from the late eighteenth century had brought the health of the community in ever more densely populated mass societies into the arena of European politics. In 1848, there was, therefore, a high profile of political discussions regarding health and disease in France and Germany: in Britain, the year was marked by the passing of the first Public Health Act.[1]

The panics generated by the arrival into Europe of killer-diseases, in particular Asiatic cholera in 1832, heightened the social disruptiveness of epidemic diseases but did not, in themselves, bring about substantial reforms.[2] The underlying conflicts of urbanization and urban health were better revealed in the indigenous, continuing problems of endemic disease—smallpox, infant diarrhoea, typhus, and typhoid fevers—and chronic sicknesses which were reproduced by insanitary living conditions and nutritional deficiencies. During the 1830s and 1840s, social movements developed across Europe, which were concerned with the health of towns, the role of medicine as a political force, with health as a right of citizenship, and with the relationship between sickness, poverty, and death.[3]

The social historian of medicine, Richard Shryock, described the movements for sanitary reform in Europe in this period as being led by individuals who were primarily interested in broad economic and social changes. Sanitarians, he suggested, viewed poverty and disease as forming a reciprocal cycle responsible for the dysfunctions of urban, industrial society.[4] Our reading of the lives and work of the central figures in the sanitary movements in Britain, France, and Germany before 1850 supports this view.

After the end of the Napoleonic wars, the major educational reforms undertaken in France included the creation of a new medical academy in Paris with a department of hygiene under the direction of Jean Noel Hallé. Hygienists studying in this department completed large scale investigations into the disease consequences of population density and dirt in the urban centres of France.[5] A socio-political analysis emerged from this work, the essential arguments of which were articulated in the

---

[1] See Shryock, Richard H. (1979). *The development of modern medicine*, pp. 211–47. University of Wisconsin Press, Madison; and Rosen, George (1976). *A history of public health*. MD Publications, New York. (3rd edn.), pp. 192–293.

[2] Pelling, Margaret (1978). *Cholera, fever and English medicine, 1825–1865*, pp. 1–33. Oxford University Press.

[3] Rosen, George (1974). *From medical police to social medicine*. Science History Publications, New York. See also Porter, D. and Porter, R. (1988). What was social medicine? An historiographical essay. *Journal of Historical Sociology*, **1**, 90–106.

[4] Shryock, op. cit., 221 (note 1).

[5] Ackerknecht, E. H. (1948). Hygiene in France, 1815–1848. *Bulletin of the History of Medicine*, **22**, 117–55.

Gazette Médicale in 1848.[6] Here, the term 'social medicine' was coined by Jules Guérin who outlined the political role of medicine in France as that of redressing the balance between industrial growth and the preservation of health.[7] The career of the leading French hygienist at this time, Louis René Villermé, illustrates these developments in medical politics.

Using demographic and statistical analysis, Villermé identified the causes of ill-health to be primarily social. Differential rates of mortality throughout Paris could be explained by the variation in the social and economic circumstances of the population. He and his colleagues in the *parti d'hygiène*, however, shared a fundamental belief in the philosophy of political economy, particularly as it had been espoused by Jean Baptiste Say. This dictated that the state should not interfere in the economic relations of the free market economy. Their solution, therefore, to the social causes of disease was not action by the state but the remoralization of the poor.[8]

In Germany, members of the medical reform movement initially believed that the politics of health had a wider mandate. Salamon Neuman, Rudolf Virchow and their associates stated clearly in their broadsheet, *Die Medizinische Reform* in 1848, that medicine is politics.[9] Virchow outlined a sociological explanation of the epidemiological patterns of disease in his essays on the outbreak of typhus in Upper Silesia.[10] Although he viewed communism as 'madness', Virchow was committed to a political ideal that the poor and the oppressed should not have to wait for heaven for their rewards; a healthful existence should be a right of citizenship in this life.[11] Throughout his career, the founder of cellular pathology rejected any unicausal etiology, even after the bacteriological explanation of disease had been well established. He maintained his heterodox view of the multicausality of disease and continued to assert that medicine should become part of a political process of change and transition to a fully democratic, welfare-based society.[12] In

---

[6] Galdston, Iago (1981). *Social and historical foundations of modern medicine*, pp. 74–8. Brunner Mazel, New York.

[7] Sand, René (1948). *Vers la médecine*, pp. 573–574. Baillière, Paris and Brussels.

[8] Coleman, William (1982). *Death is a social disease: public health and political economy in early industrial France*, pp. 277–306. University of Wisconsin Press, Madison.

[9] Ackerknecht, E. H. (1953). *Rudolf Virchow: doctor, statesman, anthropologist*, pp. 130–46. University of Wisconsin Press, Madison.

[10] Ibid., 123–37.

[11] Ibid., 166; Schlumberger, H. G. (1942). Rudolph Virchow—revolutionist. *Annals of Medical History*, 3rd Series, **4**, 147–53.

[12] Ackerknecht, op. cit., 105–18 (note 9); Pridan, David (1964). Rudolph Virchow and social medicine in historical perspective. *Medical History*, **9**, 275.

this context the role of the physician should be as 'the natural attorney of the poor.'[13]

2. The origins of public health in Britain

In Britain, Edwin Chadwick, lawyer, civil servant, and a disciple of the political philosopher Jeremy Bentham, was the leader of the sanitary movement in the 1830s and 1840s.[14] As part of his work for the Poor Law Commission from 1834, Chadwick formed a view of the relationship between poverty and disease similar to that of Virchow. In contrast to Virchow, however, Chadwick believed that the science of engineering rather than medicine should play the critical role in the development of sanitary reform. According to Chadwick's 'sanitary idea', engineering should become the handmaiden to the political economy of felicific calculus in order to achieve the greatest happiness of the greatest number. This ideology, however, was not realized in the way Chadwick had originally envisaged it. From the outset, the public health service employed medical men.[15]

While Chadwick was secretary of the Poor Law Commission in 1838, it employed three medical practitioners as inspectors to inquire into the state of health and sickness in London. Neil Arnott, James Phillips Kay (later Kay-Shuttleworth), and Thomas Southwood Smith produced a report which revealed the desperate living conditions of the poor in London. All three remained leading figures in the sanitary reform movement,[16] and Southwood Smith, in particular, became Chadwick's close ally. He, like Chadwick, had served as a secretary to Jeremy Bentham. He helped to found the Metropolitan Health of Towns Association in 1844, which became a model for many more provincial associations, and acted as a major extra-parliamentary pressure group for public health reforms.[17]

In 1839, the Poor Law Commission was instructed to undertake inquiries into the health of the working classes throughout England and

[13] Virchow quoted by George Rosen in, Rosen, G. (1941). Disease and social criticism: a contribution to theory and medical history. *Bulletin of the History of Medicine*, **10**, 15.

[14] Finer, S. E. (1952). *The life and times of Edwin Chadwick*, pp. 218–28. Methuen, London.

[15] Ibid., 1–55. For further discussion of Chadwick see Lewis, R. A. (1952). *Edwin Chadwick and the public health movement*. Longmans and Green, London.

[16] See discussion in Simon, John (1890). *English sanitary institutions*, pp. 178–87. Cassell, London. See also Frazer, W. M. (1950). *The history of English public health, 1834–1839*, pp. 12–23. Baillière, Tindall and Cox, London.

[17] Lewes, C. L. (1898). *Dr Southwood Smith*. Blackwood, London and Edinburgh.

Wales, and later also in Scotland. The result, the largest social survey completed to that date, was published by Chadwick in 1842.[18] The thrust of the 1842 Report was that epidemic diseases were caused by environmental filth and that the means of prevention were the provision of clean water supplies, effective sewerage and drainage, removal of nuisances, such as refuse from all streets and roads, control of industrial effluents, and the establishment of new standards of environmental and personal cleanliness. The Report recommended that entirely new structures of administration should be created for achieving these goals, both in local and central government, including the appointment of 'district medical officers' to inspect and report on local sanitary conditions.[19] As a result of the Report, a Royal Commission was set up in 1843 to consider the health of towns; the substance of its proposals was eventually incorporated into the Public Health Act of 1848. The Act established a central government department to deal with public health, the General Board of Health, and set up local sanitary authorities to co-ordinate the municipal responsibilities for environmental regulation, which had previously been distributed chaotically between myriad local commissions. A system for local inspection was created through the appointment of medical officers of health.[20] Because of political compromises, the power of the Act was seriously undermined by being adoptive rather than compulsory, and it thus resulted in uneven standards of public health regulation throughout the country.

Chadwick, supported by Thomas Southwood Smith's studies of fever, adopted the miasmatic theory of disease causation to legitimate an environmentalist programme of disease control.[21] This became the official orthodoxy of the first General Board of Health and governed its policies.[22] The miasmatic theory offered an atmospheric explanation of disease causation wherein pollution in the air, which arose from decaying organic matter, provided the source of infection and epidemic spread. Erwin Ackerknecht has suggested that this 'anti-contagionist'

[18] Chadwick, E. *General report on the sanitary conditions of the labouring classes of Great Britain, 1842*, edited and reprinted by M. W. Flinn, 1965. Edinburgh University Press.

[19] Ibid. For a contemporary discussion of the 1842 *Report*, see Simon, op. cit. 187–202 (note 16). See also Finer, op. cit., 209–29, 293–9 (note 14).

[20] See Frazer, op. cit., 18–37 (note 16); Finer, op. cit., 293–9 (note 14). A model of local sanitary administration had already been established under a separate Public Health Act for Liverpool in 1846 where the first Medical Officer of Health, William Duncan, had been appointed. See Frazer, W. M. (1947). *Duncan of Liverpool*. Hamilton Medical Books, London.

[21] See Southwood Smith, Thomas (1831). *Treatise on fever*. Stimpson and Clapp, Boston, Massachusetts.

[22] See Pelling, op. cit. (note 2).

theory dominated the thinking of sanitarians throughout Europe during the 1840s and 1850s.[23] It is not clear, however, how widely it was adopted among the medical profession in England. Margaret Pelling has demonstrated that the epidemiology of the sanitary era in England was characterized by a complex range of theories which incorporated both ideas of environmental pollution and explanations of disease transmission through contact.[24]

Despite variation in disease theories and policy tactics, sanitary science, both in Britain and on the continent during the 1840s, was ostensibly a political activity with social and economic change as its goal. Later, the sophistication of state medicine, at least as it emerged in England, began at mid-century to shift the emphasis of reform from legislative change to administrative implementation. A new balance of aims altered the course of disease prevention up to the early years of the twentieth century.

3. Public health in the United States

The social crises generated by industrial development did not become obvious in the United States until the late nineteenth century. Until then, epidemic diseases were believed to pose only occasional threats to an otherwise healthy social order. By the last decades of the century, however, the burgeoning social problems of the industrial cities could no longer be ignored: the overwhelming influx of immigrants crowded into narrow alleys and tenement housing, the terrifying death and disease rates of working class slums, the total inadequacy of water supplies and sewage systems for the rapidly growing population, the spread of endemic and epidemic diseases from the slums to the homes of the wealthy, and the escalating squalor and violence of the streets all demonstrated the urgent need for attention to public health. Almost all families lost children to diphtheria, smallpox, typhoid fever, whooping cough, infant diarrhoea, and other infectious diseases. Poverty and disease could no longer be treated simply as individual failings.

The early efforts of city health department officials to deal with health problems represented some attempt to mitigate the worst effects of unplanned and unregulated growth; a kind of rearguard action against the filth and congestion created by anarchic economic and urban devel-

---

[23] Ackerknecht, Erwin (1948). Anti-contagionism between 1821 and 1867. *Bulletin of the History of Medicine*, **22**, 562–93.

[24] Pelling, op. cit., 70–9 (note 2).

opment.[25] As cities grew in size, as the flow of immigrants continued, and as public health problems became ever more obvious, pressures mounted for more effective responses to the problems. New York, the largest city, and the one with some of the worst health conditions, produced some of the most active and progressive public health leaders; Boston and Providence were also noted for their public health programmes; but Baltimore and Philadelphia trailed far behind.[26]

Industrialization had meant new sources of affluence as well as of misery. America no longer fitted its self-image as a country of independent farmers and craftsmen; like the European countries, it displayed extremes of wealth and privilege, social misery and deprivation. Labour and social unrest pushed awareness of the need for social and health reforms. The great railroad strike of 1877, the assassination of President Garfield in 1881, the Haymarket bombing of 1886, the Homestead strike of 1892, and the Pullman strike of 1894 were just a few of the reminders that all was not well with the Republic. The Noble Order of the Knights of Labor—dedicated to such measures as an income tax, an eight hour day, social insurance, labour exchanges for the unemployed, the abolition of child labour, workmen's compensation, and public ownership of railroads and utilities—grew from a membership of 11 to over 700 000 within a few years. Massive strikes for better wages and working conditions revealed deep class divisions and seemed to threaten the social order. At the same time, the development of democratic machine politics challenged the dominance of the political and social élite, permitting some labour leaders to establish local bases of influence and power. The perceived social anarchy of the large industrial cities mocked the pretensions to social control of the traditional forces of church and state, and highlighted the need for more activist responses to the multiplicity of problems.

[25] Blake, John (1979). *Public health in the town of Boston, 1630–1822*. Harvard University Press, Cambridge, Massachusetts; Rosenkrantz, Barbara (1972). *Public health and the state: changing views in Massachusetts, 1842–1936*. Harvard University Press, Cambridge, Massachusetts; Duffy, John (1968). *A history of public health in New York City, 1625–1866*. Russell Sage Foundation, New York; Duffy, John (1974). *A history of public health in New York City, 1866–1966*. Russell Sage Foundation, New York; Galishoff, Stuart (1975). *Safeguarding the public health: Newark, 1895–1918*. Greenwood Press, Westport, Connecticut; Leavitt, Judith W. (1982). *The healthiest city: Milwaukee and the politics of health reform*. Princeton University Press, New Jersey.

[26] Winslow, Charles-Edward A. (1929). *The life of Hermann M. Biggs: physician and statesman of the public health*. Lea and Febiger, Philadelphia; Jordan, E. O., Whipple, G. C., and Winslow, C-E. A. (1924). *A pioneer of public health: William Thompson Sedgwick*. Yale University Press, New Haven, Connecticut; Cassedy, James H. (1962). *Charles V. Chapin and the public health movement*. Harvard University Press, Cambridge, Massachusetts; Rosenkrantz, op. cit. (note 25).

An increasing number of reform groups devoted themselves to social issues and improvements of every variety.[27] Health reformers, physicians, and engineers urged improved sanitary conditions in the industrial cities. Medical men were prominent in reform organizations, but they were not alone.[28] Barbara Rosenkrantz contrasted public health in the late nineteenth century with the internecine battles within general medicine: 'the field of public hygiene exemplified a happy marriage of engineers, physicians, and public-spirited citizens providing a model of complementary comportment under the banner of sanitary science'.[29] The most formally organized and professional body, the American Public Health Association, included scientists, municipal officials, physicians, engineers, and the occasional architect and lawyer.[30]

Physicians active in public health were often the élite of their profession, such as Stephen Smith, a founder of the American Public Health Association, or Hermann Biggs, the great public health administrator of New York State, who also maintained a highly successful private medical practice, or William Henry Welch, the Dean of the Johns Hopkins School of Medicine. More commonly, perhaps, physicians appointed to boards of health were simply respected local practitioners who might have assumed that their tasks would be undemanding; at least in the early nineteenth century, such boards met rarely and were only provoked into sudden activity by the threat of epidemics. Membership on such a board meant a certain social status and a little extra income, but had required no great burden of work. The situation was now changing; as health departments with at least some full-time staff members replaced the largely voluntary boards of health, they were expected to assume ever-increasing responsibilities.

The physicians were joined by other citizens concerned about the state

---

[27] Public health reform was a low priority for American social reformers generally. Slavery, for example, had attracted much more attention earlier. See Fee, Elizabeth (1987). *Disease and discovery: a history of the Johns Hopkins School of Hygiene and Public Health, 1916–1939*, pp. 1–30. The Johns Hopkins University Press, Baltimore and London.

[28] Charles E. and Rosenberg, Carroll S. (1968). Pietism and the origins of the American public health movement. *Journal of the History of Medicine and Allied Sciences*, **23**, 16–35; Shryock, Richard H. (1937). The early American public health movement. *American Journal of Public Health*, **27**, 965–71.

[29] Rosenkrantz, Barbara (1974). Cart before horse: theory, practice, and professional image in American public health, 1810–1920. *Journal of the History of Medicine and Allied Sciences*, **29**, 57.

[30] Smith, Stephen (1921). The history of public health, 1871–1921. In Mazyck P. Ravenel (ed.), *A half century of public health*, pp. 1–12. American Public Health Association, New York; Ravenel, Mazyck P. The American Public Health Association: past, present, future. In Ravenel (ed.) op. cit., 13–55.

of the cities. Middle- and upper- class women were especially active as sanitary reform activities gave them a respectable escape from the narrow bounds of domestic life. Such women joined in campaigns for improved housing, for the abolition of child labour, for maternal and child health, and for temperance; they were active in the settlement house movement (aiding the urban poor), trade union organizing, the suffrage movement, and municipal sanitary reform. The latter, as 'municipal housekeeping' was viewed as particularly suitable for women as a natural extension of women's training and experience as the housekeepers of the world.[31] These voluntary movements organized to support specific issues provided the organizational framework for many public health reforms. By the early years of the twentieth century, many such voluntary health organizations were established and active.[32]

The progressive reform groups in the public health movement advocated immediate change tempered by scientific knowledge and humanitarian concern. Sharing the revolutionaries' perception of the plight of the poor and the injustices of the system, they counselled less radical solutions.[33] They advocated public health reforms on political, economic, humanitarian, and scientific grounds. Politically, public health reform offered a middle ground between the cut-throat principles of entrepreneurial capitalism and the revolutionary ideas of the socialists, anarchists, and utopian visionaries. As William H. Welch expressed it to the Charity Organization Society in 1893, sanitary improvements offered the best way of improving the lot of the poor, short of the radical restructuring of society.[34]

An economic argument promoted by the progressive reformers was that public health should be viewed as a paying investment, giving higher returns than the stock market. In Germany, Max von Pettenkofer

[31] See Ryan, Mary P. (1975). *Womanhood in America: from colonial times to the present*, pp. 225–34. Franklin Watts, New York.

[32] The American Red Cross had been formed in 1882, the National Tuberculosis Association in 1904, the American Social Hygiene Association in 1905, the National Committee for Mental Hygiene in 1909, and the American Society for the Control of Cancer in 1919. See Smillie, Wilson G. (1955). *Public health: its promise for the future*, pp. 450–8. Macmillan, New York.

[33] Wiebe, Robert H. (1967). *The search for order, 1877–1920*. Hill and Wang, New York; Hays, Samuel P. (1980). The politics of reform in municipal government in the progressive era. In *American political history as social analysis*, pp. 205–32. University of Tennessee Press, Knoxville, Tennessee; Hays, Samuel P. (1968). *Conservation and the gospel of efficiency: the progressive conservation movement, 1890–1918*. Beacon Press, Boston, Massachusetts; Rogers, Daniel T. (1982). In search of progressivism. *Reviews in American History*, **10**, 115–32.

[34] Welch, William Henry (1920). Sanitation in relation to the poor. An address to the Sanitation Organization Society of Baltimore, November 1892. In *Papers and addresses by William Henry Welch*, **3**, 598. The Johns Hopkins Press, Baltimore.

had first calculated the financial returns on public health 'investments' to prove the value of sanitary reform in reducing deaths from typhoid, and his argument would be repeated many times by American public health leaders.[35] As Welch explained:

> . . . merely from a mercenary and commercial point of view it is for the interest of the community to take care of the health of the poor. Philanthropy assumes a totally different aspect in the eyes of the world when it is able to demonstrate that it pays to keep people healthy.[36]

Whether progressives stressed the humanitarian need for reform or the business efficiency of improving public health, they emphasized the need for more scientific knowledge and training for those responsible for public health activities. They argued that public health should be a profession with appropriate training and income:

> We hope that every local unit of government will have its health officer and that the iceman and the undertaker will not be considered suitable candidates, but that every health officer will be trained for his work. We hope that he will receive a reasonable reward for his services, and that the pay for saving a child's life with antitoxin will at least equal that received by a plumber for mending a leaky pipe; and that for managing a yellow fever outbreak a man may receive as much per week as a catcher on a baseball nine.[37]

The demand for centralized planning and business efficiency required scientific knowledge rather than the undisciplined enthusiasms of voluntary groups.[38] Public health decisions should be made by an analysis of costs and benefits 'as an up-to-date manufacturer would count the cost of a new process'. The health officer, like the merchant, should learn 'which line of work yields the most for the sum expended'.[39]

Existing health departments were dominated more by patronage and political considerations than by economic or administrative efficiency. Progressives regretted 'the evil of politics' and wanted to increase the pay and minimum qualifications for health officers to attract personnel on the basis of skill rather than influence. The attempt to insulate boards

---

[35] For a classic statement of this argument, see von Pettenkofer, Max (1941). *The value of health to a city*, pp. 15–52. Translated into English with an introduction by Henry E. Sigerist. The Johns Hopkins University Press, Baltimore, Maryland.

[36] Welch, op cit., 596 (note 34).

[37] Chapin, Charles (1934). Pleasures and hopes of the health officer. In *Papers of Charles V. Chapin, M. D.* Compiled by F.P. Gorham and C.L. Scamman, Oxford University Press, p. 11; Welch, op. cit., 596 (note 34).

[38] Rotch, Thomas M. (1909). The position and work of the American Pediatric Society toward public questions. *Transactions of the American Pediatric Society*, **21**, 12.

[39] Chapin, Charles (1934). How shall we spend the health appropriations? In *Papers of Charles V. Chapin, M.D.*, op. cit., 28–35 (note 37).

of health from local political control was part of a broader movement to make all forms of public administration more 'rational' and 'efficient' by reducing the influence of political bosses and by promoting a new group of professional administrators.[40] The goal was for a well-trained professional élite to conduct social reform on scientific lines. It seemed only a matter of selecting the right people and giving them the best possible training for the job. As William Sedgwick argued:

If, as I believe, we are in fact moving irresistibly towards a bureaucracy, while clinging to the ideals of a democracy, we shall do well to pause and inquire what kind of bureaucracy we are building up about ourselves . . . scientists and technicians alike . . . must be employed and paid by the people, to rule over them as well as to guide them, to constitute a kind of official class, a kind of bureaucracy constituted for themselves by the people themselves . . . what kind of scientists and technicians shall we have in our public service? . . . I honestly believe that upon our ability to solve, and solve wisely, these fundamental problems of our American life will depend in large measure our comfort and success as a people in the 20th century.[41]

By the turn of the century, public health in the United States was becoming a national and even international issue. Although the United States Congress was reluctant to enact federal health legislation, there were mounting pressures for United States attention to public health abroad. As American businessmen were seeking enlarged foreign markets, a vocal group of intellectuals and politicians argued for an assertive foreign policy. The United States began to challenge European dominance in the Far East and Latin America, seeking trade and political influence more than territory, but taking territory where they could. National defence goals included broadening control of trade routes, building a Central American canal, and establishing strategic bases in the Caribbean and Western Pacific.

In 1898, the United States entered the Spanish–American War, expanded the army from 25 000 to 250 000 men, and sent troops to Cuba. That war showed that the United States could not afford military adventures overseas unless more attention was paid to sanitation and public health: 968 men died in battle, but 5 438 died of infectious diseases.[42] Nonetheless, the United States defeated Spain, and installed an army of occupation in Cuba. When yellow fever threatened the troops

---

[40] Schiesl, Martin J. (1980). *The politics of efficiency: municipal administration and reform in America, 1880–1920.* University of California Press, Berkeley and London.

[41] Sedgwick, William T. Scientists and technicians in the public service, as cited by Jordan, Whipple, and Winslow, op. cit., 133–4 (note 26).

[42] Sternberg, George M. (1912). Sanitary lessons of the War. In *Sanitary lessons of the War and other papers*, p. 2. Byron S. Adams, Washington, DC; see also Cosmas, Graham

in 1900, the response was efficient and effective. An army commission under Walter Reed was sent to Cuba to study the disease and, in a dramatic series of human experiments, confirmed the hypothesis that it was spread by mosquitoes; Surgeon-Major William Gorgas of the United States Public Health Service then eliminated yellow fever from Havana.[43]

This experience confirmed the importance of public health for successful United States efforts overseas. Earlier efforts to dig the Panama Canal had been attended by enormous mortality rates from disease.[44] However, in 1904, Gorgas, now promoted to General, took control of a campaign against malaria and yellow fever threatening canal operations. He was finally able to persuade the Canal Commission to institute an intensive campaign against mosquitoes; in one of the great triumphs of practical public health, yellow fever and malaria were brought under control and the canal successfully completed in 1914.

United States industrialists brought some of the lessons of Cuba and the Panama Canal home to the southern United States. Socially and economically, the southern states were underdeveloped relative to the industrial northeast, and northern industrialists were beginning to invest in southern agriculture, education, and health. John D. Rockefeller thus created the General Education Board to support 'the general organization of rural communities for economic, social and educational purposes'.[45] In 1909, Rockefeller agreed to provide US $1 million to create the Rockefeller Sanitary Commission for the Eradication of Hookworm Disease, with Wickliffe Rose as Director.[46] Hookworm, a disease easily spread among agricultural labourers working under poor sanitary conditions, was endemic in the South. Hookworm were passed through the human alimentary tract into the soil, and hookworm larvae then infected children and workers who went barefoot, through the soles of the feet. Those so infected become anaemic, quickly tired, and were less productive; to the northern Yankees, hookworm was therefore aptly

A. (1971). *An army for empire: the United States Army in the Spanish–American War.* University of Missouri Press, Columbia.

[43] Kelly, Howard A. (1906). *Walter Reed and yellow fever.* Medical Standard Book Company, Baltimore, Maryland.

[44] Sternberg, George M. (1912). Sanitary problems connected with the construction of the Isthmian Canal. In *Sanitary lessons of the War and other papers*, pp. 39–40. Byron S. Adams, Washington, DC.

[45] Fosdick, Raymond B. (1962). *Adventure in giving: the story of the General Education Board*, pp. 57–8. Harper and Row, New York and Evanston, Illinois.

[46] For a detailed account of the Rockefeller Sanitary Commission, see Ettling, John (1981). *The germ of laziness: Rockefeller philanthropy and public health in the new South.* Harvard University Press, Cambridge, Massachusetts.

described as the 'germ of laziness'. The task of the Rockefeller Sanitary Commission was to eradicate hookworm by mass diagnosis, treating those infected, persuading the population to use latrines, and convincing local governments that the extension of public health services to the poor was a worthwhile social and economic investment.

The hookworm control programme spread throughout the southern states and helped create much more effective local public health organizations.[47] State health departments were strengthened and many rural areas began active health programmes. Encouraged by the success of this effort, the Rockefeller Foundation in 1914 created the International Health Board, again under the leadership of Wickliffe Rose, to extend public health efforts around the world.[48]

Meanwhile in Washington, the Committee of One Hundred on National Health, composed of such notables as Jane Addams, Andrew Carnegie, William H. Welch, and Booker T. Washington, campaigned for the federal regulation of public health.[49] Its president, the economist Irving Fisher, argued that a public health service would be good policy and good economics, in conserving 'national vitality'.[50] In 1912, the federal government made its first real commitment to public health when it expanded the responsibilities of the Public Health Service, empowering it to investigate the cause and spread of diseases, and the

[47] Rose, Wickliffe (1910). *First Annual Report of the Administrative Secretary of the Rockefeller Sanitary Commission*, p. 4, as cited in Fosdick, Raymond B. (1952). *The story of the Rockefeller Foundation*, p. 33. Harper and Brothers, New York.

[48] The Rockefeller philanthropies consisted of a number of independent trusts, each controlled by its own Board of Trustees. The General Education Board had been founded in 1902 to improve public education, especially in the southern states, and later turned its attention to the universities and to medical education. The Rockefeller Sanitary Commission was founded in 1909 to undertake hookworm control in the southern states. When it began to conduct international programmes, it was (briefly) called the International Health Commission. In 1913, when it became part of the Rockefeller Foundation, it was renamed the International Health Board. (To compound confusion, in 1927 it would be renamed the International Health Division.) Of all the Rockefeller philanthropies, those devoted to public health and medicine were probably the most successful in terms of both public relations and practical social impact. The Rockefeller Foundation initially was refused a charter by the United States Congress in 1913 because of widespread political hostility and suspicion, but gradually developed a reputation for successful public health programmes around the world. The General Education Board, with Abraham Flexner as Secretary, played a major role in the scientific transformation of American medical education.

[49] Rosen, George (1972). The Committee of One Hundred on National Health and the campaign for a National Health Department, 1906–1912. *American Journal of Public Health*, **62**, 261–3; Marcus, Alan I. (1979). Disease prevention in America: from a local to a national outlook, 1880–1910. *Bulletin of the History of Medicine*, **53**, 184–203.

[50] Fisher, Irving (1909). *A Report on national vitality, its wastes and conservation*. Bulletin 30, Committee of One Hundred on National Health. United States Government Printing Office, Washington, DC.

pollution and sanitation of navigable streams and lakes.[51] By 1915, the Public Health Service, the United States Army, and the Rockefeller Foundation were the major national agencies involved in public health activities, supplemented on a local level by a network of city and state health departments.

4. State medicine and preventive medicine in Britain

Until the early years of the twentieth century, United States public health reform had been directed largely by lay, non-professional personnel, a mixture of lawyers, philanthropists, and some concerned doctors. In Europe, the medical profession dominated events, and started to do so from a much earlier date. Virchow in Germany and Villermé in France were leading scientists and qualified physicians. In Britain, the engineering and legalistic orthodoxies of the sanitary movement declined with the removal of Chadwick from the General Board of Health in 1854. The 'sanitary idea' was replaced by the rise of state medicine during the mid-Victorian period. The domination of medicine in the English context began with the appointment of John Simon to the General Board of Health in 1854 and later at the Medical Department of the Privy Council in 1859.[52]

John Simon, a surgeon at St. Thomas's Hospital, had taken an interest in public health since he had been a founding member of the Health of Towns Association in 1844. In 1848, the City of London Corporation appointed Simon local Medical Officer of Health. Chadwick's style of management at the General Board of Health had met with political resistance from the advocates of local government autonomy; this had reached a critical point during 1854. When the Board was dissolved and reconstituted in 1855, Simon was appointed to the newly created post of Medical Officer of the Board.[53]

Before leaving the City of London, Simon published a collection of his reports to the authority. He took the opportunity 'to express . . . some thoughts on sanitary affairs in a fuller sense of the term'. He did not deal only with the City itself:

but speaking of the country in general, and pleading especially for the poorer

---

[51] For a detailed history of the Public Health Service, see Williams, Ralph C. (1951). *The United States Public Health Service, 1798–1950.* United States Government Printing Office, Washington, DC.

[52] Lambert, Royston (1963). *Sir John Simon, 1816–1904, and English social administration.* MacGibbon and Kee, London.

[53] Ibid., 221–32.

masses of the population, I endeavoured to show how genuine and urgent a need there was, that the State should concern itself systematically and comprehensively with all chief interests of the public health. I submitted, as the state of the case, that except against wilful violence, the law was practically caring very little for the lives of the people.[54]

Simon admitted that in referring to the existing evils against which there were no legal protection, such as 'uncontrolled letting of houses unfit for human occupation; the unregulated industries of sorts endangering the health of persons employed in them; the unregulated nuisance making business', he was dealing with the social questions which he 'could not pretend to discuss'. Namely:

questions as to wages and poverty and pauperism; in relation to which I could only observe, as of medical common-sense, that, if given wages will not purchase such food and such lodgment as are necessary for health, the rate-payers who sooner or later have to doctor and perhaps bury the labourer, when starvation-disease or filth-disease had laid him low, are in effect paying the too late arrears of wages which might have hindered the suffering and sorrow.[55]

Simon argued that even if the law allowed wages to find their own level 'in the struggles of an unrestricted competition' then at least it should ensure that food standards be established to prevent starvation; that conditions of lodging be regulated consistent with decency and health; and that working conditions be inspected and regulated to reduce risk. Simon had a specific vision of how these goals could be achieved. They required:

comprehensive and scientific legislation, and generally in relation to sanitary government, I urged that the supervision of the public health, in the full sense indicated, ought to be the consolidated and sole charge of some one Minister: who . . . should be responsible, not only for the enforcement of existing laws . . . but likewise for their progress . . . as the growth of knowledge would make desirable.[56]

In 1858, a new Public Health Act moved Simon's medical department to the Privy Council, where its main function was to be 'Inquiry and Report'.[57] It had direct powers only with regard to the enactment of the vaccination acts and the Disease Prevention Act for control of epidemics. Apart from the special place that the administration of vaccination had in Simon's responsibilities, he perceived that the task of his department at the Privy Council was to:

[54] Simon, op. cit., 253 (note 16).
[55] Ibid., 254.
[56] Ibid., 254–5.
[57] Ibid., 279.

develop a scientific basis for the progress of sanitary law and administration . . . we had to aim at stamping on public hygiene a character of greater exactitude than it had hitherto had.[58]

Thus began the period of 'blue-books' wherein Simon and his inspectorate produced annual reports of investigations into disease prevalence in the country, 'measured and understood with precision . . . in respect of their causes and modes of origin'. The investigations fell, said Simon, into two basic categories. The first studied the '*Excesses of Disease*, epidemic or endemic, in particular districts or particular classes of the population'. The second focused on the 'distribution of the common *Necessaries of Health* among the population, and into the effect of deficiencies which were found existing'.

To realize his broad mandate, Simon employed the leading medical, epidemiological, and scientific experts of the day: Edward Seaton, John Burdon Sanderson, Henry Greenhow, William Thudicum, Robert Barnes, and John Syre Bristowe. Their reports, completed between 1858 and 1871, examined epidemic and endemic sicknesses: diphtheria, famine diseases, meningitis, yellow fever, cholera, cattle-plague, pulmonary diseases, mortality of infants, and ague. Inquiries were also completed at the same time on 'standards which in great part were those of common social experience', such as the report on *Elementary requisites for popular healthiness* which investigated the provision of food supply, house accommodation, physical surroundings, industrial circumstances, and local precautions against the most notorious dangers in common life—'local nuisances, and the contagions of disease from man and beast'. Further reports followed: *Dangerous industries, Hospitals of the United Kingdom, Accidental and criminal poisoning, Dwelling of the poorer labouring classes in town and country, Specialised mortuary statistics,* and the *Average annual proportions of deaths.*[59]

During the first six years at the Privy Council, Simon and his inspectorate had amassed sufficient evidence to launch an appeal for a review of the law. This was achieved through a new Sanitary Act in 1866, which imposed a 'duty' upon local authorities to provide for proper inspection of their districts and the removal of nuisances. It gave local authorities new powers to intervene in the provision of clean water supplies, to regulate the tenements of the poor, and to impose penalties for those infected. Most importantly, the new 'grammar of common sanitary legislation' contained in the Act extended the power of the central government to coerce local authorities. The Act covered defaults of all

[58] Ibid., 286.
[59] See Lambert, op. cit., 289–371 (note 52); and Simon, op. cit., 281–322 (note 16).

kinds by local authorities and placed the power of determining faults and ordering action into the hands of the Home Secretary. The Act was passed without the outrage and opposition which had been met by Chadwick for attempting the same thing earlier, largely because of the support of Parliament's medical adviser, Simon.[60]

Simon had realized the ideals of a centrally administered state medical policy as envisaged in 1856 by Henry Rumsey.[61] Between 1858 and 1871, Simon expanded his office from a single appointment to a state department with its own parliamentary secretary; the department occupied two buildings with a staff of over thirty. But state medicine, which arose at mid-century, did not long survive. In 1867, the British Medical Association pressured Parliament for an inquiry into the chaotic multiplicity of the public health laws, and the Royal Sanitary Commission was subsequently appointed in 1868. The end result of the inquiry was the great codifying legislation, the Public Health Act of 1875, and the establishment in 1871 of the Local Government Board to co-ordinate the administration of both the Poor Law and public health into one government department. Simon transferred to the Local Government Board but found the restriction of Poor Law administration upon his department made it impossible to function with the same breadth. He resigned the medical officership in 1876 and, as his excellent biographer, Royston Lambert, pointed out, his resignation signalled the eclipse of state medicine.[62]

The declining fortunes of state medicine in central government led to a shift in emphasis in public health matters. The subsequent development in disease control has been characterized as an era of 'preventive medicine'.[63] This was a much broader movement, outside the central corridors of power and beyond the élite provinces of the medical and scientific communities. It was not, however, a 'lay' movement, but was associated with the growth of prevention as a professional practice distinct from cure. It centred around doctors whose primary function was the provision of health in the community and who relinquished the treatment of illness in individuals.

The struggle for economic and social security by Medical Officers of Health in the 1880s helped them to develop an identity as practitioners of preventive medicine separate from the clinical profession as a whole.[64] At the same time, a group of professional associations

[60] Ibid., Lambert, 377–91; Simon, op. cit., 298–302 (note 16).
[61] Rumsey, Henry W. (1856). *Essays on state medicine.* Churchill, London.
[62] Lambert, op. cit., 347–77 (note 52).
[63] Sand, op. cit., 557 (note 7).
[64] See Dorothy Porter, Chapter 3.

dedicated to the advancement of preventive medicine were established, such as the College of State Medicine, the Royal Institute of Health, the Institute of Hygiene, and the Royal Sanitary Institute. They started their own journals, held annual conferences, and provided facilities for research. The Royal Sanitary Institute provided education and qualifying examinations for sanitary engineers. The membership of these institutions and the membership of the Society of Medical Officers of Health could be described as the professional community of preventive medicine in the late Victorian period. Preventive medicine crystallized within this professional context and represented an ideological transition away from the 'sanitary idea' of the 1840s.[65]

In 1881, Chadwick addressed the Social Science Association, of which he was a long-time member, on the relative merits of prevention and cure. He praised the achievements of preventive science and bemoaned its poor standing in the eyes of the medical profession, government, and public at large. He defined prevention in 'sanitary' terms and focused on the deaths avoided by the environmental regulation of water pollution, sewage disposal, street widening, and other civil engineering works.[66]

A decade later, those concerned with preventive medicine thought such views characterized an outdated era of disease control and a form of knowledge which, for future progress, must be unlearned.[67] The first Professor of Hygiene at the Royal Army Medical School in Netley, Edmund Parkes, declared in his *Manual of practical hygiene*, that prevention had, in the past, worked with generalized assumptions about the nature of disease causation and had used generalized methods, moving haphazardly in the dark. The scientific future of prevention, he said, lay in the discovery of the specific causes of individual diseases. Without the principle of specificity the science of hygiene was only 'working with shadows'.[68]

5. The impact of bacteriology

The historiography of medicine and science has rightly warned against assuming that what looks, with hindsight, to have been a revolution in

[65] See Watkins, D. E. (1984). The English revolution in social medicine. Ph. D. thesis. University of London.

[66] Chadwick, Edwin (1881). Progress of sanitation: prevention as compared with that of curative science. *Transactions of the National Association of Social Science*, 625–49.

[67] See, for example, the presidential addresses of Joseph Ewart to the Epidemiological Society in 1891–92, *Transactions of the Epidemiological Society*, New Series, **10** (1890–91), 1–21; and **11** (1891–92), 1–26.

[68] Parkes, Edmund Alexander (1873). *A manual of practical hygiene* (4th edn.), pp. 443–4. Churchill, London.

knowledge, was perceived as such at the time.[69] The developments in bacteriology, which took place in the 1880s, were, however, embraced by the preventive community in Britain from the 1890s. In the United States, the advent of bacteriology may have been even more important in helping to weld a new professional, scientific identity for public health.

The 'sanitary idea' in Britain, and the 'old public health' in the United States, had attempted to procure the health of an undifferentiated 'public' with generalized methods of prevention. Towards the end of the nineteenth century, a shift in public health ideology began to categorize individuals into 'risk populations' based on what Edmund Parkes had termed 'the great principle of specificity'.[70] Bacteriology introduced the principle of specificity into understanding disease processes, and it also presented a powerful new way of differentiating scientific experts from mere social reformers. The response to the new scientific basis of preventive medicine diverged, however, in the United States and Britain. New policy directives in both national contexts shared some common features, but in other policy areas differed widely.

In the United States, in the period immediately following the brilliant experimental work of Pasteur, Koch, and the German bacteriologists, the bacteriological laboratory became the primary symbol of a new, scientific public health. The clarity and simplicity of bacteriological methods and discoveries gave them tremendous cultural importance: the agents of particular diseases had been made visible under the microscope. The identification of specific bacteria had cut through the misty miasmas of disease and had defined the enemy in unmistakable terms. Bacteriology thus became an ideological marker, sharply differentiating the 'old' public health, mainly the province of untrained amateurs, from the 'new' public health, which belonged to scientifically trained professionals.

Young Americans who had studied in Germany brought back the new knowledge of laboratory methods in bacteriology and started to teach others: William Henry Welch and T. Mitchell Prudden in New York, George Sternberg in Washington, and A.C. Abbott in Philadelphia were among the first to introduce the new bacteriology to the United States. These young scientists were convinced that other physicians spent too much time squabbling over medical ethics and politics, while they exemplified commitment to the purer values of laboratory

[69] See, for example, the discussion in Porter, Roy (1986). The scientific revolution: a spoke in the wheel? In Roy Porter and Mikulas Teich (ed.), *Revolution in history*, pp. 290–316. Cambrige University Press.

[70] Parkes, op. cit. (note 68).

research. The laboratory ideal rapidly influenced leading progressives in public health. By the 1880s, Charles Chapin had established a public health laboratory in Providence, Rhode Island; Victor C. Vaughan had created a state hygienic laboratory in Michigan; and William Sedgwick had used bacteriology to study water supplies and sewage disposal at the Lawrence Experiment Station in Massachusetts.[71] Sedgwick demonstrated the transmission of typhoid fever by polluted water supplies and developed quantitative methods for measuring the presence of bacteria in the air, water, and milk. Sedgwick, enthusiastic about the potential of bacteriological discoveries to solve public health problems, described the decade of the 1880s as 'a glorious ten years'.[72]

The powerful new methods of identifying diseases through the microscope drew attention away from the larger and more diffuse problems of water supplies, street cleaning, housing reform, and the living conditions of the poor. The approach of locating, identifying, and isolating bacteria and their human hosts was a more elegant and efficient way of dealing with disease than worrying about environmental reform. Because of its rapid early successes, many assumed that bacteriology would show the way to conquering all diseases. The public health laboratory thus demonstrated the scientific and diagnostic power of the new public health. However, when public health officials began requiring the reporting of infectious diseases, challenging physicians' diagnoses, producing their own antitoxin, and even treating patients, they quickly came into conflict with private medical practitioners, many of whom preferred that public health not trespass on what they regarded as their own territory.

The use of bacteriological laboratory techniques also emphasized the importance of scientific training for public health workers. Bacteriology thus narrowed the focus of public health, distinguished it from more general social and sanitary reform efforts, set the stage for potential conflicts with the medical profession, and reinforced the importance of scientific knowledge as the basis for public health practice.

A new epidemiology developed, based on the new bacteriology, and like it, firmly oriented to the control of specific diseases. Charles Chapin, the Superintendent of Health of Providence, Rhode Island, was one of the leading proponents of the new epidemiology. Chapin had published a comprehensive text on municipal sanitation in 1901, but soon concluded that much of the effort devoted to cleaning up the cities was wasted; instead, public health officers should concentrate on controlling

---

[71] For Sedgwick's rather lyrical view of bacteriology, see Sedgwick, William T. (1901). The origin, scope and significance of bacteriology. *Science*, **13**, 121–8.

[72] As cited in Jordan, Whipple, and Winslow, op. cit., 57 (note 26).

specific routes of infection.[73] In 1910, Chapin published a new text, *The sources and modes of infection*, which became a gospel of infectious disease control.[74]

Hibbert Winslow Hill, director of the division of epidemiology of the Minnesota Board of Health, popularized Chapin's work in a lively series of articles first printed in 1 100 newspapers across the United States, and later published as a book, *The new public health*.[75] Hill likened the epidemiologist to a hunter trying to find a sheep-killing wolf. The old-fashioned amateur hunter covered the mountains with his assistants, and told them to follow all wolf trails until they found the one that led to the slaughtered sheep. The new professional hunter, however, took a different approach:

Instead of finding in the mountains and following inward from them, say, 500 different wolf trails, 499 of which must necessarily be wrong, the experienced hunter goes directly to the slaughtered sheep, finding there and following outwards thence the only right trail . . . the one trail that is necessarily and inevitably the trail of the one actually guilty wolf.[76]

The new epidemiologist, Hill argued, started with the 'slaughtered sheep'—the sick patient. From there, he traced back the single trail to the source of disease. All other unrelated environmental trails—decaying milk, flies in the marketplace, outdoor privies—were irrelevant.

Hill explained that modern scientific methods were more efficient in the control of disease than old-fashioned approaches of social reform. To control tuberculosis, for example, it was not necessary to improve the living conditions of the 100 million people in the United States, only to prevent the 200 000 active tuberculosis cases from infecting others. He contrasted the expense and difficulty of trying to secure good food, decent housing, and safe working conditions for the entire population with 'the expense of supervision of two hundred thousand people *merely to the extent of confining their infective discharges* . . . Need any more be said to indicate the superiority of the new principles, as practical business propositions, over the old?'[77] The vital statistician, Hill said, would be the future scientific and financial manager of public health:

Much abused, laughed at, neglected, he is or will be, like the cost-of-production scientific manager of modern business, 'the most indispensable man on the

[73] Chapin, Charles V. (1901). *Municipal sanitation in the United States*. Snow and Farnham, Providence, Rhode Island.

[74] Chapin, Charles V. (1910). *The sources and modes of infection*. John Wiley and Sons, New York.

[75] Hill, Hibbert Winslow (1916). *The new public health*. Macmillan, New York.

[76] Ibid., 69.

[77] Ibid., 19–20.

staff' . . . a man who knows costs in each department in proportion to production, and where to save time, unnecessary work, and waste in general.[78]

The dominance of the disease-oriented approach to public health was
evident in the first handbook for practising public health officers,
Manual for health officers, published in 1915 by J. Scott MacNutt, and
echoing the views of Chapin and Hill.[79] MacNutt devoted approxi-
mately half of his 600-page handbook to the infectious diseases, four
pages to industrial hygiene, and gave only passing notice to housing,
water supplies, public education, and environmental health.

However, although the narrow bacteriological view was dominant,
there were several competing models for public health research and
practice extant at the same time. Public health was characterized by a
diversity of views and approaches. Compare, for example, Hill's narrow focus with the broad and expansive gaze of Charles-Edward A.
Winslow, a public health spokesman who would become head of Yale's
department of public health:

Public health is the science and art of preventing disease, prolonging life, and
promoting physical health and efficiency through organized community efforts
for the sanitation of the environment, the control of community infections, the
education of the individual in principles of personal hygiene, the organization of
medical and nursing service for the early diagnosis and preventive treatment of
disease, and the development of the social machinery which will ensure to every
individual in the community a standard of living adequate for the maintenance
of health.[80]

Winslow's was not the only alternative view. In the same year that
Hill published his book on the new public health, Alice Hamilton, in
Illinois, conducted a survey of industrial lead poisoning and established
the fact that thousands of American workers were being slowly killed
by white lead.[81] Hamilton's method was not that of following the single
trail to the guilty wolf, but of following hundreds of trails to find the
many guilty wolves in pottery glazing, bath tub enamelling, cut glass
polishing, cigar wrapping, can sealing, and dozens of other industrial
processes. Unaided by legislation, Alice Hamilton argued, persuaded,
shamed, and flattered individual employers into improving working

[78] Ibid., 134–5.

[79] MacNutt, J. Scott (1915). *A manual for health officers*, p. 85. John Wiley and Sons,
New York.

[80] Winslow, Charles-Edward A. (1920). The untilled fields of public health. *Science*,
51, 23; see also Winslow, C-.E.A. (1923). *The evolution and significance of the modern public
health campaign*. Yale University Press, New Haven, Connecticut.

[81] See Sicherman, Barbara (1984). *Alice Hamilton: a life in letters*, pp. 153–83. Harvard
University Press, Cambridge, Massachusetts.

conditions. Almost single-handedly, she created the foundations of industrial hygiene in America.

Joseph Goldberger's brilliant epidemiological studies of pellagra for the United States Public Health Service offer an example of yet another approach to public health. In 1914, Goldberger announced that pellagra was due to dietary deficiencies and not, as many believed, to some unknown micro-organism; he and his colleagues had cured endemic pellagra in a Mississippi orphanage by feeding the children milk, eggs, beans, and meat. He then teamed up with the economist, Edgar Sydenstricker, to survey the diets of southern wageworkers' families. They showed how the sharecropping system had impoverished tenant farmers, led to dietary deficiencies, and thus produced endemic pellagra.[82] That guilty wolf—the economic system of cotton production and the pattern of land ownership—had swallowed much of the South.

Alice Hamilton, Joseph Goldberger, and Edgar Sydenstricker were minority voices in America amid the growing majority focusing exclusively on bacteria. Only the minority continued to relate the problems of ill-health and disease to the larger social environment. As most bacteriologists and epidemiologists concentrated on specific disease-causing organisms and the individuals who harboured them, the larger social environment became almost irrelevant.[83]

Although the broader conceptions of public health required an understanding of economics and politics, the dominant model of public health knowledge was based almost exclusively on the biological sciences. In the United States, this latter definition of the problems of health and disease in bioscientific terms reinforced the medical profession's claim to a dominant influence in the field—a claim that had long been accepted in Britain, but that was actively contested in the United States.

In Britain, knowledge of specific modes of transmission of different diseases encouraged new lines of preventive action. A new emphasis upon notification, isolation, and disinfection had a high profile amongst Medical Officers of Health in the 1890s. A list of the most common infections spread by social contact was made notifiable under an adoptive act in 1889 and the law became compulsory in 1899.[84]

---

[82] Terris, Milton (ed.) (1964). *Goldberger on pellagra.* Louisiana State University Press, Baton Rouge. See especially Goldberger and Sydenstricker, Ch. 13, Pellagra in the Mississippi flood area, pp. 271–91.

[83] For a detailed examination of this point in the case of tuberculosis, see Kantor, Bonnie (1985). The new scientific public health movement: a case study of tuberculosis in Baltimore, Maryland, 1900–1910. Sc.D. dissertation. School of Hygiene and Public Health, The Johns Hopkins University.

[84] For discussion of the development of notification and the response of the public health service, see Watkins, op.cit., 214–38 (note 65).

Discussions of infectious disease control dominated the preventive journals up to 1900.[85] All the preventive journals included bacteriological sections. Bacteriological diagnosis was used in incidents of notified infections and district public health officers increasingly demanded laboratory facilities from their sanitary authorities.[86]

One consequence of the new concern with notification was a growing awareness of the need for systematic and comprehensive planning of disease control by health officers in Britain. In the early 1900s the Society of Medical Officers of Health discussed the desirability of adding tuberculosis to the list of notifiable diseases. Arthur Newsholme, when Medical Officer of Health for Brighton, had established an efficient system in his district. He warned the Society, however, not to act hastily in demanding the notification of tuberculosis. He pointed out that a notification system could not work without the full co-operation of a sanitary authority in providing sufficient hospital and ambulance services for isolating sufferers. Newsholme thus articulated the need to plan health care provision for a locality on the basis of its projected needs.[87]

Identification of specific diseases led preventive medicine in Britain to identify specific populations 'at risk'. This concept shaped the subsequent expansion of public health policy in different ways. The debates that surrounded the popular concern with national fitness and efficiency in Britain before the First World War paid special attention to the groups identified as 'unfit'.

6. Public health and medicine

In Britain, after the defeats of the British Army by South African farmers during the Boer War, concern over the physical fitness of the troops spilled over into a wider panic about physical deterioration in the nation as a whole. The Select Committee on Physical Deterioration was set up in the midst of a public and political alarm about national efficiency. Following the publication of their report in 1904, which highlighted acute health deficiencies amongst certain sections of the population, the Edwardian social and political consciousness became preoccupied with the degeneration of the Imperial Race by virtue of the

[85] Ibid., 276–333.

[86] For discussion of public health laboratories see Davies, D.S. (1898–99). Bacteriology in public health work. *Public Health*, **11**, 187–192.

[87] Society of Medical Officers of Health (1890). *Minutes of an ordinary meeting of the Society*. 11 April; see also *Public Health* (1890–91). **3**, 2–9.

Darwinian principle of natural selection.[88] By far the greatest response to the question of national efficiency, however, was the extension of the sociological classification of the health of the population.[89] A new focus emerged on the health of the school child, ante-natal care, infant welfare, and the diseases of occupations.[90] The 1911 census provided the data for Thomas Stevenson to devise the first socio-economic classification of occupations for the Registrar General, which was then used as a basis for calculating mortality rates, thus extending the statistical tabulations of health risks to include occupation and social class.[91]

These estimates of health risks by social class enhanced the development of comprehensive planning for disease prevention and health preservation. Nowhere was this trend more pronounced than amongst the medical officers of health. Closer allegiance grew up between medical officers of health and the advocates of town planning, for example, in the search for integrated systems of municipal management which would ensure health efficiency.[92] But corporatism found its clearest expression in the increasingly strident demands amongst medical officers of health for a national system of health provision. Up to 1911, numerous articles and editorials in *Public Health* discussed proposals for the nationalization of health care, structured around the existing public health organization. Many envisaged a national system administered through public health departments and co-ordinated by a new single government ministry to which all health authorities would be directly responsible. Influential medical officers of health argued for a national system of preventive health care in which they would play the crucial organizing role, no longer as local government officers, but as civil servants financed and salaried directly from the Exchequer.[93] Medical officers of health in Britain by this time had not only well-developed

---

[88] Searle, Geoffrey (1971). *The quest for national efficiency*. Basil Blackwell, Oxford. For discussion of degeneration in the development of concepts of social hygiene in England during the Edwardian period, see Jones, Greta (1986). *Social hygiene in twentieth century Britain*. Croom Helm, London. For discussion of the intellectual origins of degenerationism, see Chamberlin, J. E. and Gilman, Sander (1985). *Degeneration, the dark side of progress*. Columbia University Press, New York.

[89] See discussion in Watkins, op. cit. 291–322, (note 65), and in Armstrong, David (1983). *The political anatomy of the body: medical knowledge in Britain in the twentieth century*. Cambridge University Press.

[90] See Porter and Porter, op. cit. (note 3); Wohl, A. (1984). *Endangered lives: public health in Victorian Britain*, pp. 329–41. Methuen, London; Armstrong, op. cit. (note 89).

[91] Szreter, Simon (1988). The importance of social intervention in Britain's mortality decline c.1850–1914: a reinterpretation of the role of public health. *Social History of Medicine*, **1**, 1–37.

[92] Porter and Porter, op. cit. (note 3).

[93] Watkins, op. cit., 214–38 (note 65); Porter and Porter, op. cit. (note 3).

professional control over preventive medicine, but had aspirations to direct the future development of medical care in the nation.

By 1911, the medical profession in Britain had dominated public health for over 50 years. Because Britain had industrialized before the United States, public health activities had started earlier, and the medical profession had welcomed the prospect of state positions. Fifty years later in the United States, the medical profession, in a situation of growing economic and professional power, was less eager to accept salaried employment. The American Medical Association, in particular, was dubious about any form of physician payment that might restrict physicians' autonomy. At the same time, the prospects for physicians in private practice had never been brighter. Only a small minority would want to turn down such possibilities for the sake of a career in public health.

In the United States, other professional groups were interested, active, and involved in public health, and often more willing to accept salaried employment than the physicians. Civil and sanitary engineers were creating clean city water supplies and new sewerage systems and probably deserve the lion's share of the credit for the decline of infectious disease mortality and morbidity in the late nineteenth century. Indeed, sanitary engineers resented the physicians' assumption that they were automatically the best qualified to direct public health departments.[94] The professional competition between sanitary engineers and physicians became intense in the early years of the twentieth century as the sanitary engineers vociferously complained about the increasing 'medical monopoly' of public health.

By 1912, 15 states required that all members of their boards of health be physicians, 23 states required that at least one member be a physician, and 10 states had no professional requirement for eligibility.[95] The medical profession was well organized and making a strong claim for dominance in public health. The sanitary engineers' counter-claim was an uphill battle; the physicians were willing to concede their responsibility for public sanitation and water supplies, but little else.

[94] On the estimation of mortality rates for the period, see Meeker, Edward (1972). The improving health of the United States, 1850–1915. *Explorations in Economic History*, **9**, 353–73; Haines, Michael R. (1976). The use of model life tables to estimate mortality for the United States in the late nineteenth century. *Demography*, **16**, 289–312; Hoffman, Frederick L. (1906–1907). The general death rate of large American cities, 1871–1904. *Publications of the American Statistical Association*, **10**, 1–75. For a general discussion of the social impact of infectious diseases, see Duffy, John (1971). Social impact of disease in the late nineteenth century. *Bulletin of the New York Academy of Medicine*, **47**, 797–811.

[95] Knowles, Morris (1913). Public health service not a medical monopoly. *American Journal of Public Health*, **3**, 111–22.

A less powerful but nonetheless numerous and important group were the public health nurses. In the cities, tuberculosis nurses visited both rich and poor in their homes, giving advice about diet, rest, fresh air, the disposal of sputum, and the protection of other family members from infection. Maternal and child health nurses visited new mothers, giving advice about infant care, breast-feeding, the boiling of milk, and ways to protect children from ubiquitous infections. Community support for such activities was strong and led to the creation of the federal Children's Bureau in 1912—the first federal governmental agency to be run by a woman, and with women's interests and concerns specifically in mind.

Other professional groups also contributed to public health: bacteriologists, chemists, biologists, social workers, educators, statisticians, and sanitary inspectors. The central task in creating a unified profession of public health would be to weld unity of training, purpose, and function from these diverse and often competing interests.

Some resolution would have to be achieved between the different visions of public health, and some position taken with respect to the tensions between public health and medicine, between the biological and social views of public health, between the physicians, sanitary engineers, and nurses, and between the bacteriologists and those who sought a broader definition of the field. Ideally, the resolution of these issues would be inclusive, providing space within public health for the intellectual and practical contributions of a diversity of voices—yet result in co-operation and effective programmes rather than intra-professional squabbling. In order to create a more unified profession, decisions would have to be taken about the proper scope and content of public health, the kinds of knowledge and skills required of public health practitioners, the kinds of training to be provided, and the kinds of credentials to be offered.

In the United States, these questions would be worked out in the context of new schools of public health, largely founded and funded by the Rockefeller Foundation. These schools were open to physicians, but not limited to them. Indeed, when physicians displayed relatively little interest in public health training, the doors of public health were gradually opened wider to admit members of many other professions and those trained in a great variety of scientific disciplines. Some degree of professional unity was created among this diverse group through specialized public health training and the awarding of public health degrees. The experience of different professional groups—physicians, nurses, engineers, and later, sociologists, economists, lawyers, and health educators—studying and working together within schools of public health, helped prepare them for co-operative relationships in their subsequent careers. Although physicians were usually preferred for public health administrative positions, non-physicians came to occupy important positions within public health departments, especially in specialized technical and research positions.

In Britain, there would continue to be a sharp divide between the medical officers of health on the one hand, and the public health nurses, the public health inspectors, and the sanitary engineers on the other; the latter group held a singularly low status and tended to be regarded merely as employees of the medical officer of health. In Britain, the training and socialization of these groups was completely distinct from that of medical officers of health, a point which is elaborated by Roy Acheson in Chapter 8.

Conclusion

A comparative analysis of the development of public health in Britain and the United States has revealed both parallels and contrasts. The philosophy of public health in Britain was born in the 1830s and 1840s amidst a Europe having wide concern about the political dimensions of the role of medicine in ameliorating the ill health produced by urbanism, industrialism, and the free market economy. Public health in the United States also emerged as a social response to the disastrous health conditions of the industrial working class in the cities.

In both the United States and Britain, the sanitary reform movements were initially dominated by non-medical personnel who pursued the prevention of disease within the broad framework of preventing poverty and social distress. From the mid-nineteenth century in Britain, however, medicine moved to centre stage through the establishment of a medical department and a senior civil service medical appointment. The career of John Simon signalled the domination of the public health system by the medical profession. The transition from political philosophy to technical policy was assisted by Simon's strategy of supplementing legislation with administrative planning. A medical ideology of prevention was established with the rise of a new medical specialty which consolidated its identity through claims of legitimate authority in a new field of expertise, preventive medicine.

In the United States, public health remained somewhat separate from medicine. Public health as a profession only developed in the second decade of the twentieth century, at a time when reforms in medical education had already consolidated the professional identity and incomes of physicians. Relatively few were now interested in salaried public health positions. At least in part as a response to the relative disinterest of the medical profession, public health schools were open to non-physicians: to engineers, statisticians, biologists, and others interested in specialized public health disciplines. The schools of public health thus provided a route for non-physicians into public health careers and helped make the definition and boundaries of public health more flexible by providing room for new areas of concern such as environmental health, the social and behavioural sciences, and health economics. Public health tended to retain a broad definition of goals and interests, extending well beyond the boundaries of 'preventive medicine'. Relative to private medical practice, public health enjoyed less status and prestige than clinical medicine, and certainly less wealth. By retaining a separate identity from medicine, it also preserved some elements of the social reform impulse that marked its origins. As in Britain, public health became scientific, and its methods were moulded by the constraints of scientific and statistical methodology, but its relative independence from medicine represented an advantage as well as a constraint. In the United States, public health was never absorbed by the medical profession; the close but often strained relationship between the two would continue to influence, but not determine, the future development of public health as a profession.

2

The British Diploma in Public Health: birth and adolescence

ROY ACHESON

1. Introduction

The Diploma in Public Health was born in Dublin on 12 June 1871, and lived for 103 years. This was only 13 years after the General Council for Medical Education and Registration had been created, and at a time when there was neither structure nor organization in medical education. Much of clinical practice was unethical and unsafe. The Diploma died on 1 October 1974, when the National Health Service, in place for 25 years, was bringing high quality health care, free of direct cost, to everyone who sought it. The occasion of the Diploma's death was the first of a series of Acts of Parliament which restructured the health service. With this restructuring, the post of Medical Officer of Health ceased, and with it the need for a Diploma in Public Health. Neither had sustaining relevance in a changing world.

In mid-nineteenth century Britain, the idea that medical practice should be based on scientific principles was new. There were four established universities in Scotland and one in Ireland, which provided pre-clinical and clinical education along lines that would be recognizable to us today. In England from the 1840s, Cambridge, and shortly afterwards a very small number of students in Oxford, received BA degrees by studying chemistry, physics, anatomy, pathology, and materia medica in preparation for a clinical apprenticeship in one of the London teaching hospitals. When that was complete they returned to their mother university to be examined by honorary consultants from London (some of whom had probably taught them there) to receive bachelor's degrees in medicine and surgery. The majority of those studying medicine in England did not enter a university at all, however. In London, students did their pre-clinical studies in University College or King's College, or in a school in one of the older teaching hospitals before walking the wards with their colleagues from Oxford and Cambridge. Their pre-clinical, clinical knowledge, and skill were tested by one of the medical Royal Colleges, or the Society of Apothecaries, which issued a licence to the successful, and in turn enabled them to enrol in the Medical Register.

There was little training for specialization in medicine. All but a very few ceased to study the day they registered, and those few set themselves apart by being elected to the Fellowship of the Royal College of Physicans or Surgeons, or by submitting a thesis to their university and being awarded an MD. Fellows of the College of Physicians were unlikely to perform operations, whereas those of the College of Surgeons were, but in most instances both were generalists. At a humbler level, licenciates certainly were generalists. The identification of a unified profession of medicine, its structure, its training, its standards, and its proper role in society were all in a state of flux.

It was against this background of change and uncertainty that terms, such as sanitary science, state medicine, preventive medicine, and public health itself came to be discussed and increasingly used during the 1850s and 1860s. It is hardly surprising that when the medical profession brought pressure to bear on the government, not only to establish public health as a specialty in a profession where no definitive specialty had been recognized, but also to take detailed responsibility for the nature and standards of training, that the decision was made to rely on existing institutions, in particular the newly created General Medical Council. Within the very strict limits that the Council set for it, the Diploma in Public Health (DPH) and the training procedures established for it were successful. Inevitably, however, the time came when these limits no longer matched requirements. Cultural, organizational, political, scientific, and other factors inexorably changed, and the DPH became first a misfit and then an anachronism. By the time it had made its final contribution, other methods for establishing new, and nurturing old medical specialties, and training men and women for them had evolved. Each specialty is now responsible for setting and keeping its own standards, and the role of the General Medical Council is to act as co-ordinator. The story of the DPH is one of victories and defeats, and is unlikely to be repeated.

2. The origins of medicalization of public health in Britain

In Britain, public health as a specialty requiring medical skills can be traced to the Public Health Act of 1848. Among other things this legislation authorized local health boards to appoint a legally qualified medical practitioner as officer of health. Today this may seem the natural thing to do, but in the eighteenth century this was not the case. Edwin Chadwick had previously argued that civil engineers were better suited to do the job of organizing the prevention of illness than the physician: 'who has done his work when he has pointed out the disease that results from the neglect of proper administrative measures . . . '.[1] In crude and simple terms, Chadwick's line of thinking was as follows:

> . . . stench from excrement and rotting animal and vegetable matter causes miasma and miasma causes disease; remove the stinking material through properly constructed pipes and disease will be prevented—not only that, but there would be a healthier people who would also be better off economically and socially . . .[2]

Indeed, in similar vein the *Lancet* went so far as to describe the medical members of what in 1831 was the Central Board of Health as 'drones, sycophants, courtiers and titled imbecility' and cynically to postulate 'that no two of those gentlemen are agreed upon the point, whether (cholera) is infectious or not . . . '.[3] Nevertheless, when the Act came to be drafted Chadwick changed his position and conceded that he saw an important new public responsibility for 'members of the medical profession'. But it was not as easy as that. The *Lancet* pointed out that unless it was made abundantly clear that the medical officers were 'legally qualified', 'any quack or impostor who is actually practising as a physician or surgeon may lawfully receive the appointment'.[4]

Thus was thrown down a gauntlet which was soon to be picked up by Henry Wyldebore Rumsey,[5] a general practitioner and surgeon from Cheltenham. In 1856, he published a treatise, *Essays in state medicine*,[6] which set out what he considered state medicine to be, how it should be practised and administered, and how state physicians should be trained and paid. His suggestions in turn found support from three long-established universities, Oxford, Cambridge, and Trinity College, Dublin, together with the British Medical Association.[7,8]

[1] Finer, S.E. (1952). *The life and times of Sir Edwin Chadwick*, p. 218. Methuen, London.

[2] Flinn, M.W. (ed.) (1965). Introduction. In *Edwin Chadwick: first report of the Poor Law Commissioners on the sanitary condition of the labouring population of Great Britain*, p. 11. Livingstone, Edinburgh.

[3] *Lancet* (1831). Leading article, 'The Board of Health'. **ii**, 433–4.

[4] *Lancet* (1848). Leading article, 'The Public Health Bill'. **i**, 616.

[5] Acheson, Roy M. (1988). Henry Wyldebore Rumsey and the case for state medicine. *Public Health*, **102**, 217–25.

[6] Rumsey, Henry Wyldbore (1856). *Essays in state medicine*. Churchill, London.

[7] Stokes, William (1867). Presidential address to the 35th annual meeting of the British Medical Association, Dublin, 6 August. *British Medical Journal*, **ii**, 101–2.

[8] Acheson, Roy M. (1986). Three Regius Professors, sanitary science, and state medicine: the birth of an academic discipline. *British Medical Journal*, **293**, 1602–6.

In the meantime, the work to be done by the new medical officials had been set out in a circular issued in 1851 from Whitehall by the General Board of Health; these, the Board directed, were to be limited to:

the detection, the promulgation, and as far as may be practicable the removal and prevention of the common localising causes of disease, and more especially of those causes, on the existence and extent of which the . . . outbreak and intensity of epidemic diseases . . . mainly depend. This . . . forms no part of the ordinary duty of private medical practitioners.

They were not, therefore, to be concerned with the treatment of disease.[9] Nothing was said about how they were to earn their living.

It would seem that the term 'state medicine' was coined by Rumsey himself, and one can appreciate how important the name must have been to the medical profession at a time when the case was being argued as to whether public health should be a specialty of medicine. The related issue of how its practitioners should be paid was also being debated. Rumsey stressed that public health was a specialty of medicine, and that its practitioners should be paid state salaries.[10]

Little of the material upon which the treatise was based was original to Rumsey but his use of it was. He drew in particular from the writings of Chadwick but also from William Farr, and pulled together ideas from other apparently disparate sources, and moulded them into a fairly coherent whole, albeit a bulky and indigestible one. He argued that the practitioner of state medicine, who in Germany had been the *Kreisphysikus*, should care for a defined population, should be medically trained to a nationally acceptable standard for the purpose, and should be paid an adequate full-time salary from public funds so that he could afford not to have to undertake private clinical practice.

His book, *inter alia*, influenced the decision to establish the Royal Commission on the Public Health (subsequently to be known as the Royal Sanitary Commission),[11] and more locally, George Paget's efforts,[12] only partially successful, to persuade the University of Cambridge that it should be the first to help to develop the subject. This they

[9] Fraser Brockington, C. (1965). *Public health in the nineteenth century*, p. 175. Livingstone, Edinburgh.

[10] Acheson (1986), op. cit. (note 8).

[11] *British Medical Journal* (1868). State medicine: conference of the Committees of the British Medical Association and the Social Science Association, **1**, 489.

[12] *Cambridge University Reporter* (1874). Remarks by Professor Paget made before members of the University Senate, 8 December, 135–6.

did by instituting an MD in State Medicine in 1868,[13] to be followed seven years later by what was to be called the Certificate of Sanitary Science.[14]

Two years after the publication of the *Essays*, the Medical Act of 1858, which had been nascent for over a decade, created a new statutory body, the General Medical Council on Education and Registration. Its responsibilities, as the name implies were, and still are, to keep a register of all medical practitioners who have been properly trained, and are competent to practice, and to supervise the content and conduct of all medical education; in other words to protect the public from quackery. This it did by controlling the content and standards of basic medical practice, and by keeping a register of those whose training had conformed with their regulations and whose behaviour accorded with an accepted code of medical practice. Most of its members were nominated by educational and examining bodies in medicine throughout the country, but a few were chosen by the Privy Council. In November 1863, Rumsey was chosen, and, coincidentally, in the same month George Paget was nominated to it by the University of Cambridge.[15] The Council has always been answerable to the Privy Council.[16]

The medicalization of public health stemmed immediately from these events. But the force behind them was the fear of cholera and the Chadwick's realization that, despite their success, engineering and social reform were insufficient to allay this fear, let alone totally to control the great epidemics. Success could not be achieved without an informed

---

[13] University of Cambridge Archives (1868). *Grace of the Senate*, 7 May, [Min VI 53].
[14] *Cambridge University Reporter* (1874). 1 December, 118–20; Acheson, Roy M. (1987). Sir George Paget and postgraduate medical education; state medicine, the M.D. degree and the Diploma in Public Health. *Cambridge*, **21**, 51–8.
[15] General Medical Council (1864). *Minutes of General Council*, 13 January, 4, 5.
[16] The Privy Council is derived, through the 'Permanent Council', from the Norman–Angevin *Curia Regis*, and so, apart from the monarch, is the oldest arm of government in England. It became powerful under Henry I at the beginning of the twelfth century and so remained until Tudor times at the end of the fifteenth century. It pre-dated parliament by some 200 years and unlike parliament consisted of advisers chosen by the monarch. The Lord President of the Council, its titular leader, is now a Member of Parliament and of the Cabinet. Although the membership of the Council is large, including among others, several hundred present and past Members of Parliament, its quorum is only three. In this form it meets the monarch regularly to seek Royal approval for certain routine acts of government such as the appointment of government ministers, commissions and promotions in the Armed Forces, changes of statutes of bodies with a Royal Charter, actions of the General Medical Council, etc. The proceedings of these Royal audiences are published in the *London Gazette*. The General Medical Council is one of the councils directly answerable to it; the most important of these, however, is the Cabinet itself. Its affairs are managed by two senior government officers, the Clerk and the Assistant Clerk to the Privy Council, and they are assisted by a staff of civil servants.

contribution from the medical profession.[17] The newly created General
Medical Council was not slow to accept responsibility for postgraduate
state medicine in addition to its *raison d'être*, which was the control of
standards of clinical medical practice.[18] By so doing it set the scene for
the recruitment and training of a cadre of doctors competent in public
health.

An important consequence of the decision to establish an effective
new public health service was the rationalization of the system of local
government, which outside the large cities was poorly structured and
inefficient. The Public Health Acts of 1872 and 1875 provided a sound
structure, not only for the administrative aspects of public health, but
also for local government. The proper definition of county boundaries,
together with the Registration of Births and Deaths Act of 1874 also
made possible the institution of an effective national system for vital
statistics. Thus in Britain public health became a specialty in the profession of medicine and at the same time in a real but limited sense, a
national health service was provided.

In our study of how a system of training and education for those who
were to work in public health evolved we shall concentrate on the
experience of the first five universities to offer an examination to them,
namely, as Sir Henry Acland put it in his presidential address to the
General Medical Council in May 1875: ' . . . the universities of Dublin,
Edinburgh, Cambridge, Oxford and London, [which] have successfully, instituted Examinations . . . bearing on Public Health'.[19] In
addition, we shall consider an examination board established conjointly
by the Royal Colleges of Physicians and of Surgeons in London. The
combined contribution to the training of public health doctors of these
five bodies was great and the differences between them revealing.

In 1870 and 1871, before an educational system got underway, three
authoritative bodies defined state medicine. The most prestigious and,
chronologically, the last of these was the Royal Sanitary Commission[20]
which did this in the following terms: 'State Medicine shall be taken to

[17] General Medical Council (1868). *Minutes of General Council*, 27 June, 197, 198. On
23 April, the Chairman and Secretary of the British Medical Association had written a
Memorial to the General Medical Council asking for a recognized plan to be developed
for a special qualification for Medical Officers of Health, and for regulation of its standards. The Council received the Memorial and appointed a committee: 'to report on the
steps . . . to be taken . . . for granting Diplomas or Certificates of Proficiency in State
Medicine, and for recording the same in the *Medical Register* . . . '. The Committee was
known as the State Medicine Committee.
[18] General Medical Council (1869). *Minutes*, 7 July, 62–5.
[19] Ibid. (1875). Presidential address, 24 May, 13.
[20] Royal Sanitary Commission (Royal Commission on Public Health) (1871). *Report*,
ii, 61.

mean the application of the Physical and Medical Sciences to the safety and well-being of the community; it shall include Medical Jurisprudence and the care of the Public Health.' The second, more attractive, definition was drafted by the State Medicine Committee of the General Medical Council and was: 'the expression "state medicine" shall be taken to mean the application of the physical and medical sciences to the safety and wellbeing of the community and it shall include medical jurisprudence and the care of the public health'.[21] The first to be written, but the most austere of the three was drafted for internal use by the University of Cambridge by Paget on 27 January 1870, and reads: 'The term State Medicine, as used in the Communication from the Medical Council, comprehends Forensic Medicine and Sanitary Science as applied to the Community at large, and therefore includes all the details of Vital and Sanitary Statistics, Medical Topography, Preventive Medicine, Psychological Medicine & etc.'[22] The why is merely hinted at, only the means are set out.

An emphasis on science was, as we shall see, of great importance if Paget's democratically governed scientific university was to offer its first professional diploma. This qualification would be broadly influential for 40 years in the establishment of national standards.

3. The General Medical Council attempts to establish a curriculum in state medicine

The medical profession had to learn to live with the new General Council of Medical Education and Registration which the nation had established to ensure that the standards of education and practice of those who provided medical attention were high. It is not surprising, therefore, that the British Medical Association, at its annual meetings in the years following the first Medical Act, continued to pay a good deal of attention to education. In 1864, the Association met in Cambridge and heard George Paget describe in his Presidential Address how he had introduced science rather than Latin, Greek, and mathematics as the basis for medical education in Cambridge and added: 'I have the satisfaction of remembering that . . . the *clinical*[23] examination, the most efficient test of practical knowledge, was first introduced here by myself

---

[21] General Medical Council (1870). *Minutes*, 1 March, 48.

[22] University of Cambridge Archives (1870). *Memorandum in state medicine for the consideration of the Medical Questions Syndicate*. 27 January [Min VI 53].

[23] Author's italics. The importance of this innovation to medical education in general cannot be overemphasized.

three and twenty years ago',[24] that was to say 1841. This new emphasis on practical experience and expertise was to be faced by those responsible for training in state medicine and was to create difficulties for them. As well as considering these innovations in medical education, the meeting gave Rumsey, Paget, and William Stokes[25] the opportunity to lay plans for a further educational meeting of the Association, the theme of which was to be postgraduate training in state medicine.[26]

The meeting, which was probably the most important single event in the development of the DPH, was held under Stokes' presidency in Trinity College, Dublin in August 1867. There, Rumsey gave the principal paper, which was a synopsis of his *Essays*,[27] and together with Paget and Acland (Regius Professor of Medicine at Oxford), received an honorary MD from the University of Dublin.[28] The Association unanimously moved that government support should be sought to ensure that a high standard of postgraduate training should be made available for doctors wishing to follow a career in state medicine.[29] Accordingly, on 22 May 1868, a group of distinguished people, among them the three honorary graduands, and William Stokes, John Simon,[30] William Farr, and Edwin Chadwick requested and received an audience from the Lord President

[24] Paget, George E. (1864). Presidential address to the thirty-second annual meeting of the British Medical Association, Cambridge. *British Medical Journal*, **2**, 141–6.

[25] William Stokes was Regius Professor of Physic in the University of Dublin. He was a leading member of the distinguished group of physicians and surgeons who made Dublin one of the most important medical centres in Europe in the 1820s and 1830s. He is credited with being the first to bring Laennec's stethoscope from Paris to the United Kingdom. Among his eponyms are Stokes–Adams syndrome and Cheyne–Stokes breathing, which are still part of the clinical nomenclature today.

[26] *British Medical Journal* (1867). Report of 35th annual meeting of the British Medical Association held in Dublin, 6–8 August, 197–204.

[27] Rumsey, Henry Wyldbore (1867). State medicine in Great Britain. *British Medical Journal*, **2**, 197–201.

[28] University of Dublin Calendar (1868). Later, because it seemed that there was nothing to prevent an honorary receptor of the MD from registering such a degree, and so becoming eligible to practice clinical medicine, perhaps without proper training, Paget, President of the General Medical Council at the time, retrospectively declined this honour as did Acland, Paget's successor to the Presidency. Rumsey who, unlike the other two, was not a university graduate, but had been licensed by the Royal College of Surgeons, retained his. William Farr was also at the meeting; he was an active proponent of the concepts associated with state medicine, and was honoured with an honorary MD by the Royal College of Physicians of Ireland. Although the College subsequently conceded that it had no right to make such an award, Farr wrote the letters after his name for the rest of his life.

[29] *British Medical Journal* (1867). Thirty-fourth annual meeting of the British Medical Association. State medicine; general discussion of Dr Rumsey's paper. **2**, 201–4.

[30] John Simon subsequently contributed to the development of training in state medicine, later public health, in two chief ways. The first was that between 1855 and 1871, in his role as Chief Medical Officer to the Board of Health, he had direct access to the government and its ministers. Secondly, he was one of the Privy Council's nominees on

of the Council, the Duke of Marlborough. Chadwick was representing the National Association for the Promotion of Social Science[31] which had also been addressed by Rumsey.[32] The petition was agreed at a joint meeting of the Social Science Association under Chadwick and Acland respectively, but Rumsey had drafted it in the first place.[33] The audience was granted and the petition sought the establishment of a Royal Commission to consider the matter of state medicine, and in particular the matter of training medical men to practice it. There was no question about the dominance of medicine now. The publication of the names of the commissioners was one of the last actions taken by Disraeli before the resignation of his first government.[34]

A second direct consequence of the Dublin meeting was that on 27 June 1868, the General Medical Council considered a letter which had been written on 23 April by the British Medical Association. The letter asked that a plan be developed for education towards a special qualification for medical officers of health and that the Council should regulate standards at an appropriate level. The Council proceeded to appoint a State Medicine Committee, under Acland's chairmanship: 'to inquire into the proper steps to be taken, if any, for granting Diplomas or Certificates of proficiency in State Medicine and for recording the same in the Medical Register'.[35] It consisted of eight leading members of the profession including George Paget (President 1869–74), Edmund Parkes (the great military hygienist), Sir Robert Christison (representative for Scotland nominated by the Queen and Member of Parliament for the

the General Medical Council from 1876, where he was always active in debates which related to the subject; he remained a member until 1895.

[31] Chadwick's disdain for the medical profession has already been mentioned. Here, however, we see him associating himself with a delegation which was conceived in the British Medical Association. A few years later, on 14 June 1871, he was to accept, together with the Earl of Shaftesbury, the Honorary Vice-Presidency of the Epidemiological Society of London. This, from its foundation in 1850, until it was finally disbanded half a century later, was exclusively medical apart from these few honorary officers. Margaret Pelling maintains that Chadwick's reaction to doctors was part of a general antipathy to the kind of inertia that is derived from professional self-interest. [*Cholera, fever and English medicine, 1825–1865* (1978), Ch. 1. Oxford University Press.]

[32] *British Medical Journal* (1868). State medicine. **1**, 33; State medicine: memorandum adopted by the Joint Committee of the British Medical Association and the Social Science Association, ibid., 513.

[33] *British Medical Journal* (1868). State medicine. Memorandum drafted by the Joint Committee of the British Medical Association and the Social Science Association. **2**, 513, 514.

[34] See *The London Gazette* (1868). 23 November, 6107; *British Medical Journal* (1868). **2**, 23 November, 513–14, 541–3. The Commission did not actually meet until the spring of the following year when, after some foot-dragging and changes in its membership, it was convened by Gladstone.

[35] General Medical Council (1868). *Minutes*, 27 June (note 17), and 6 July, 300.

University of Edinburgh), William Stokes, Aquilla Smith (a physician with statistical interests, also from Dublin), and Henry Rumsey.[36] It had to face the task of drawing up sound national guidelines for postgraduate medical training. This was a totally new challenge and faced with such a radical innovation it decided to seek the opinions of authoritative people in many walks of life; it surveyed 29 correspondents at home and five abroad.[37]

Eight questions were asked in the questionnaire and an analysis of the results was reported to the Council in 1869. Five of them were concerned with creation of the curriculum and syllabus, the standard to which the examination should aspire, and the type of examining board which would be required. The other questions addressed the inefficiencies of medical witnesses and a means of remedying them. These reflected a potential relationship between legal and state medicine that had been posited by Chadwick and Rumsey as well as by the Scots.[38]

The first question sought comment on the appropriateness of a series of subjects which the Committee believed might be included in a course for a diploma in state medicine. These were forensic medicine, morbid anatomy (human and comparative), psychological medicine, laws of evidence, preventive medicine, vital and sanitary statistics, medical topography, and portions of engineering science and practice. No respondent thought that all of the subjects were suitable, nor did any consider that all were unsuitable. Many added suggestions of their own, such as: dietetics, vegetable physiology, hydrostatics, chemistry, meteorology, the effects of overcrowding, unwholesome foods, trades, impure water, etc., experimental philosophy, laws of human economy, the principles of inductive and deductive logic, the laws of actuary, and epidemiology.[39] Only one respondent disapproved of a diploma (or a certificate) in state medicine altogether, Dr Douglas Maclagan, who was soon to become responsible for a two-year course in Edinburgh:[40] in the University and city there had been a strong and continuous tradition of medical police and public health dating back to the end of the eighteenth

---

[36] Ibid. (note 35).

[37] The debate of the General Medical Council which followed Acland's proposal that a group of distinguished people should be approached in an inquiry seeking guidance about the curriculum and teaching procedures in state medicine is reported *in extenso*, see *British Medical Journal* (1868). **2**, 57–60.

[38] A relationship assumed also by French sanitarians and exemplified in the journal series *Annales d'Hygiène Publique et Médecine Légales*; for discussion see Coleman, William [1982]. *Death is a social disease: public health and political economy in early industrial France*, pp. 14–24. The University Press, Madison, Wisconsin.

[39] General Medical Council (1869). *Second report of the Committee on State Medicine*, xi–xvi.

[40] Ibid., 39–43.

century.[41] The term 'medical police' meant the surveillance of the health of a population.

Information was also sought about appropriate course length and suggestions ranged between 6 and 36 months.[42] Some replies outlined very specifically defined timetables, such as that by Professor Samuel Haughton, who was a member of the General Medical Council and Registrar of the Medical School at Trinity College, Dublin. He thought that the first year should be devoted entirely to practical study in chemistry, botany, meteorology, actuarial tables, and sanitary engineering; and that the second year should cover medical jurisprudence, pathology, toxicology, and epidemiology. At the other extreme, some believed that there should be no fixed order of study at all: 'or [it] should be left unreservedly to the candidates option',[43] a course of action which was to be adopted eventually in Trinity College, Dublin.

The important issue of practical instruction was totally ignored by seven correspondents, but all of those who did comment agreed that practical laboratory study and its examination were necessary. William Guy, one of the proponents wrote: 'All study of the natural sciences is utterly useless without a practical acquaintance with the facts on which they rest. This should be ascertained by examination.'[44] The issue of gaining a practical acquaintance with the duties of office was to become a source of aggravation, and we will return to it later.

The correspondents were generally indecisive about the setting of standards but showed a good deal of agreement as to which books would be valuable.[45] Among the several objections put forward to the whole concept of postgraduate training in state medicine was that the General Medical Council should not do anything to: 'encourage specialism when there were already too many qualifications entered on the

---

[41] Crewe, F. A. E. (1949). Social medicine as an academic discipline. In *Modern trends in public health* (ed. Arthur Mascie) pp. 46–79. Butterworth, London.

[42] Op.cit. xv–xvi (note 39).

[43] Ibid., xvi–xviii.

[44] Ibid., 32, and xviii–xix, 42.

[45] Ibid., xx–xxi. The books most frequently cited were: Edmund Parkes, *Manual of practical hygiene*; E. D. Mapother, *Lectures on public health*; Ambrose Tardieu, *Dictionnaire d'hygiène publique et salubrité*; Michael Levy, *Traité d'hygiène publique et privée*; A. S. Taylor, *Treatise on medical jurisprudence*. There were some more unusual suggestions such as that of Henry Maudsley that Mills' *System of logic* was an essential basic text, and Dr J. A. Simmonds of Clifton who believed that Neill's *Logic*, Bain's *Psychological treatises*, and Lewes' *History of philosophy* should be the mainstay of any reading programme in a public health curriculum. Nowadays, attempts to teach logical reasoning to aspiring members of the medical profession are rarely made beyond such instruction as is offered in courses on 'scientific methods' which are based, of course, on logic. It was not until the years following the Second World War, however, that the elements of logic ceased to be a required course for every freshman medical student in Trinity College, Dublin.

Register'.[46] As a consequence of the wide diversity of views that they received from their canvass, the Council's State Medicine Committee had no option but to be indecisive, and the universities took the law into their own hands. Therefore, a wide range of curricula and of procedures for examining slowly developed: standardization was achieved in 1895 when the General Medical Council formally enforced resolutions and rules which, with consultation, it had drafted and negotiated over six years.

4. A curriculum is created and implemented by Dublin Trinity College

Public health in Victorian England differed from other professional pursuits. As its importance became recognized, so a national movement was initiated within medicine to ensure that those who were to practice it should be properly trained to undertake the tasks which faced them. This realization of a need for education and training was in turn unusual for another reason: public health, unlike anatomy, was not concerned with structure; unlike physiology, it was not solely concerned with process; unlike pathology, it was not concerned with degenerative tissue change: it was an endeavour by any legitimate means that could be marshalled to ameliorate the circumstances of living in order to improve the health of the people. In this section we describe how, by stratagem and fecit, a curriculum was adopted, and an examination based on it was established. The responsibility for this achievement lay solely with medical academics.

Rumsey's treatise was taken as the basis of the first curriculum, which was to be consolidated in Trinity College, Dublin, and recognized by the General Medical Council. Rumsey found inspiration in the work of Chadwick and Farr when he compiled his list of the tasks which he felt a state physician should discharge. He and his colleagues included anything and everything of an administrative nature which they believed could be done better by someone with a medical training than by a layman. The tasks he suggested included: creating a Register of illness attended at the public expense; giving legally acceptable evidence in courts of law in claims for compensation; control and examination of all water supplies; and supervising the registration of births and deaths.[47]

The Royal Commission of 1869–72 paid no attention to these details, and it was to be the last decade of the century before the role of a

---

[46] Ibid. (note 39).
[47] Rumsey, op.cit. (note 6).

Medical Officer of Health, whose title related more closely to Chad-wick's officer of health than to Rumsey's idea of what a practitioner of state medicine might do, was to emerge and a generally agreed training programme was to be established. The most important difference from Chadwick's or Rumsey's concepts was that, although the officer received copies of death certificates, he held no responsibility for their issuance.[48] The forces which in the first place determined what was to be taught included the independent examining boards established by the Royal Colleges of Physicians and of Surgeons in England, in Scotland and in Ireland, the medical profession, the universities, and within the universities, the interests of the various professors and teachers whose fields might have a possible bearing on the training of the medical officer of health. At the outset, the General Medical Council had no legal auth-ority to enforce its recommendations but could only issue guidelines. There follows a brief description of how the first five examining boards came to make their contributions between 1871 and 1875.

Dublin

The first initiative to achieve something concrete in the way of provid-ing a qualification in state medicine was taken by George Paget, with his State Medicine MD at Cambridge University in 1868. As part of a general scheme to introduce basic qualifications in their own univer-sities, he, together with Acland, helped Stokes in Dublin to persuade his university to introduce an examination for a Certificate in State Medi-cine which was held in Trinity College, Dublin. Certificates were awarded to four successful candidates on 14 June, 1871.[49] 'The Institu-tion of this examination does great honour to the University of Dublin', wrote the British Medical Journal.[50] However, only one of the four gra-duands registered his certificate with the General Medical Council and became a medical officer of health and general practitioner in Bedford. Of the others, one became Professor of Physiology at King's College, London, and two became honorary consultants to the Meath Hospital, as physicians with fashionable Dublin practices.[51]

In 1870, Stokes had called a series of meetings of all the medical pro-fessors at Trinity College, Dublin, before whom he laid, not the report of the General Medical Council's survey, but the proposals which Rum-

---

[48] Registration of Births and Deaths Act 1874: [37 & 38 Vict. Ch. 87], Clauses 1, 9, 28.

[49] Acheson (1986), op. cit. (note 8).

[50] British Medical Journal (1870). University of Dublin: a new qualification in state medicine, 2, 343–4; ibid. (1871). The new qualification in state medicine, 2, 18.

[51] Acheson (1986), op. cit. (note 8).

sey set out in his treatise.[52] The outcome was a written examination consisting of a set of nine question papers as follows:

1. Law (including the law of epidemics).
2. Engineering.
3. Pathology.
4. Vital and sanitary statistics.
5. Chemistry.
6. Meteorology.
7. A general paper set by the Regius Professor of Physic (William Stokes) which after Stokes' retirement came to be called State Medicine.
8. Medical jurisprudence.
9. Hygiene.

The questions were based on the extensive and detailed syllabus of some 2000 words, covering five pages, which the professors had prepared, and which had been published in the Dublin University Calendar in 1871.[53] The University *per se* made no attempt to teach the candidates, although presumably they sought instruction for themselves on a private basis, and presumably in some instances at least this was offered by the examiner. This failure to teach was common to most universities in the early years but was slowly to change.

Several other facets of this examination are worthy of comment. Of interest here is the way it reflects ignorance of the causes of epidemics in the period immediately before the advent of bacteriology. It would perhaps be misleading to think of Stokes as an apostle of Farr but he evidently subscribed to many of Farr's views concerning the laws of epidemics and statistics. It seems curious, nevertheless, that the law of the land and the law of epidemics were to be grouped in the same paper; in the event, no questions on the latter were set. The title of the paper subsequently became 'Law'.[54] There was no examination question solely on epidemiology: the statistics paper dealt with the procedures of what we would now call basic demographic analyses including those of mortality and natality which Farr had been developing. Apart, however, from a reference to zymotic diseases no questions related these to nosology, or the specific diseases about which Farr had been writing for 30 years. It is difficult, now, for us to judge what answers Stokes

[52] Archives of Trinity College, Dublin (1870). Letter from Stokes to Registrar of College, 3 February, [MUN/v/5/12]: Minute Book of Meetings of Medical Professors, December 23, 1869 to June 24, 1870, 26–34.
[53] Dublin University Calendar (1871), 93–7.
[54] Ibid. (1874), 368.

expected to some of his own 15 widely ranging questions. For example: 'How far is the history of cholera in Europe confirmatory of, or opposed to, the doctrine of its contagious nature ?' and 'Can you offer any explanation as to why malaria, productive of intermittent fever, is not observed in the bogs of Ireland?'[55] Our only clue is that, like Farr, Stokes accepted the theory of miasma.

Of the eight papers, other than that set by Stokes, four (Hygiene, Chemistry, Pathology, and Medical jurisprudence) were set by medically qualified examiners. The recruitment of scientists and lawyers to examine the other subjects created difficulties, both in Dublin and elsewhere, because their questions did not always have an obvious relevance to public health medicine. In April 1873, the General Medical Council passed an elaborate motion proposed by Stokes that power should be granted to the Council to Register a Qualification in State Medicine according to Regulations approved by the Council, and that the curriculum stipulated by Trinity College, Dublin, as a basis for certification, should be forwarded to every Council member. As we have noted, it was not until 1895 that the Council was able to enforce its rules. From then on the Diploma in Public Health as a certificate of specialist skill was at last a reality, and it was only then that an agreed curriculum emerged, but until then the Dublin examination of 1871 stood as a take-it-or-leave-it guideline, fully minuted by the Council.

In 1874, the University of Edinburgh and in 1875, that of Cambridge, offered their first examinations and it is difficult to say how much either was influenced by the Dublin model. Unquestionably there were similarities but in both Edinburgh and Cambridge the examination was more structured. It was divided into two parts, the first being concerned with the basic sciences, and the second with the practice of public health. It was also more searching because candidates were required to subject themselves to practical and oral examinations. These differences probably reflect the interests and history of each of the three universities more than any direct influence of the General Medical Council.

Edinburgh

The University of Edinburgh chose to offer a B.Sc.in Public Health, not in the Faculty of Medicine, but in the Faculty of Science. The first examination was in October 1874, and until 1892, when a candidate registered an MD in State Medicine he had obtained from the University of London, was the only public health *degree* in the country. There were

---

[55] Ibid. (1871), 174–81.

papers on Chemistry, Physics, Vital statistics and Sanitary law in Part 1, and one on Medicine in Part 2.[56] The University set itself apart from the others in the field in two ways.

Since the early years of the century it had appointed a series of distinguished Professors of Medical Jurisprudence and Medical Police, such as William Pultney Alison,[57] who held his chair from 1820 to 1827, when he became Professor of Medicine. He was preceded by Andrew Duncan and followed by Sir Robert Christison. Christison in turn was succeeded in 1875 by Sir Douglas Maclagan; and after Maclagan's retirement in 1897, by Sir Henry Littlejohn at the age of 71, who, since 1862, had been Edinburgh's first Medical Officer of Health.[58] The last three of these contribute directly to the story of the Diploma in Public Health. They were authorities on medicine and the law, and Andrew Duncan had contributed to the genesis of teaching in public health as early as 1798, when the undergraduates there received their first course in 'medical police' from him.[59]

That four such outstanding men should successively be professors in the field is a measure of the medical profession's interest in public health, over the whole of the nineteenth century. Three of them were knights of the realm. The titles of the chairs they held were as changeable then as they are now in Britain. For Alison, it was Medical Jurisprudence; for Christison, Medical Jurisprudence and Medical Police; for Maclagan, Medical Jurisprudence and Public Health; and for Littlejohn (who was succeeded by his son Harvey), it was Forensic Medicine. All of them had joint appointments with the Faculty of Law. One of the four was

[56] University of Edinburgh: *Minutes of Senatus Academicus 1873–1875*, **V**, 158, 203, 206, 218, 238–41 and 437–8.

[57] Brotherston, Sir John (1958). William Pultney Alison: Scottish pioneer of social medicine. *Medical Officer*, **99**, 331–6; see also Flinn, op.cit., 63–6 (note 2). Alison was a vigorous antagonist of the miasma theory and engaged in a public debate with Chadwick on the matter.

[58] Obituaries are to be found as follows: Sir Robert Christison, *Edinburgh Medical Journal* (1882). **XXVII**, 852–62; Sir Douglas Maclagan, ibid. (1900). **VII**, 515–17; Sir Henry Littlejohn (1914). *British Medical Journal*, **2**, 648–50.

[59] I am grateful to Dr Alistair Nelson who drew my attention to this course given by Andrew Duncan and informed me that it had the following content:

- Hospital administration (to which most emphasis was given, since the hospitalization of the all too numerous sick poor constituted one of the major administrative problems of the day).
- The elements of epidemiology (at a time when the responsible pathogenic organisms were still unknown).
- The rudiments of vital statistics, of occupational hygiene, and of personal and environmental sanitation.
- The definition of human needs in respect of air, water, food, clothing, heat, light, and a consideration of the means of their satisfaction.

President of the College of Surgeons, one of the College of Physicians, and Maclagan was serially President of both.

Secondly, although candidates did not need to be graduates of the University they were required to submit evidence of having attended courses of instruction in public health and analytical chemistry given by a teacher formally recognized by the University before entering the examination.[60] Some years were to elapse before these were to become 'two courses of instruction scientific or professional [in the university] and bearing on the subjects of the examinations'.[61] This was an important first move towards training and education in the field by teaching rather than by examination. Candidates had to be graduates in medicine of a recognized university, and had to give evidence of attending a relevant course as matriculated students of the University of Edinburgh. There were, from the outset, written, oral, and practical components to the examination. Each paper was set and marked, as they were in Dublin, by a single examiner who generally was a member of the University. The reliance on a single examiner, some medically qualified and some not, competent though they may all have been, to 'value' a paper both in Dublin and Edinburgh (and indeed elsewhere), was subsequently to attract the unfavourable attention of George Duffey, who was the Council's first inspector.[62] 'Such procedures', he wrote 'may be contrary to the views of the Council'.

The Edinburgh examination papers were, in general, very pertinent to the practice of public health. There were only three questions on chemistry and sanitary law in Part 1 of the examination: there was a question in the former about the detection of impurities in a village well, and in the latter about the constitution and function of the 'Local Government Board'. In contrast, there were 14 questions in the physics paper, which included meteorology, but these too, in the early days, were immediately practical. One, for instance, was the nature and value of information given by wet and dry bulb thermometers. Part 2 comprised two papers one of which was entitled 'Medicine' (this subsequently changed its name to the more appropriate one of Medicine as applied to Public Health); and the other Practical Sanitation. The syllabus for the former included topics, such as the origin, nature, and pro-

[60] University of Edinburgh Calendar (1880–88). *Regulation, 3*, 124–5.

[61] University of Edinburgh (1874). *Minutes of Senatus Academicus*, 10 July, 238–41.

[62] General Medical Council (1895). *Report of the Public Health Committee*, Appendix XVIII. Report on examinations for the degree in Science in the Department of Public Health in the University of Edinburgh, 631; ibid., Appendix XXI. Report on the qualification in State Medicine in the University of Dublin, 713; ibid. (1896). Appendix 6, 395, 400.

pagation of epidemic and contagious diseases; the prevention of contagion and infection; the geographical distribution of disease; epidemiology and fevers. The paper on Practical Sanitation was concerned with the duties of a Health Officer. Candidates sat Part 2 at least six months after passing Part 1. In short, in terms of content, methods of teaching and examination and general standards, the degree in Public Health compared very favourably with a degree course in any other scientific subject at that time.

Cambridge

Cambridge offered its first examination four years after Dublin. In the early years, like Dublin, successful candidates obtained a certificate. In abbreviated form it should, according to the University regulations, be written 'S.Sc.Cert.Camb.' denoting holders of the Certificate in Sanitary Science. It was, however, generally referred to as the Certificate in State Medicine. The recurring and persistent emphasis on sanitary science in the internal regulations and documents was presumably to placate the dons in Cambridge who were uneasy about the appropriateness or otherwise of a Certificate in State Medicine. As Dr Mayo, an eccentric of the time, was later to say in a debate in the Senate House: ' . . . the subject of hygiene was absurdly restricted, as the professors provided for the protection of one only out of the five senses, namely the olfactory sense'; eccentric or not, Mayo amused the gallery by pithily presenting the popular view in Senate debates.[63]

It was not until 1976, a century later, that there was a clinical school in Cambridge. Before that the University considered its responsibility to provide a scientific grounding for students who would go to the London hospitals to gain their clinical experience. It was in this tradition that they believed that a sound and appropriate basis could be provided for the practice of state medicine. This philosophy is evident from their definition quoted in the first section of this chapter which is just a little more generous than the Certificate itself, drafted in 1875 and which can be found on the following page.

Two days were devoted to each part of the Examination. Part 1 comprised physics and chemistry, and their applications to sanitary matters. Part 2 comprised ' . . . the causes and prevention of epidemic and infectious diseases, the circumstances and conditions of life which are injurious to health and the Laws of the Realm which relate to Public

---

[63] *Cambridge University Reporter* (1906). 14 May, 891. For an amusing description of the "extreme eccentricities" of James Mayo, see Venn, J. A. (1953). *Alumni Cantabrigiensis*, Part II, **V**, 378. Cambridge University Press.

KNOW ALL MEN by these presents that:

having been duly examined:

the Examiners in that behalf appointed by the CHANCELLOR MASTERS and SCHOLARS of the UNIVERSITY of CAMBRIDGE and having approved himself to the aforesaid Examiners by his Knowledge and Skill in Sanitary Science to wit Chemistry and Physics in the causes and prevention of Epidemic and Infectious Diseases and in the means of remedying or ameliorating those Circumstances and Conditions of life which are known to be injurious to health as well as in the the Realm relating to Public Health is CERTIFIED to be well qualified in respect of his Knowledge and Skill aforesaid to fulfil the Duties of a Medical Officer of Health IN TESTIMONY whereof the Vice Chancellor of the said University by the authority of the CHANCELLOR MASTERS and SCHOLARS has hereto set his hand and Seal the

day of one   thousand eight hundred

and

seal

VICE CHANCELLOR[64]

Health'.[65] Apart from the fact that Parts 1 and 2 could be taken in immediate sequence, and passed in any order, this was broadly similar to Edinburgh. The policy about examiners differed, however.

In each part two papers of questions, each of which had to be submitted to all four Examiners, were set, to which written answers were required; in each part the Candidates were also questioned orally by two of the Examiners sitting together, and in each part the Candidates were tested by practical work.[66]

It would seem that the four examiners also contributed questions to each of the four papers because neither at the outset, nor in the following 20 years, was it usual for a paper to be devoted to any single subject. Three of the examiners in the first year were doctors of medicine, namely Paget as the Regius Professor of Physic; Edmund Parkes, author of the leading textbook of the day; A. W. Barclay, a practising medical officer of health,[67] and James Dewar, a Cambridge physicist. Parkes and Barclay were external to the University and as such were early examples of what was to become a very important aspect of British academic assess-

[64] Ibid. (1875), 42.
[65] Ibid., 71.
[66] Ibid.
[67] A. W. Barclay was a Cambridge graduate and one of the leading practising health officers of the day. Barclay was an honorary consultant physician at St. George's Hospital and Treasurer to the Royal College of Physicians. The role he played in helping to create a public health specialty around the work of the Medical Officer of Health is described by Dorothy Porter in Chapter 3.

ment, not only in public health, but in all aspects of higher education. Not until the turn of the century did a generation of examiners in public health emerge who had themselves taken the examination. The need for experienced and competent examiners was an issue to which the Council would give its attention during the years following the Second Medical Act of 1886, but although opinions differed about the curriculum they caused little contention because without proper legislation *laissez faire* ruled the day.

No reference was made in the Cambridge regulations as to whether, where, or how candidates should seek help in preparing themselves for the examination. Like Edinburgh, the syllabus was less diffuse than in Dublin. Between 1875 and the introduction of the Second Medical Act, courses of lectures and practical laboratory work were slowly developed in Cambridge under the aegis of the Professor of Chemistry, for those who paid the necessary fee.[68] They were simply available on a help-yourself basis: indeed, during the nineteenth century, courses were never obligatory there, nor anywhere else.

Oxford and London

The Universities of Oxford and London both had, for internal reasons, difficulty in initiating examinations for certificates. Details of these are not relevant to this book. In brief, in Oxford they were due to the fierce resistance of a large proportion of senior members of the university to Acland's efforts, successful if painfully slow, to introduce any form of science including a modern medical school to the university. Until 1895, only graduates of the University's small pre-clinical school were eligible to take the Certificate of Public Health and Preventive Medicine. In London, the problem was that the University was federal, and at that time prevented by law from offering any registrable medical qualification. It was not until the passing of the Medical Amendment Act (University of London) in 1873 that this was changed,[69] and not until the end of the Edwardian era that the University could teach medicine

---

[68] Professors of Chemistry were to play a leading role in the introduction of an examination for the DPH in other universities, for instance, Arthur Ransome in Victoria University, Manchester, Alfred Hill in Queen's College, Birmingham, and after Acland's retirement at Oxford, Benjamin Brodie, Wayneflete Professor of Chemistry, contributed to the establishment of the high standard of the examination there. These men differed from Liveing in Cambridge inasmuch as they were all registered medical practitioners and he was not, nor was his successor Purvis *vide infra*. Indeed, as Dorothy Porter shows in Chapter 3, Hill and Ransome became embroiled in the political issues which surrounded the social and professional establishment of the Medical Officer of Health.

[69] *Medical Act Amendment (University of London)* (1873). [36 & 37 Vict., c. 55].

or any other subject. The majority of the students of the great London teaching hospitals took a licence to practice medicine in one of the Royal Colleges of Physicians or of Surgeons and a few of the more privileged took bachelors' degrees in Oxford and Cambridge.

By May 1876, however, Oxford had advertised its first examination for a Certificate in Preventive Medicine and Public Health, and the University of London, a similar Certificate in State Medicine. Later, on 24 May, Acland was able to say in his annual presidential address to the General Medical Council: 'It may be remarked, that the Universities of Dublin, Edinburgh, Cambridge, Oxford and London, have successfully instituted examinations with a bearing on Public Health.'[70,71]

However, the thoroughness and high standards of the instruction and examining of Maclagan in Edinburgh University were not emulated by Dublin, where the numbers of candidates were small; Cambridge, which for over 50 years had attracted more candidates than any other examining body; or Oxford with its problems in finding candidates.

Conjoint Boards

Initially, universities alone offered certificates or diplomas, as well, of course, as degrees. Under pressure from the General Medical Council, the London Royal Colleges separately instituted examinations.[72] The first of these was a Certificate of Hygiene in the Royal College of Physicians which was available for two years before they joined forces with the Royal College of Surgeons to create the Diploma in Public Health of a Conjoint Examining Board.[73] This meant that candidates could meet the General Medical Council's requirement of qualifying in medicine

[70] General Medical Council (1877). *Minutes of Council*, Presidential address by Sir Henry Acland, 24 May, 13; see also Watkins, Dorothy (1984). Licensed to practice: the Diploma in Public Health, 1868–1911, Ph.D. thesis. University of London.

[71] Acland had indeed advertised the Oxford Certificate on 10 May, and had appointed Farr and Simon as examiners, but he was to be frustrated because, like Dublin (but neither Edinburgh nor Cambridge), Oxford University had disallowed him from admitting candidates who were not graduates of his University. As a mere handful of candidates for the Bachelor of Medicine were admitted to Oxford each year it is not surprising that only two Certificates were awarded over the 29 years this constraint was in operation.

[72] The Committee established to negotiate the formation of the Conjoint Examining Board, which was primarily concerned with the needs of students requiring a qualifying licence to register with the General Medical Council, sat under the chairmanship of Sir James Paget who was President of the Royal College of Surgeons and younger brother of Sir George. James was a most distinguished medical scientist. He was the first to describe no less than six diseases, the best known of which are osteitis deformans and Paget's disease of the nipple, a form of carcinoma of the breast. He was, *inter alia*, President of the Royal College of Surgeons and Vice-Chancellor of the University of London.

[73] Cooke, A. M. (1972). *A history of the Royal College of Physicians of London*, Vol. 3, pp. 885–6. Oxford University Press.

and surgery by sitting a single rather than separate examinations.[74] Thus the London Conjoint Examining Board, which was primarily brought into existence to provide a combined qualifying examination, was the last of the six examining bodies with which we are principally concerned. The Royal Colleges in Scotland and Ireland followed suit some years later in forming conjoint boards to offer 'Sanitary Certificates'.

When the Medical Act became imminent there was a rush among other universities to instigate an examination so that by the end of 1886, 14 different licensing bodies were providing qualifications in sanitary science, state medicine, and public health. These included the Edinburgh College of Physicians which had previously been against the whole idea.[75] (See table 2.1.)

The domination of the pioneer universities and the conjoint board

The Diploma in Public Health was to remain as the statutory qualification for the practice of public health for 103 years. During that time, although their relative importance changed consistently, the five pioneer universities and the London Conjoint Board dominated training, as Fig. 2.1 shows.

Before the turn of the century Cambridge awarded most certificates; subsequently, in succession, the London Conjoint Board and the London School of Hygiene and Tropical Medicine, through the University of London, superseded them as leaders.

5. Changes and developments in the curriculum

We have already noted how long it took Parliament to give appropriate powers to the General Medical Council to control the Diploma in Public Health, and we shall show, at the end of the chapter, that when the legislation was eventually passed it was poorly put together, and further delay resulted. However, over the years there was another insidious obstruction to change and progress, for curricula are notorious for their facility to become static. To take two examples: on the one hand for a full decade, the importance of bacteriology was ignored, and on the other, meteorology need not have been retained in the curriculum for 60 years.

---

[74] General Medical Council (1884). *Minutes*, 81–9.
[75] Ibid. (1887), 304. One may assume that fiscal realism won the day against conservative purism.

Table 2.1. List of Licensing Bodies granting Diplomas or Certificates for proficiency in Sanitary Science, Public Health, or State Medicine, and the Designation of such Diplomas or Certificates, with Abbreviations under which they may be Registered.

Licensing Bodies.	Titles.	Abbreviations for Registration.
Royal College of Physicians of London and Royal College of Surgeons of England	Certificate in Hygiene★ Diploma in Public Health†	{ Cert. Hyg. R. Colls. Phys. Surg. Eng. Dip. Publ. Health, R. Coll. Phys. Surg. Eng.
Royal College of Physicians of Edinburgh	Certificate of Qualification in Public Health	Cert. Publ. Health, R. Coll. Phys. Edin.
King and Queen's College of Physicians in Ireland	Diploma in State Medicine	Dip. State Med. K. Q. Coll. Phys. Irel.
Faculty of Physicians and Surgeons of Glasgow	Qualification in Public Health	Qual. Publ. Health, Fac. Phys. Surg. Glasg.
Royal College of Surgeons in Ireland	Diploma in Public Health	Dip. Publ. Health, R. Coll. Surg. Irel.
University of Oxford	Certificate in Preventive Medicine and Public Health	Cert. Publ. Health, Oxfd.
University of Cambridge	Certificate in Sanitary Science★ Diploma in Public Health‡	Cert. San. Sci. Camb. Dip. Pub. Health, Camb.‡
University of Durham	Licence in Sanitary Science	Lic. San. Sci. Durh.
University of London	Certificate in Subjects relating to Public Health	Cert. Publ. Health, Lond.
University of Edinburgh	Bachelor and Doctor of Science in Department of Public Health	B.Sc. D.Sc. (Publ. Health) Edin.
University of Glasgow	Qualification in Public Health	Qual. Publ. Health, Glasg.
University of Dublin	Qualification in State Medicine	Qual. State Med. Dubl.
Royal University of Ireland	Diploma in Sanitary Science	Dip. San. Sci. R. Univ. Irel.

★ Present Title.   † Proposed New Title.   ‡ New Title.

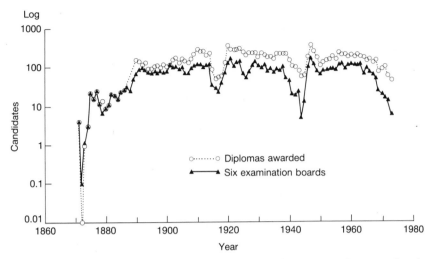

Fig. 2.1 The secular trend in the total numbers of Certificates, Diplomas, and registrable Degrees awarded in State Medicine, Public Health, etc. from 1871 to 1973 (upperline); the lower line indicates the numbers awarded by the Universities of Dublin, Edinburgh, Cambridge, Oxford, and London together with the London Conjoint Board. Note that for the first 15 years, before the Board came into existence, all the qualifications were awarded by these five universities. Thereafter there were very few years when the six pioneering bodies did not award 50 per cent of the qualifications, and overall they awarded nearly 60 per cent.

Epidemiology and meteorology

It is not easy to assess correctly the way epidemiology, meteorology, and bacteriology were taught between 1850, when the Epidemiological Society of London was formed, and 1895, when the General Medical Council formally required bacteriology to be examined for the Diploma in Public Health. Nevertheless, it is worth attempting because these were the three subjects which at the turn of the century were expected to provide a basis for the understanding of the causes of disease, and especially epidemic disease. At one of its early meetings, in November 1850, the Epidemiological Society drew up its 'objects' in eight paragraphs. From these it can be surmised that the Society's definition of epidemiology was in broad terms a: 'Rigid examination into the causes and conditions which influence the origin, propagation, mitigation, and prevention of epidemic diseases in order to throw light into the whole question of epidemics'.[76] Thus, this science, so defined, pre-dated bacteriology by some 30 years and was included in the curricula of all the examinations we have considered in detail, with the exception of the

[76] *Journal of Public Health and Sanitary Review* (1885). Transactions of the Epidemiological Society of London, **1**, Supplement 2.

first Dublin examination. In this, 'The Laws of Epidemiology' were to be included in the paper on the law of the land (but in the event were omitted). For a short time in the 1880s the Royal College of Physicians of Edinburgh offered a diploma of its own which included a paper in Epidemiology and Endemiology,[77,78] otherwise the word was one of many which appeared, without special emphasis, in the detailed syllabuses of the time. Epidemiological questions usually sought description of disease patterns and were often concerned with clinical aspects of the management of fevers. However, a very few looked for comprehension of epidemiological method, such as: 'If sent to enquire into a supposed outbreak of enteric fever, how would you set about the investigation?'[79] Epidemiology was not to be recognized as a science in its own right until after the First World War.

Meteorology, in contrast, received a great deal of emphasis, even though it cannot have been looked upon as more than an adjunct to and for a time perhaps, a substitute for, epidemiology. The contagionists and the miasmatists might contest the relative merits of their pet theories, but neither group questioned that on a local level weather, and on a global one climate, were frequently closely related to outbreaks of epidemic diseases. It followed that if weather could be understood and predicted, then epidemics might be predicted and perhaps understood as well. This was doubtless in part because weather measurement is simpler than disease measurement in populations, but William Farr's influence is clear. From his earliest days in the Registrar General's Office he had been interested in the relationship between the climate and the weather on the one hand, and the health of the people and the mortality they suffered on the other.[80]

Farr was a miasmatist, but he accepted that some diseases were contagious. Stressing the importance of the most detailed meteorological data as a basis for understanding the pathogenesis of what he called endemic disease he wrote:

The temperature, weight, humidity of the atmosphere, and other physical forces should not be masked under mean values, but laboriously traced throughout their course from day to day and if it were possible from morning

[77] An example of what was expected of the candidates is to be found in the question: 'Give the chief circumstances that precede and accompany an epidemic of ergotism together with the symptoms of the disease'.
[78] Edinburgh University Calendar (1883). Department of Public Health second examination for the B.Sc. degree, 9 April, paper entitled "Medicine", Question 3.
[79] University of Oxford (1885). Examination papers for the Certificate in Preventive Medicine and Public Health, Paper 2, Hygiene (General Portion), Question 9.
[80] Registrar General (1840). *Second annual report of the Chief Statistician*, 86–8; ibid. (1841). 3rd, 102–9; ibid. (1863). 23rd, xxv–xxvi; ibid. (1868). 28th, xvii–xix.

to night and from night to morning, and observed in connexion with the contemporaneous facts that relate to human life, these also are successively recorded, if the sway with which they exercise is to be appreciated in its full significance.[81]

Farr always published summaries of meteorological readings over a year with his annual statistical tables, and this practice was not discontinued until 1973, nearly 100 years after he died. Their extraordinary longevity illustrate how the authority of a truly great man, even though he was not recognized as such by his contemporaries, can bridge time. He had made an important contribution to the creation of a new curriculum; but we have also seen how later his authority may have stultified change and development.

In the Dublin examination, a complete paper was assigned to meteorology for the first 17 years until Stokes ceased examining; thereafter, there was a compulsory viva but no longer a separate paper. The other five examining bodies, with which we are concerned, continued to set written questions on it. For example, in 1885, Oxford candidates were asked to: 'Describe a rain gauge and its use. What is a pluviometer? How much rain falls on one acre if the rain gauge shows 3 inches?' The relevance of the third part of the question to the practice of public health is not immediately obvious, but that perhaps is why in the three following examinations (1887, 1896, and 1897), meteorology was omitted.[82] After that, the rules of the General Medical Council required that the subject should be included and it continued so to be. Thus, in 1930–31 the last examination ever to be held in Cambridge included the question: 'Describe the mercurial barometer, its units of graduation and its use. How does the atmospheric pressure affect the working of (a) the common pump (b) the siphon?'.[83] It was a long haul from such material to the interests of the new social medicine movement which by then, in the early 1930s, was beginning to gather impetus among a new generation of medical students, particularly in Cambridge but also elsewhere.[84]

The introduction of bacteriology

By the end of 1875, which was the year that Koch set out his postulates, and so qualifies to be looked upon as the beginning of the bacteriological

[81] Ibid. (1868). *28th annual report*, 18–19.

[82] University of Oxford (1885). Examination in Preventive Medicine and Public Health, Paper II, Hygiene, Question 5.

[83] University of Cambridge (1931). Examination papers, examination for the Diplomas in Public Health etc., 30 March, Part I, Paper I, Question 5.

[84] Three distinguished members of the British social medicine movement who were medical students in Cambridge in the 1930s were, in alphabetical order, Archie Cochrane, Charles Fletcher, and Alice Stewart.

era, there were 10 medical schools in Britain (four in England, four in Scotland, and two in Ireland). At that time three, Dublin, Edinburgh, and Cambridge offered examinations, together, in the case of Edinburgh, with teaching. Because the General Medical Council had no legal authority to insist on the introduction of new subjects or to enforce changes, and because of vested interests in the *status quo*, important advances in related fields passed public health by. The establishment of microbes as a basic cause of epidemic diseases was by far the most important of these. The acceptance, or otherwise, of this innovation can be looked upon as a bell-wether of the ability of a nationally controlled curriculum for public health professionals to stay apace with scientific and technical developments in the field. The Cambridge examiners had from the outset expected candidates to be aware of the importance of bacteria, not it must be said, as pathogens, but as components of the health environment. In 1876, examinees were required to: 'Describe succinctly the present state of knowledge regarding the relation of Bacteria to the processes of putrefaction and fermentation',[85] which, of course, were themselves thought by miasmatists to be pathogens. A similar question was asked in Oxford[86] the following year, where the examiners asked for a description of five organisms including *Bacillus subtilis* together with any 'hygienic operation' each performed. Bacteriology this certainly was, but it had little direct relevance to the pathogenesis of disease. In April 1894, the stasis of the syllabus notwithstanding, a question appeared in Cambridge which asked how a bacteriological examination would be undertaken in a case of cholera to satisfy oneself with the: 'existence of the organism usually associated with cholera'.[87] Thirty years had passed since Budd and Snow had adduced, in their own ways, epidemiological evidence of the bacteriological origins of cholera. The ambivalence of the times is evident from a question in another paper in the same examination: 'Give an account of the influence, if any, of soil, season and climate on pulmonary consumption, scarlet fever and diphtheria . . . '.[88] This was set presumably by a miasmatist with the approval of the other three examiners who, in compliance with the internal regulations, had to approve mutually all questions. This paper contains more on bacteriology than did the October examination of the

---

[85] University of Cambridge (1876). Examination papers, Sanitary Science, Paper 2, Question 3.
[86] University of Oxford (1877). Examination papers, examination in Preventive Medicine and Public Health, Paper 2, Hygiene, Question 1. Archives of Bodleian Library, Oxford.
[87] University of Cambridge (1894). Examination papers, Sanitary Science examination, 17 April, Part I, Paper 1, Question 4. Cambridge University Library.
[88] Ibid. (1894). 19 April, Part II, Paper 1, Question 4.

same year which was inspected by Sir George Duffey for the General Medical Council, and evoked his stern criticism because of the serious lack of questions on bacteriology.[89] He pointed out that even the practical on microscopy was directed towards the description and identification of particles in fluids and powders.

Thirteen years after Koch had published his postulates, Edinburgh took the radical step of revising its syllabus and requiring knowledge of 'Micro-organisms in relation to epidemic and other diseases'.[90] More years were to pass before other schools followed suit. In Edinburgh from 1888, practical laboratory work in bacteriology was required where the candidates were examined as well as being subjected to written and oral tests. The work undertaken included the examination of: water; air; foods; beverages (i.e. tea, coffee, cocoa, alcohol, and aerated waters); condiments; sewage; soils (including micro-organisms); disinfectants and deodorizers; building materials; clothing; and last, but by no means least, bacteriology. Physics was separated from chemistry and its syllabus became of less obvious relevance to public health. Duffey observed this in July 1894 when he challenged the purpose of the question: 'Show how the mass of Jupiter can be compared with that of the Earth'. He was favourably impressed, however, by the extent to which bacteriology was taught, both as a laboratory science, and as a basis for understanding the aetiology of infectious diseases—or as they were then known—zymotic diseases.

Over and above the inertia which resists change, two forces stood against the acceptance of bacteriology as a basic science of public health in the universities. One was the vested interest in the teaching of the natural sciences, particularly by the chemists. For instance, Liveing, the Professor of Chemistry in Cambridge, whose classes on contributions to the analysis of water, air, food, etc., would be threatened.

The second was the concept of zymosis. In 1888 in Cambridge the examiners postulated that in a population of a given magnitude there were in the four quarters of the year a given number of deaths from typhoid fever, from infantile diarrhoea, and from scarlatina; they went on to ask candidates to calculate the zymotic death rate for the year and by quarter.[91] The term zymosis, coined by Farr, had been helpful to him in his attempts to bring reason to the perplexing world of what are now

---

[89] General Medical Council (1895). *Minutes*. Report on the examination in Sanitary Science for the Diploma in Public Health in the University of Cambridge, 29 November, Appendix XII, 508.

[90] University of Edinburgh Calendar (1887–88), 313; ibid. (1888–9), 449.

[91] University of Cambridge (1888). Examination papers, Sanitary Science examination, 5 October, Part II, Paper 1, Question 6.

known as infectious diseases. The term appears in early examination papers in Dublin, Edinburgh, and Oxford. He attributes the word 'zymosis' to Sydenham who wrote of: 'humours worked up into a substantial form or species that discovers itself by particular symptoms, agreeable to its peculiar essence'.[92] He used the terms 'Zymin' and 'Zymine' to describe facets of the process of pathogenesis as he saw it, and the diseases they caused, zymotic diseases. Farr's modification of this was to think in terms of zymotic molecules which he named 'zymads'.[93] The diseases he considered as being zymotic were not confined to the miasmata, although they included them. Farr nevertheless believed that: 'the mere aggregation of people together generates or diffuses the zymotic matter', so that:

to limit the operation of zymotic diseases overcrowding in towns must be absolutely prohibited: the mere accumulation of people living within narrow limits either generates or ensures the diffusion of epidemic disease.[94]

He observed that: 'epidemics appear to be generated at intervals in unhealthy places, spread, go through a regular course, and decline'. These predictable patterns he considered to be in accord with the laws of epidemics.[95] His subdivision of the zymotic diseases he described in the following terms:

The tendency of zymotic diseases to increase and decline in activity is indicated by the terms epidemic and endemic; the latter serving to designate diseases which are excited by miasmata, and prevail in proportion to the quantity of miasm developed; the former, epidemic, denoting the diseases transmitted by man to man, independently of locality, or only dependent on locality, temperature, and moisture as adventitious circumstances. For statistical purposes the epidemic, endemic, and contagious diseases have been classed under one head.[96]

To this day the same diseases are grouped under the heading 'Infective Diseases'; a grouping that was to prove apposite for so long it was hardly surprising that there were many who could see no need for the bacterial theory of disease.[97] The theories of miasma and zymosis had

[92] Wallis, G. *Sydenham's work*, translated from Latin; cited by Farr in his *Fourth annual report to the Registrar General*.
[93] Farr, William (1875). *Supplement to 35th annual report of the Registrar General*, iv, lxv.
[94] Ibid. (1870). *30th annual report*, 213, 214.
[95] Ibid., 212.
[96] Ibid., [1868]. *28th annual report*, xviii–xix.
[97] Eyler, John M. (1979). *Victorian social medicine: the ideas and methods of William Farr*. Johns Hopkins University Press, Baltimore. A critical exposition of Farr's views of the zymotic theory of disease is to be found among John Eyler's collection of essays on William Farr. Eyler's concern is to examine, in the retrospect of a century, how Farr's conceptions of the causation of what we now recognize as infectious diseases developed and matured through his long career. This contrasts with our object which is to consider

found wide support in 1875 and for a long period seemed perfectly adequate to many thinking and influential men—why worry about bacteria?[98]

When great scientific strides are taken, many people are concerned with how they came about and the intolerance of those who resisted their acceptance. However, there may be much sense in the opposition's point of view. The weight of Farr's opinions about aetiology which were based on carefully collected and analysed statistical data must have made people reconsider the importance of bacteria. It was against this background that in 1884 Henry Younger, a leading brewer, invited Pasteur to Edinburgh.[99] Maclagan and his colleagues were evidently inspired by Pasteur's visit and were sufficiently far-sighted to break away from the traditions which had grown from 17 years of teaching public health and subsequently, introduced bacteriology into the syllabus. In Cambridge, the only change of note during those years was the reluctant decision to rationalize the name of the S.Sc.Cert.Camb. to the Diploma in Public Health. Even this was done under pressure from alumni. In Dublin where, as we have shown, the miasmatic influence was strong, there was no change at all.

Chemistry and physics

By the end of the First World War, the usefulness of chemistry and physics was also under question. In a Special Syndicate in Cambridge, which sat briefly early in 1923, to consider the future of the DPH in the University, G.H.F. Nuttall, Professor of Parasitology, is recorded as saying that he had heard that chemistry teaching: 'was not always satisfactory'. He added that: 'a good deal of this work could be left to the analyst'.[100] Here again, as with measuring the weather, there were two fundamental underlying questions. The first was the extent to which a medical practitioner, highly trained in a responsible specialty of his profession, could reasonably be expected to master technical minutiae which were remote from tasks appropriate to his special skills. The

the extent to which Farr's early work in the Registrar General's office influenced medical professors, *aves rarae* in those days, when they sat down to construct a curriculum which would provide a satisfactory basis for training of officers of health, and how subsequently these same ideas have impeded progress.

[98] For further consideration of these issues see Pelling, op.cit. (note 31).

[99] Maclean, Una (1975). *The Usher Institute and the evolution of community medicine in Edinburgh*. Usher Institute Library, Edinburgh. (Limited edition, not generally published.)

[100] University of Cambridge Archives (1923). Minutes of Syndicate appointed by grace of the Senate, January 19, (also unminuted manuscript notes taken by Syndicate secretary of meeting 26 April) [Min vi 53 & 53 A]; see also Chapter 8 (note 46).

second, as we have seen, related to flexibility and modification of the curriculum in response to scientific advance. After all, many chemical procedures, such as aspects of water and food analyses, had already been outdated by the contributions of bacteriologists. Between 1887 and 1893, when every examining body still had freedom to manage its own affairs, chemistry and physics both ceased to be specified in the Oxford curriculum.[101] Technical training should be concerned with the future, but all too often it has simply told of the past.

6. The road to legitimacy

In Sections 2–5 of this chapter we have seen how a national need for a cadre of medical practitioners specially trained to care for, and promote, the health of the public was perceived. Chadwick and the sanitarians, Simon and Rumsey, who carried the infant British Medical Association, all had a part to play. We have seen too how four of the oldest universities in the British Isles ultimately pursued the same cause with success. We have discussed a few of the many problems which were encountered in establishing a sound curriculum, and why, once established, it resisted change.

By the early 1880s, when the examination had existed for 10 years, and some 120 certificates and diplomas had been awarded,[102] a variety of interests was being brought to bear on how practical training should be conducted. Although between them the universities and Royal Colleges had accepted responsibility for turning out an accredited specialist, they differed in their views as to how this was to be done. The General Medical Council had accepted the charge of ensuring that the overall programme was of a high standard, but was impotent without statutory legal support. Also, of growing importance were the new specialists themselves, the medical officers of health, many of whom had obtained the qualification, and some, depending on the mood of the times (see Fig. 2.2), had entered it in the Medical Register. In Chapter 3, Dorothy Porter describes the successes and difficulties met by this group as they struggled to create their identity. Our attention in the rest of this chapter is concentrated on how the examining bodies went about their business,

[101] General Medical Council (1887). *Minutes*, 15 February, 70–1.

[102] The data shown in Figs 2.1 and 2.2 have been obtained from many sources including: *Minutes of the General Medical Council*; *Archives of General Medical Council*; *Cambridge University Reporter*; *Oxford University Gazette*; *Minutes of the Council of the Royal College of Surgeons*, and *Calendars* of all universities which have offered degrees or diplomas in public health, etc. A few of these calendars are extraordinarily primitive and uninformative.

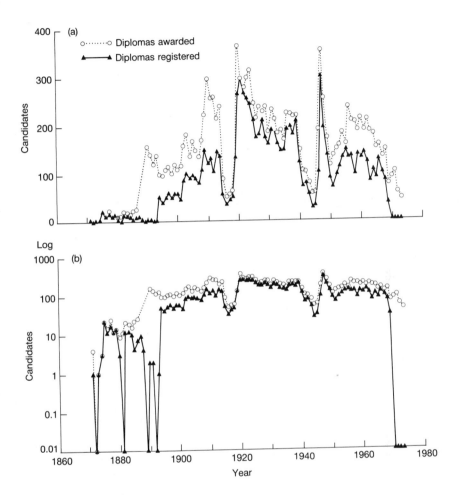

Fig. 2.2 A comparison between the numbers of qualifications in public health awarded and the numbers registered over the years when the DPH (or equivalent) was a registrable qualification. Registration of this qualification was a requirement for practice as a Medical Officer of Health in all but the smallest local authorities. The data are displayed both in arithmetic (a) and logarithmic plots (b). During the 1870s almost all diplomas awarded were registered. However, in the 1880s, when the Medical Act of 1886 was being drafted and debated, the registration rate fell to zero. The reason for this is not evident from readily available information. Presumably it was because of impending legislation that the State Medicine Committee of the Council rarely sat during the 1880s. Awards were all made by the five pioneer universities during those years and details are shown in Fig. 2.1. Although the registration rate was maintained at a high level during the 1920s and the 1930s, it never again reached 100 per cent. This also is the period during which the award rate was highest so it seems that it was then that the qualification was being put most consistently to the purpose for which it was designed.

whether they offered classroom and laboratory instruction, and if they did, how it was carried out.

Education by examination has been a peculiarly British phenomenon. Wickliffe Rose of the Rockefeller Foundation, a pioneer in education in public health, dryly recorded without obvious enthusiasm, when he came to London for the first time, that he was interested to see this system at first hand. Nevertheless, until the 1880s this was how the programme was conducted in the universities of Dublin, Cambridge, Oxford, and London. Indeed, as late as 1920 Professor Henry Kenwood of University College London, the leading academic in public health in England at that time, told Rose that he had abandoned lectures in public health and hygiene and that instead he told the students what to read and offered them quizzes.[103]

Apprenticeship to a medical officer of health

The 1895 General Medical Council inspector's report on teaching and examining in the DPH, to which we shall return, was very critical of the examining bodies' failure to offer and examine in practical experience— be it clinical, epidemiological, laboratory, or 'outdoor work' (the last was the term used at the time for practical experience as an apprentice to a medical officer of health).

However, this was not a new idea. Twenty years earlier, the General Medical Council had unsuccessfully attempted to establish a curriculum, by a consensus survey. Only three of 34 respondents recommended that candidates should have: 'Practical instruction by an Officer of Health in the duties of his office'.[104] These were William Guy, Vice-President of the Royal Society, and Professor of Hygiene in Kings College London, Maclagan of Edinburgh, and Mapother the Medical Officer of Health in Dublin. Maclagan clearly specified a need for experience in what came to be known as 'outdoor work'; Mapother recommended: 'six months with a medical officer of health' and Maclagan, who was directly responsible for the two-year Edinburgh course, wrote that, of this time: 'six months should be spent in the laboratory and one year as assistant to an officer of health'. It was the latter, the supervised apprenticeship, that examining boards found to be a difficult pill to swallow.

However, the value of apprenticeship training in clinical practice had long been recognized in England. To walk the wards of the London

---

[103] Archives of the Rockefeller Foundation (1920). Diaries of Wickliffe Rose. January 1, 20.

[104] General Medical Council (1869). *Minutes of Council*. Second Report of the Committee on State Medicine. 3 July, 3–5.

teaching hospitals under the tutelage of Fellows of the Royal College of Physicians or Surgeons had been, for centuries, the hallmark of English medical education. This experience provided important training components which led up to the qualifying degrees offered in Oxford and Cambridge—the only universities in England until the early nineteenth century. Alternatively, this clinical experience could lead directly to a licence to practice from the Royal College of Physicians or to membership of the Royal College of Surgeons, both registrable by the General Medical Council. The 'clerking' the apprentices did for the physicians, and the 'dressing' they did for the surgeons, were critical contributions to the work of the hospitals, which depended upon voluntary support for their income. Practical work in public health was, as far as the Colleges were concerned, of far less obvious relevance. It was an administrative nuisance to the examination boards, and precious few of the mentors were Fellows. There clearly was, nevertheless, a broadly based concern to ensure that the newly graduated diplomate in public health would be fully prepared to assume with confidence the tasks which were to fall on his shoulders; he should have first hand experience of how they ought to be discharged. Otherwise, the newly qualified officer would have less knowledge of sanitary inspection than sanitary inspectors who would be working under his authority in a district health department.[105]

Laboratory work

Not only the colleges, but also the universities, had to be self-supporting. Few of the professors who were not practising professionals had, apart from their own private means, sources of income other than from endowments and the fees of their pupils, fees which now had to meet the costs of laboratories as well as staff incomes. These economic realities coloured both the wide interest displayed by all the examining bodies throughout the country in offering the DPH, and their attitude to any impediment there might be to the flow of candidates.

There is no reason to believe that any motive other than the furtherance of his subject, which was chemistry, not state medicine or sanitary science, underlay the possessiveness of Professor G. D. Liveing in his teaching and management of the examination in state medicine at Cambridge. In the early 1870s, chemistry offered the most important scientific basis for public health. It was therefore natural that he should be the first secretary of the State Medicine Syndicate, which held total responsibility for the examination and, later, teaching, and was answerable through its chairman, the vice chancellor, directly to the Council of the

[105] Ibid. (1896). 9 June, 387, 388.

Senate. Liveing continued to be a diligent member when he stood down from the secretaryship, and remained a member for 34 years, until his retirement at the age of 81 in 1908.[106] The introduction of bacteriology was smothered and chemistry was promoted until 1895 when the General Medical Council enforced change. Liveing ensured that, on his retirement, his loyal demonstrator, J. E. Purvis, was appointed to a tenured university post and secretaryship of the Syndicate.[107] The bench fees paid by generations of public health students contributed usefully to the support not only of technical staff and the purchase of reagents and other equipment in the Department of Chemistry, but also to the stipends of lecturers, such as Purvis and his predecessors.[108] Accommodation used by public health students was also available for other purposes. Thus, the universities favoured laboratory experience for reasons which were not simply altruistic, and derived long-term benefits which the Conjoint Boards did not. By the late 1870s, Edinburgh, Cambridge, and Oxford all offered such instruction.[109] We shall return to this issue in Chapter 8.

Delay in effectively controlling standards

The early growth of interest in the Certificate in State Medicine was followed by stasis (see Fig. 2.2), and as we have seen, disorder was widespread. Over 20 years were to elapse between the publication of the Report of the Royal Sanitary Commission and 1895 when the General Medical Council legitimately and effectively was able to control standards. The failure of the Commission to take an assertive line and firmly to state that medical officers of health should be properly trained explained this delay in part only. What the Commission had had to say on the matter of state medicine (over and above the definition quoted in the first section of this chapter), was brief: 'inducement should be provided for the study of "State Medicine" . . . It is probable that the large towns would select for the appointments of Officers of Health, men possessing due qualification in "State Medicine"'[110]

[106] *Cambridge University Reporter* (1908). 109.

[107] Ibid. (1909). 1144, 1145.

[108] *Cambridge University Reporter* (1923). Report of the Syndicate on the duties and responsibilities of the Syndicate on State Medicine, 29 April; for drafts see Archives of the University of Cambridge (1923). Special Syndicate on State Medicine, [Min VI 53 A]; see also Chapter 8 (note 42).

[109] Ibid; see also Acheson, Roy M. (1987). The origins, content and early development of the curriculum in State Medicine and Public Health, 1856–1895. *Community Medicine*, **9**, 372–81.

[110] Royal Sanitary Commission (1871). Observations, *Report ii*, 61.

From the government's viewpoint, other reasons were first, the final form of a qualification in state medicine would depend on the working environment, and the terms of reference of the post of Medical Officer of Health. These were derived from the Public Health Acts of 1872 and 1875 (the latter sometimes referred to as the Local Government Act), and the Registration of Births and Deaths Act 1874, referred to in Section I, all of which preceded the Medical Act of 1886. In addition to clarification of the tasks which were expected of the Medical Officer of Health, they described the circumstances in which he would work. Secondly, the Medical Act itself had to deal with other important matters such as the education of medical students and, in particular, their entry on the Medical Register, the registration of women, and the creation of the Conjoint Boards. But the Act, through careless phrasing, occasioned several further years' delay.[111]

The Commissioners' term 'due qualification' was taken to mean a new examination, which would ensure a high standard of preparation of public health doctors and offer benefits to the welfare of the general population. In effect, no demands were to be made on an examining board other than the not too taxing task of administration, a state of affairs which must have been welcomed by treasurers of the Royal Colleges.

During the months immediately before and after the Medical Act became law, interest returned and the number of examining bodies doubled so that by February 1887, as Table 2.1 shows, the diversity of names of qualifications was nearly as great as the number of bodies offering them, and so, to a lesser extent perhaps, was the diversity of the curricula.[112] The former must have been deliberate. One can only assume that this was a means of advertising the individualities of the various examining boards. Their agents would have been their proud alumni who would certainly have written the appropriate series of letters after their names, because such was the style of the times (and indeed still is the style in Britain today.) Indeed, it would seem that the legislators were so preoccupied with the problems of primary registration that they did not give due thought to Section 21 of the Act, the only Section which dealt with postgraduate examinations in state medicine and public health. It was couched as follows:

Every registered medical practitioner to whom a diploma for proficiency in sanitary science, public health or state medicine has after special examination been granted by any college or faculty of physicians or surgeons or

---

[111] Medical Act (1886), [49 & 50 Vict., c. 48], 12, 13.
[112] General Medical Council (1887). *Minutes*, 14 February, 364, 390.

university in the United Kingdom or by bodies acting in combination, shall if such a diploma appears to the Privy Council or to the General Council to deserve recognition in the Medical Register be entitled on payment of such a fee as the General Council may appoint to have such a diploma entered upon the said register.[113]

Nothing was said about the means the Council might use to determine whether a 'body' should deserve recognition nor how it should be considered worthy of having it. Thus, there was no way whereby the Council could maintain the high standards it had already stated were necessary to ensure that the country would have competent health officers.[114] The Council had been given power to inspect qualifying examinations, but the DPH was certainly not such an examination. The examining bodies had only their own interests at heart and saw inspection as a threat to their independence; they stood their ground with the hope of avoiding control, and denied inspectors access. The General Medical Council was therefore compelled to wait until the legal advisers to the Privy Council had obtained a formal ruling on the anomaly, which finally was given in these arcane terms:[115]

The power conferred on the General Medical Council to inspect . . . Examinations refers only to . . . the right for Registration and does not extend to . . . granting Diplomas in State Medicine, but that having regard to the statutory powers and duties of the Council to inquire and consider the Examinations and courses . . . for Diplomas in Sanitary Science . . . and not to give [them] recognition . . . unless satisfied that [they] ensure the standard of proficiency which the Council considered necessary [by inspecting the Examinations] the Council are doing what is convenient and in no way are exceeding their duty.[116]

This opinion is repeated in the minutes more than once[117] so it would appear that despite the Council's acceptance of it—there was resistance elsewhere—the examining bodies themselves were unlikely to have relished the prospect of inspection. All this difficulty in bending a poorly prepared law to meet the recognized needs of those for whom it had been introduced in the first place took another seven years. Whereas there was good cause for the delay involved in introducing the Act itself, in the lack of evidence of malfeasance, bungling seems to be the only

---

[113] Op.cit., para. 21 (note 111).

[114] General Medical Council (1889). *Minutes of Council*, 1 June, "Diplomas . . . deserve recognition in the Medical Register [when] in the judgement of the Council the possession of a distinctively high proficiency scientific and practical in all branches of studies which concern the Public Health."

[115] Ibid. (1887), 131.

[116] Ibid. (1891). Appendix V, 8–9.

[117] Ibid. (1887), 131.

explanation for the further delay of nearly a decade in its implementation.

As Fig. 2.2 shows, about 20 diplomas were awarded annually from 1882 to 1886, but the number who registered fell from 12 of 27 (44 per cent) to 4 of 21 (19 per cent). There follows the three-year period, immediately after the Act had been passed, for which there is no readily available information about diplomas awarded in the country at large. However, by 1890, immediately after the Act had been passed, there was a six-fold increase in the number of diplomas awarded from 26 in 1886 to 155 in 1890. This was due in large part to the doubling of the number of examining boards between 1884 and 1887. The number registering fell to zero in 1889 and again in 1892, but rose slowly thereafter, and continued to rise until the turn of the century when the halcyon days of the DPH began. Both the numbers of awards and the proportions registering sustained their highest levels during the years between the two World Wars.

Inspection at last

On 5 December 1893, immediately after the Privy Council had accepted the legal opinion that permitted inspection of the DPH examination, Dr George Duffey was appointed. The Council was at last placed in a position where, when it chose, and at first hand, it could commission independent information to be collected about the content and standard of any examination for the Diploma.[118]

Duffey was a Dubliner born and bred, who did his medical training and took his Certificate in State Medicine in Trinity College. He practised as a physician in fashionable Merrion Square, the Harley Street of his native city.[119] He had a penetrating eye and a mordant wit. Of the public health examination in his *alma mater* he observed, because there were only two candidates and both failed, that the standards should be high. His detailed comments cast some doubts on whether he really believed this to be the case. He inspected every one of the 13 examining bodies in Britain starting with Edinburgh in July 1894 and finishing with Oxford in November 1895. So far as the substance of the examinations was concerned his first and most forcible criticism was of the lack of emphasis directed towards bacteriology. His recommendations rapidly put this right. Centralized control of the DPH had at last been achieved and was to have the effect of enabling the General Medical

---

[118] Ibid. (1898), 168.
[119] *Dublin Journal of Medical Science* (1903). In memoriam; George Frederick Duffey, **CXVI**, 405–8.

Council to monitor its development more closely, and when clarity was needed to eliminate any ambiguity of purpose. In the long run, however, the stultifying effect of the system was such that the shadows of some ambiguity would have been welcome.

In the next chapter, Dorothy Porter tells of how a new and at times unhappy, medical specialization struggled into existence. She discusses how, during the last 15 years of the century, the General Medical Council came to formulate its first set of Recommendations and Rules, and how it demonstrated that it could and would enforce standards.

Duffey's inspection can be looked upon as a turning point in the development of the Diploma in Public Health. It marked the beginning of the second of the three phases in its existence. The first had been its growth, from seeds which had been sown early in the nineteenth century, and developed through the flowering of the Certificate in State Medicine to maturity in the late 1890s. The story is told in Chapter 8 of how the situation seemed to be well nigh perfect during the Edwardian era; how standards fell as numbers rose; and how demands both at home and abroad for diversification led to a weakening of purpose and the decline of the DPH; but also to the evolution of training in Community Medicine and to the establishment of the professional diploma now known as the Membership of the Faculty of Public Health Medicine.

3

Stratification and its discontents: professionalization and conflict in the British public health service, 1848–1914

DOROTHY PORTER

1. Introduction

The role of the professions is central to an understanding of the development of community health care in Britain.[1] Since the mid-nineteenth century, the construction and execution of health policy has increasingly been determined by professionals legitimated by the authority of specialized knowledge and services.[2] One professional group crucial to Victorian public health administration was medical officers of health. Both Edwin Chadwick and John Simon believed that district health officers were indispensable to an effective system of disease prevention.[3]

The compulsory appointment of medical officers of health, first to metropolitan sanitary districts in 1855 and later to provincial districts throughout England and Wales in 1872, led to the creation of a national service of doctors who were responsible for the health of the community rather than the treatment of individuals.[4] They were employed by local sanitary authorities to monitor health conditions through inspection and report. They were responsible for the removal of nuisances, and implemented the sanitary regulation of overcrowded lodging houses, building standards, the condition of bakeries, dairies, and

---

[1] See, for example, Lewis, Jane (1986). *What price community medicine? The philosophy, practice and politics of public health since 1919.* Harvester, Sussex; Watkins, D. E. (1984). The English revolution in social medicine 1889–1911. Ph. D. thesis, University of London.

[2] Watkins, op. cit. (note 1).

[3] Finer, S. E. (1952). *The life and times of Edwin Chadwick*, pp. 218–28. Methuen, London; Simon, John (1890). *English sanitary institutions*, pp. 334–52. Cassel, London.

[4] *Metropolitan Management Act* (1855) [18 Vict]; *Public Health Act* (1875) [38 & 39 Vict].

slaughter houses, etc. From 1889, they enforced prevention of infectious diseases through notification and isolation procedures. By the turn of the century they increasingly supervised local services such as health visiting.[5]

The annual reports of medical officers of health are a rich historical source of information on the 'people's health' during the nineteenth and twentieth centuries. Karl Marx was one of the first to use this material in his analysis of the living conditions of agricultural workers.[6] Modern social and economic historians have used the same materials to analyse the impact of social policy upon Victorian health and the role of state intervention upon local economies.[7] Jeanne Brand and Ruth Hodgkinson have examined the role of state doctors, working in both the Poor Law and public health service, in terms of their contribution to policy development and execution.[8] However, no analysis has yet been made of medical officers of health as a professional group. The function of public health officers was structured by Parliament, but the interpretation of policy was governed by professional ideology. Thus, examining the emergence of professionalism amongst public health doctors explores not so much what they did as why.

Max Weber identified bureaucratic and professional forms of social organization as the defining characteristics of modern industrial society.[9] Weber suggested that professionalization resulted in the operation of power by certain occupations by creating market monopolies on the supply of specialized labour. Emile Durkheim, on the other hand, suggested that the secularization of the moral order of modern society would be achieved through the rise of professional ethics. Durkheim regarded professional practice as the foundation of a new moral order which would replace waning religious values as the basis for social cohesion.[10]

[5] Frazer, William (1950). *History of English public health 1834–1939*, pp. 121–5, 131, 198. Baillière, Tindall & Cox, London.

[6] Marx, Karl (1887). *Das Kapital*. Trans. from 3rd edn. by S. More and E. Aveling (ed. Frederick Engels), 2 volumes, Vol. 1, pp. 484–95. Sonnenschein, London.

[7] See, for example, Wilkinson, Anne (1982). The beginnings of disease control in London. The work of medical officers of health in three parishes. Ph. D. thesis. University of London.

[8] Hodgkinson, Ruth (1956). Poor Law medical officers of England. *Journal of the History of Medicine and Allied Sciences*, **11**, 229–38; Brand, Jeanne (1965). *Doctors and the state: the British medical profession and government action in public health, 1870–1912*. Johns Hopkins University Press, Baltimore, Maryland.

[9] Weber, Max (1964). *The theory of social and economic organisation*. Trans. A. M. Henderson and Talcott Parsons. Free Press, New York.

[10] Durkheim, Emile (1957). *Professional ethics and civic morals*. Trans. Cornelia Brookfield, pp. 10–29. Routledge & Kegan Paul, London.

During the 1930s, Carr-Saunders and Wilson extended the Durkheimian model in an analysis of the 'traits' which characterized the professions as 'a collective orientation', 'altruism', and 'a commitment to service'.[11] Talcott Parsons reinforced the idea that the professions realized common social goals and aims. Parsons claimed that professional occupations embodied the 'primacy of cognitive rationality', thus making them the standard bearers of the institutionalization of science in social organization. In the medical profession, Parsons traced the expression of cognitive rationality through mechanisms, such as affective neutrality and the functional specificity of the professional role. In this way, he argued, doctors were able to emphasize the technical basis of their role to manage relationships of potential tension with patients.[12] Both the trait model and functional analysis of the professions have been severely criticized by modern sociologists. Terence Johnson, for example, has pointed out that both of these models were ahistorical. He suggested that the social status and function of occupational groups changed in relation to much broader social conditions which prevailed at any particular time.[13]

Taking up a number of themes from Johnson, Elliot Freidson has recently indicated that the term professionalism has assumed a generic meaning, but that it actually represents the development of specifically Anglo-American professions, such as the law and medicine. He suggests that this static model of professionalism should be replaced by an historical typology of occupations. Occupational groups should be examined with broader reference to changing patterns of social stratification. Like Rueschemeyer, Freidson emphasizes the need to follow the historical development of occupational autonomy through the social control of expert knowledge.[14]

In this context, Freidson has suggested that some of the concepts developed by Everett Hughes in his analysis of 'The making of the physician' are important. Specifically, he suggests that 'licence and mandate' as a means of achieving market monopoly over the supply of expert knowledge are especially useful concepts for understanding

[11] Carr-Saunders, A. M. and Wilson, P. A. (1933). *The professionals*. Oxford University Press.

[12] Parsons, Talcott (1951). *The social system*. Free Press, New York.

[13] Johnson, Terence J. (1972). *Professions and power*, pp. 9–47. Macmillan, London.

[14] Friedson, E. (1983). The theory of professions: state of the art. In *The sociology of the professions* (ed. R. Dingwall and P. Lewis) pp. 19–37. Macmillan, London; Rueschemeyer, D. Professional autonomy and the social control of expertise. In ibid., pp. 38–58.

professional development.[15] This chapter is a historical study of medical officers of health as an occupational group. It traces the origins of stratification and its importance to the establishment of professional identity, aims, and goals up to the First World War. Equally, the chapter concentrates on the function of licensing in the labour economy of preventive medicine and its role in securing the professional consolidation of medical officers of health.

2. Social and occupational stratification

Charles Webster recently pointed out how medical officers of health could vary widely in their occupational orientation. During the 1930s, some medical officers of health strangled schemes for distributing free milk to school children while other officers maximized them.[16] Such contrasts, it would seem, were not simply the result of the philosophy of individual officers but were determined by the structure of the occupational group as a whole.

From their initial appointment under the 1848 Public Health Act all medical officers of health were medical practitioners even though the Act itself was ambiguous about qualifications. The first two officers were employed before 1848 under local public health acts passed by the City of Liverpool and the City of London. William Duncan in Liverpool, and John Simon in the City, had established prestigious and élite medical careers before entering public health service.[17]

The Lancet had expressed fears that the ambiguity of the 1848 Act would allow the new appointments to be taken up by ill-qualified

[15] Hughes, E. (1956). The making of the physician. *Human Organisation*, **14**, 22–5. The history of the sociology of the professions presented here is necessarily brief and incomplete. For additional discussion of history and sociology of the medical profession see Parry, N. and Parry, J. (1976). *The rise of the medical profession: a study of collective social mobility*. Croom Helm, London; Merton, R. K. (1960). *Some thoughts on the professions in American society*, Brown University Papers, **37**, Providence; id., Some preliminaries to a sociology of medical education. In Merton, R. K., Reader, G., and Kendall, P. L. (ed.) (1957). *The student physician*, pp. 3–79. Harvard University Press, Cambridge, Massachusetts; Reader, W.J. (1966). *Professional men: the rise of the professional classes in nineteenth-century England*. Weidenfeld & Nicolson, London; Rueschemeyer, D. (1964). Doctors and lawyers: a comment on the theory of the professions. *Canadian Review of Sociology and Anthropology*, **1**, 17–30; Ben-David, Joseph (1971). *The scientist's role in society: a comparative study*. Prentice-Hall, Englewood Cliffs, New Jersey.

[16] Webster, Charles (1985). Health, wealth and unemployment during the depression. *Past and Present*, **109**, 204–30.

[17] Frazer, W. M. (1947). *Duncan of Liverpool*. Hamilton Medical Books, London; Lambert, Royston (1963). *Sir John Simon 1816–1904 and English sanitary administration*. Macgibbon and Kee, London.

Table 3.1. Metropolitan medical officers of health appointed in 1855

Highest qualification	Place where qualification obtained					Total
	London	Scotland	Oxford and Cambridge	Dublin	Europe	
FRCP/ FRCS	13 (27.1)	2 (4.2)		1 (2.1)		16 (33.4)
University degree	3 (6.2)	10 (20.8)	1 (2.1)		1 (2.1)	15 (31.2)
MRCS/LRCP and LSA	16 (33.3)	1 (2.1)				17 (35.4)
Total	32 (66.6)	13 (27.1)	1 (2.1)	1 (2.1)	1 (2.1)	48 (100.0)

Source: Medical directory for England and Wales, 1856–1900. Allan, F. J. (1906). *Public health*, Jubilee number.

quacks.[18] Colin Fraser Brockington, however, has shown that the first officers were all fully qualified medical men and some enjoyed reputations equivalent to those of Simon and Duncan.[19] When the first compulsory appointment of officers was established in London by the Metropolitan Management Act in 1855, the recruitment of élite medical men continued. Although few had Oxford or Cambridge degrees, a third of the first 48 London officers were Fellows of the Royal medical corporations.[20]

Some were members of the London hospital élite, such as Andrew Whyte Barclay (1817–84). Barclay, who was the son of one of Nelson's officers, studied medicine in Edinburgh, Berlin, and Switzerland before entering Cambridge in 1843. His first apppointment was at St. George's Hospital and, on the retirement of Bence-Jones, he became a consultant

[18] Brockington, C. F. (1965). *Public health in the 19th century*, p. 141. Livingstone, Edinburgh. See also discussion by Simon, op. cit. (ref. 3), 244–78.

[19] Brockington, op. cit. (note 18), 141–63, 187–91, and Appendix IV.

[20] For discussion of the structure of the medical profession in mid-Victorian England see Peterson, Jeanne (1978). *The medical profession in mid-Victorian England.* University of California Press, Los Angeles; Loudon, I. (1983). The origin of the general practitioner. *Journal of the Royal College of General Practitioners,* **33**, 13–18; id. (1986). *Medical care and the general practitioner, 1750–1850.* Clarendon Press, Oxford; Waddington, Ivan (1977). General practitioners and consultants in early 19th century England: the sociology of intra-professional conflict. In *Health care and popular medicine in nineteenth-century England,* (ed. J. Woodwood and D. Richards), pp. 164–85. Croom Helm, London.

physician there. He was treasurer of the Royal College of Physicians in
1883.[21]

Other medical officers of health were members of the scientific medical élite. Frederick Pavy, John Burdon Sanderson, William Odling and
Edwin Lankester were all distinguished members of the Victorian scientific community. Lankester was already a Fellow of the Royal Society,
President of the Royal Microscopical Society and member of the Darwinian scientific circle when he took up the appointment of Medical
Officer of Health to St. James's district in London.[22] Pavy, Odling, and
Sanderson were, however, at the outset of their careers when they
became metropolitan public health officers. Earlier in the decade they
had all been students of Claude Bernard. All three were subsequently to
make significant contributions to medical chemistry. Pavy continued to
work on the theory of diabetes. He opposed Bernard's theories and
maintained an ongoing controversy with his contemporary William
Thudichum. Both Pavy and Thudichum completed research for the
Medical Department of the Privy Council and the Local Government
Board. Odling succeeded Faraday as Fullerian Professor of Chemistry at
the Royal Institution and later replaced Benjamin Brodie as Waynflete
Professor of Chemistry at Oxford. John Burdon Sanderson became the
leading Victorian chemical pathologist and experimental physiologist.[23]

The first Metropolitan Medical Officers of Health were also recruited,

[21] *Lancet* (1884). **i**, 872; Brown, G. F. (ed.) (1955). *The lives of the Fellows of the Royal
College of Physicians of London, 1826–1925 (Munk's Roll)*, 6 volumes, vol. 4, pp. 62–3.
Routledge & Kegan Paul, London. For discussion of the distinguished career of Henry
Bence-Jones see Rosenbloom, Jacob (1919–20). An appreciation of Henry Bence-Jones.
Annals of Medical History, **2**, 262–4; Bence-Jones, H. (1929). *An autobiography with elucida-
tions and dates.* Crusha, London.
[22] Lankester was a leading natural historian and President of the Natural History
Society. His son, Edwin Ray Lankester, became Linacre Professor of Anatomy at
Oxford, and was later the Director of Natural History at the British Museum. See *Dic-
tionary of national biography* (1959). 22 volumes, Vol. 11, pp. 578–80. Oxford University
Press. *Lancet* (1874) **ii**, 616–627. He also replaced Thomas Wakley as Coroner for Central
Middlesex. The Coronership was a controversial office during the mid-Victorian period.
Wakley had led a campaign to improve the quality of expert medical evdence in the court
room. Lankester continued Wakley's aim to retain a medical man as the Coroner for Central Middlesex. See Anderson, Olive (1987). *Suicide in Victorian and Edwardian England*,
pp. 15–40, 107–47. Clarendon Press, Oxford.
[23] *Lancet* (1911). **ii**, 976–80; ibid. (1874). **ii**, 578; Burdon Sanderson, Lady (1911). *Sir
John Burdon Sanderson. A Memoir.* Clarendon Press, Oxford. See also Pavy, F.W. (1869).
Researches on the nature and treatment of diabetes. Churchill, London. For controversy
between Pavy and Thudichum see Pavy, F.W. (1860). On experimental glycosuria.
British Medical Journal, **1**, 202–6. For discussion of Thudichum and Pavy see Simon, op.
cit. (note 3), 285–95. For an example of J. B. Sanderson's pioneering research see: On the
intimate pathology of contagion, *Twelfth report of the Medical Officer of the Privy Council
with appendix, 1869*, pp. 229–56. Eyre & Spottiswoode, Her Majesty's Stationery Office,
London.

both from amongst university trained doctors and from amongst those with basic licensing qualifications only. Although officers had trained in a wide variety of locations, a predominant pattern was the combination of a London licence and a Scottish MD. Many of the earliest public health doctors had thus experienced the combined practical and theoretical education available at the Scottish schools.[24] Subsequent recruitment to the Metropolitan public health service came largely from this middle level of university-trained doctors. The élite physicians, scientists, and surgeons disappeared from the public health profession in London and were increasingly replaced by what Charles Newman described as the 'safe general practitioner'.[25] This is not the place to reiterate the history of English medical education. It is important to mention, however, that new trends after the passing of the 1858 Registration Act which encouraged joint qualification—manifested in the establishment of joint licences, such as the English Conjoint Board LRCP, LRCS, founded in 1884—were reflected amongst new officers appointed in London.[26] The officers taking up appointments between 1856 and 1887 were less likely to be either élite doctors or by contrast only minimally qualified men. Those from the middle stratum swelled the ranks of the profession.[27]

Two new laws changed the pattern of recruitment in the 1890s. The 1888 Local Government Act was designed to reorganize local government through the creation of County Authorities. It also created a new layer of public health administration with a county health department and officer. Clause 21 of the Act stated that no officer should be appointed to a district with a population of more than 50 000 without possessing a registered qualification in public health.[28] This ensured that only qualified officers would be employed in the new county service and in large, urban, densely populated districts. In 1891, the Public Health (London) Act made specialist qualifications compulsory for all

---

[24] For discussion of medicine and enlightenment in Scotland see Lawrence, C. (1984). *Medicine as culture: Edinburgh and the Scottish enlightenment*. Ph. D. thesis. University of London.

[25] For discussion of medical education in the Victorian period see Newman, Charles (1957). *The evolution of medical education in the nineteenth century*. Oxford University Press; McMenemey, W. H. (1966). Education and the medical reform movement. In *The evolution of medical education in Britain*, (ed. F.N.L. Poynter), pp. 138–53. Pitman, London; Holloway, Sidney (1964). Medical education in England, 1830–1858: a sociological analysis. *History*, **49**, 299–324.

[26] For the history of the formation of the Conjoint Board and its role in medical education see Cooke, A. M. (1972). *A history of the Royal College of Physicians of London*, Vol. 3, pp. 860–6. Clarendon Press, Oxford.

[27] For prosopographical analysis, see Watkins op. cit. (note 1), 72–80, 100–3.

[28] Parliamentary Papers (1888). *Local Government (England and Wales) Bill, as amended in Committee*, [51 & 52 Vict.], [Bill 338], Vol. IV, 136ff.

Table 3.2. Metropolitan medical officers of health appointed 1855–1914

Highest qualification	Place where qualification obtained					Total
	London	Scotland	Oxford and Cambridge	Dublin	Europe	
FRCP/ FRCS	1 (3.2)					1 (3.2)
University degree	3 (9.7)	7 (22.6)	6 (19.3)	3 (9.7)	3 (9.7)	22 (71.0)
MRCS/LRCP and LSA	4 (12.9)	4 (12.9)				8 (25.8)
Total	8 (25.8)	11 (35.5)	6 (19.3)	3 (9.7)	3 (9.7)	31 (100.0)

Source: *Medical directory for England and Wales, 1888–1900.*

metropolitan appointments. The Act also changed the employment status of metropolitan officers providing them with security of tenure. Up to that point all were employed on annually renewable contracts.[29]

This changed recruitment to the metropolitan service dramatically. Even an officer who was in post in 1890 could be required to obtain a specialist qualification when his contract was renewed in 1891. Thus, the great majority of metropolitan officers in the 1890s possessed a specialist postgraduate qualification in preventive medicine. Almost half of them had obtained a postgraduate Diploma in Public Health from Cambridge, and the others had specialist qualifications from the London Conjoint Board or the Universities of Oxford, Durham, or Edinburgh.

The post–1888 recruits had a different pattern of occupational distribution from that of previous metropolitan officers. The initial metropolitan medical officers of health frequently had hospital appointments in the large teaching hospitals and were in general practice. General practitioners coming into the service held fewer hospital posts but more often worked in local dispensaries. Although pre-1888 officers clearly continued to practice curative medicine, very few of them held appointments as Poor Law medical officers. Subsequently, most officers were full-time and were obliged to abandon general practice. Frequently, however, the post–1888 recruits had never practised curative medicine at any stage of

[29] Parliamentary Papers (1890–99). *Public Health (London) Law Amendment Bill,* [54 Vict.] 1, Vol. III.

their professional career. They did continue to hold other appointments, but these were usually in public health, such as that of a public analyst, or teaching university courses in preventive medicine.[30]

From 1855, the metropolitan public health service contained well-qualified doctors, but by the end of the century these were largely specialists in preventive medicine. Late nineteenth century London officers had abandoned the practice of curative medicine and had a distinct professional orientation and an identity with community health.

In 1875, the Public Health Act made the appointment of medical officers of health to provincial sanitary districts compulsory. There were no clauses in the Act specifying special qualifications. In his evidence to the 1868 Royal Sanitary Commission, Henry Rumsey, the prominent mid-Victorian spokesman for the medical profession, had suggested that the medical officer of health should be a physician or surgeon who had discontinued general practice. He believed that hospital work was not, however, incompatible with public health service.[31] In the second reading of the Public Health Bill itself, Lyon Playfair, the most prominent parliamentary representative of the medical profession, clarified the conflict of interests which could arise between a public health office and private practice:

And what class of men does the Bill look to for so much independence? To the Poor-Law medical officers? That is a meritorious hard worked and poorly paid class of medical men; but they are already borne down by the extent of their curative duties. If you add extensive preventive duties to these, and even pay them well for the new work, what chance is there that both the curative and preventive functions will be efficiently executed? It would have been possible if local authorities were united into county areas to have obtained medical men who relinquished the cure of disease in order to have no conflict between the interests of his patients and those of the public; for a medical man must be well paid to secure independence of action when he devotes his whole time to the health of communities instead of individuals.[32]

The failure of the 1875 Public Health Act to compel small districts to combine their resources in order to obtain full-time officers remained a thorn in the flesh of the public health service and played an important role in subsequent professional conflicts. Once the Act was in force, the

---

[30] See Watkins, op. cit. (note 1), 80–7.

[31] Parliamentary Papers (1868–69). *First report of the Royal Sanitary Commission, minutes of evidence*, Vol. XXXII, 283. For Rumsey see Power, Sir D'Arcy (1930). *Plarr's lives of the Fellows of the Royal College of Surgeons of England*, 4 volumes, Vol. 2, pp. 252–4. Simkin Marshall, London. *British Medical Journal* (1876). **2**, 638–9.

[32] Hansard (1872). *Parliamentary debates, Commons*, 4th series, Vol. CCX, 857–8. For Playfair see *Dictionary of national biography* (1959). 1st Supplement, pp. 1142–4. Oxford University Press; Reid, Sir T. Wemys. *Memoirs and correspondence of Lyon Playfair*. Cassell, London.

size and population levels of districts determined the range of appointments. At one end of the scale there were large urban districts which
appointed full-time officers qualified in preventive medicine. At the
other extreme there were small, sparsely populated rural districts where
the appointment of a medical officer of health and his salary were simply
nominal, a token gesture to comply with the law. Thus, the 1875 legislation created a differential structure in the provincial public health service, divided between full- and part-time appointments. The career
histories of two samples of provincial officers, appointed between
1875–1914, are examined here in order to identify variations in professional orientation. The two samples are those holding 'nominal
appointments' as medical officers of health and those holding full-time
posts.[33]

First, it is clear that recruitment of part-time officers decreased after
1900, whereas the number of newly employed full-time officers
increased almost by the same ratio. The type of doctors recruited to
part-time nominal appointments remained consistent throughout the
period up to 1914. Predominantly they obtained their licence to register
as medical practitioners from the London Conjoint Board and a small
proportion had obtained an MD either from Edinburgh or Glasgow.
Hardly any possessed a Diploma in Public Health.

By contrast, few full-time officers had not received a university education. A small proportion had been trained in English provincial
medical schools and this proportion increased after 1900. Ninety-three
per cent of officers appointed after 1900 possessed a DPH. Although
many of them would be required by law to have a specialist qualification, it was still possible for full-time officers to be appointed on the
basis of previous experience and then obtain a DPH once in post. It is

---

[33] The sample of 'nominal appointments' was derived from the *Medical directory for
England and Wales* (1875–1914). It is a list of all medical officers of health receiving £25 or
less per year during that period. An original list of such appointments, as they existed in
the year 1899, was drawn up by T.W.H. Garstang. Garstang's list was, however, of only
limited value. It was quite accurate for the year 1899. For all other years it was inaccurate
because of the combination of districts from year to year. See Garstang, T.W.H.
(1899–1900). Security of tenure for medical officers of health. *Public Health*, **12**, 63–79.
The total sample of 'nominal appointments' presented in this essay is 207 officers. The
sample of full-time officers was also derived from the *Medical directory for England and
Wales* (1875–1914). These were officers who were listed as 'not in private practice'. The
salaries of these officers ranged between £350 and £1000 a year. There could have been
officers who were not in private practice but who were not listed as such in the *directory*.
The sample of full-time officers listed, however, was large enough for the preliminary
analysis presented here. The total number of full-time officers analysed was 245. It is clear
from the *directory* that the majority of provincial officers were neither in full-time nor in
'nominal appointments'. Most officers were 'half-time' or 'part-time'. These officers
received between £26 and £400 a year.

clear, however, that provincial full-time officers had specifically trained for full-time public health service. Few of them had drifted from general practice into public health. The majority of such full-time provincial officers obtained their DPH at Cambridge but after 1900, more of them had taken their DPH in London and at the new provincial medical schools.

Nominal part-time provincial officers had a significantly different professional orientation from full-time medical officers of health. The former were often low-qualified general practitioners who took up an appointment as a medical officer of health for the small extra salary it would add to a meagre income. Taking up a state appointment also prevented outside competition coming into the local medical market-place. Full-time provincial officers, however, had more in common with their metropolitan colleagues. They were university-trained doctors who had specialized in preventive medicine with a view to full-time employment in public health.

Professional identity was equally reflected in patterns of medical employment. Part-time medical officers of health held a wide variety of government medical appointments, most frequently being a local Poor Law officer and public vaccinator. Some were factory inspectors. Often, they held appointments in local voluntary hospitals and dispensaries. A part-time officer in an isolated rural district was often the only registered medical practitioner available and thus filled all the local state medical posts. This was not the case, however, amongst part-time officers in small urban districts. Here, there would be much greater competition amongst local general practitioners for government and hospital appointments. The part-time officers who took up multiple medical appointments in this context must have been able to mobilize enough prestige and influence to compete successfully against their local rivals. Holding a public health office could have been a major stepping-stone to establishing a superior reputation and enlarging a practice within the local medical market-place. Thus, part-time public health officers who also remained in private medical practice were often bitterly resented by other local general practitioners.[34]

Full-time provincial officers were not allowed to remain in private practice but could hold other appointments. As was the case with metropolitan districts, very few were Poor Law medical officers and hardly any worked in dispensaries. Occasionally they were factory inspectors and some were local public analysts. Full-time officers increasingly became responsible for administrating local isolation

[34] See Crawford, Thomas (1895–96). The position of medical officers of health in regard to the administration and working of the Infectious Diseases Notification Act. *Journal of the Sanitary Institute*, **16**, 353–61.

Table 3.3. Provincial medical officers of health holding nominal appointments, 1875–1900 (occupational distribution)

	Hospital	Teaching post	School officer	Dispensary appointment	Medical officer	Public vaccinator	Public analyst	Factory inspector	Auxiliary employment
FRCS and FRCP	2			1	2			1	3
University degree	11			4	20	10		2	15
MRCS/LRCP and LSA	22	1	4	8	66	35	2	17	63
DPH					3	2			4

Note: Individual officers often held more than one appointment at the same time.
Source: Medical directory for England and Wales, 1875–1900.

Table 3.4. Provincial medical officers of health holding nominal appointments, 1901–14 (occupational distribution)

	Hospital	Teaching post	School officer	Dispensary appointment	Medical officer	Public vaccinator	Public analyst	Factory inspector	Auxiliary employment
FRCS and FRCP					**None**				
University degree	14	2	1	3	15	10		4	14
MRCS/LRCP and LSA	7	1	1	1	13	13		5	14
DPH					**None**				

Note: Individual officers often held more than one appointment at the same time.
Source: Medical directory for England and Wales, 1901–1914.

hospitals as more authorities provided them. The most pronounced trend amongst full-time provincial officers, however, was to have no additional employment at all. Full-time office often meant exactly that, with no time for additional occupations.

Salary levels were crucial to the question of how much time an officer devoted to his public health appointment. As Lyon Playfair pointed out, the state could purchase the independence of a doctor from private practice only with a substantial salary. How much did independence cost? A list of salaries of full-time provincial officers prepared as an internal memorandum for the local government board in 1885 showed that the lowest was about £350 and the highest was £900. Most salaries actually ranged between £400 and £600.[35] The range of salaries for full-time officers recorded in the *Medical directory* from 1875 to 1914 remained largely within this range. After 1900 some salaries increased substantially. Dr M. K. Robinson, Medical Officer of Health for Dover (excluding the Port Authority) was receiving £1300 a year by 1914. After 1900 there were very few full-time officers who received less than £500 per year. Part-time salaries ranged between £10 and £350, depending on the amount of time a medical officer of health devoted to his office and the size of the district. Some part-time medical officers of health held more than one such part-time appointment and the combination of salaries was equivalent to the salary of a full-time officer. This type of officer has not been considered in this chapter and it is not known whether medical officers of health in this group devoted their whole time to public health work or whether a proportion of them continued in private practice even though they were receiving a high aggregate salary from separate local sanitary authorities.[36]

There was considerable occupational mobility between the provincial and metropolitan services. Forty-six per cent of recruits to the metropolitan boroughs between 1875 and 1914 had previously held full-time posts in provincial districts. Very few London medical officers of health left to become provincial officers and those who did took up appointments as county medical officers of health.[37]

A tripartite structure of stratification emerged in the English public health service at the end of the nineteenth century. Metropolitan medical officers of health were employed under ideal conditions by the end of the century and their career histories reflect their specialist professional orientation. They were employed full-time on high salaries and had security of tenure. Full-time provincial officers often shared many of the

[35] Local Government Board. Correspondence with Poor Law unions and sanitary districts, MH12/2947/74704.
[36] *Medical directory for England and Wales* (1875–1914).
[37] Ibid.

Table 3.5. Provincial medical officers of health holding full-time appointments 1875–1900

	Asylum	Vol. hosp.	Fever hosp.	Teaching post	Dispens. appt.	Medical officer	Public vacc.	Factory insp.	Public analyst	Auxiliary employ.	Bact. lab.
FRCS and FRCP		4	8	2	3	2	1		5	7	
University degree	1	11	9	4	4	6	4	2	4	11	1
MRCS/LRCP and LSA	1		3	2		1	2		1	3	
DPH	1	5	11	6	3	2	3	1	6	8	1

Note: Individual officers sometimes held more than one appointment at the same time.
Source: Medical directory for England and Wales, 1875–1900.

Table 3.6. Provincial medical officers of health holding full-time appointments, 1901–14 (occupational distribution)

	Asylum	Vol. hosp.	Fever hosp.	Teaching post	School officer	Dispens. appt.	Medical officer	Public vacc.	Factory insp.	Public analyst	Auxiliary employ.	Bact. lab.
FRCS and FRCP			1		2				1	1	1	
University degree	2	13	47	10	60	1	4	4	8	2	27	4
MRCS/LRCP		4	16	2	12							4
DPH	1	8	54	11	59		3	2	6	5	23	7

Note: Individual officers sometimes held more than one appointment at the same time.
Source: Medical directory for England and Wales, 1901–1914.

professional attributes and orientations of metropolitan officers. They were not, however, employed under the same terms. They had no security of tenure and had to face reassessment each year by their employers, the local sanitary authority.

Part-time officers in nominal appointments received the lowest salaries and had no professional orientation toward preventive medicine. They were general practitioners in the fullest sense, who took up multiple part-time public health appointments but remained primarily private family doctors. Such officers were by far the greatest majority within the public health service in England and Wales up to the First World War.

Although professional medical officers of health were thus in a small minority, they succeeded in dominating the public health system by uniting to pursue their collective interests. They mobilized a market monopoly upon the supply of specialized services and established a powerful political voice in Victorian health care.

3. Licensing and legitimacy

The young aspiring professionals within the public health service were the product of new patterns of clinical and preventive medical education. After the Medical Act of 1858, medical training became organized and was increasingly based in the universities. Education in preventive medicine mushroomed during the 1890s.

Specialist training was significant for the professionalization of the medical officer of health. It became a mandatory licence to practice preventive medicine in community health. The meaning of medical licensing qualifications differed according to the educational values which they represented. Similarly, the value of the DPH as a licence was determined by the regulation of curricula, rules of study, and examination.

The development of a diploma in state medicine began within the General Medical Council in 1868.[38] The history of the intrigues behind setting up the first diplomas, their content and early development, has been discussed in the last chapter.[39] This chapter draws out the function of the DPH as a means of economic monopoly in the medical labour

---

[38] General Council for Medical Education and Registration (1868). *Minutes of the General Council*, **6**, 27 June.

[39] See also Watkins op. cit. (note 1), 105–59; Acheson, Roy M. (1978). Medicine, the community and the university: a century of Cambridge history. *British Medical Journal*, **2**, 1737–41; *idem* (1986). Three Regius Professors, sanitary science and state medicine: the birth of an academic discipline. *British Medical Journal*, **293**, 1602–6.

market. The role of curricular manipulation through state regulation is crucial to this analysis. The initial certificates and diplomas were offered by examination in the 1870s and 1880s and were characterized, from the outset, by a wide variation in standards between different licensing institutions.[40] For example, at neither the University of London nor the Conjoint Board of the Royal Colleges of Physicians and of Surgeons could candidates enter the examinations unless they had been registered practitioners for at least one year. Nor could they, in the case of the Board, until they were at least 23 years old when taking Part I, and 24 when taking Part II of the diploma. Thus, the candidate could obtain the DPH only after completing his medical licensing examinations.[41] This was not universally the case at that time. In the University of Durham, for example, candidates could take a public health diploma before sitting the final examinations of the medical licence. This was also the case at the University of Glasgow and at all the Irish Licensing Boards.[42] The English Conjoint Board had an interval of six months between Parts I and II of the diploma, but elsewhere two-part examinations, such as those at Cambridge, could be taken simultaneously, which meant that candidates who failed the first part could still take the second.[43]

During the 1870s and 1880s, the reform of medical education moved closer towards dual licensing, which was finally established under the 1886 Medical Act. The Act also included a clause which created a register for qualifications in sanitary science.[44] Within two decades of this new specialism being created, the postgraduate diploma in public health became the first (and last) such qualification to be registrable by the state. The registrable status of the DPH was a prerequisite to its becoming an effective licence, as it gave the General Medical Council the same power to police the regulation of its standards that it already possessed for clinical medical education. This, together with the clauses of the Local Government Act of 1888 discussed earlier, which abolished unqualified appointments in densely populated sanitary districts, created a stratum of specialist officers employed in the provincial districts. The licence to specialize in 'preventive' rather than 'curative' medicine was the basis of a new

[40] The first four certificates in state medicine were awarded by Trinity College, Dublin in 1871. In England, an examination for certificates was instituted by the University of Cambridge in 1875, and the next year by the Universities of London and Oxford. Licensing authorities throughout England established examinations during the 1870s and 1880s. See Watkins, op. cit. (note 1), 144.

[41] *Medical directory for England and Wales* (1887), 227.

[42] General Medical Council for Education and Registration (1888). *Minutes of Executive Committee*, **25**, 27 February, para. 13.

[43] Ibid.

[44] *The Medical Act 1886* [Vict 49–50], c. 48, 12–13.

professionalism amongst community physicians, who no longer engaged in the restorative treatment of sick individuals.

The General Medical Council had not at that time exercised the power granted to it to remove unsatisfactory clinical licensing bodies from the register.[45] This power was used, however, in the regulation of licences in preventive medicine. In 1889, the General Medical Council instructed its Education Committee to investigate the regulations of the licensing authorities in respect of their public health certificates. The Committee's first report highlighted many discrepancies between authorities.[46] Only six of them made sure that candidates already possessed a medical licence. Some universities allowed their regulations to be suspended for their own graduates. None of those licensing boards which held two-part examinations, except for the Conjoint Board, required candidates to pass Part I before entering Part II. The lack of uniformity of regulations jeopardized the postgraduate status of the diploma. The Education Committee reported that the situation could not be allowed to continue given the importance which the DPH had acquired: 'The possession of a diploma in state medicine must therefore be held to imply higher and special qualification and it must be for the public interest that all such Diplomas should really signify what they appear to signify'.[47]

The Education Committee of the General Medical Council presented a second report to the General Council on 31 May 1889. As a result, the Council drew up eight rules on 1 June and issued them to the licensing authorities on 19 June. Failure to comply with the new regulations would disqualify any examining board from having its qualification registered.[48] The new rules specified age and qualifications necessary for candidature; stated levels of practical and sanitary work to be obtained; and specified the rules of study and examination of the diploma.[49] Thus, for the first time the Council threatened to use its power to 'sanction' rather than follow a policy of 'suasion' to regulate standards. They sought support for their action from the Local Government Board. In 1891 they worked together with the Board to ensure that practical instruction would be included in the DPH curriculum. Later, this became a central issue, but initially the Council requested that the Board simply provide enough medical officers of health to supervise and certify apprenticeship and outdoor practical study.[50]

---

[45] Charles Newman, op. cit. (note 25), 243–5.
[46] General Medical Council (1889). *Minutes of Council*, **26**, 70–1.
[47] Ibid. Remarks of the Education Committee, 72.
[48] General Medical Council (1889). *Minutes of Council*, **27**, 1 June.
[49] Ibid., Appendix.
[50] Local Government Board. *Miscellaneous correspondence*, MH25/86/47244/91.

George Buchanan, who in 1876 replaced John Simon as Medical Officer to the Local Government Board, responded to the General Medical Council's initial request for assistance.[51] Buchanan sat on the fence. He acknowledged the need to regulate the DPH but was also concerned that it should not be made too difficult for part-time students to obtain it. Like the rest of the public health service, he wanted the diploma only to be taken by candidates who wanted to follow a career in public health. However, he did not want to place too many obstacles in the way of getting the degree altogether.[52] The final letter from the Board to the General Medical Council (May 1891) was cautiously worded, and promised little practical support. The Board, it suggested: 'would approve a proposal to require from Candidates some evidence of their familiarity with actual sanitary business'. It qualified this, however, by saying that the Board: 'see reasons for not formulating with this object any appointed course of instruction and they apprehend difficulties in the way of selecting, as certifiers for this purpose, any particular class of persons'.[53]

The General Medical Council's regulations of 1889 generated disputes with the licensing bodies. In-fighting amongst the Scottish authorities provided the Council with the first test of its resolve. In 1890, Glasgow University granted 55 certificates, which constituted almost 17 per cent of the entire number issued by all licensing bodies throughout Scotland between 1871 and 1887.[54] Fifty-seven candidates had entered the Glasgow examination and 55 passed. This gave a pass ratio which, compared to the Scottish average, suggested an entirely dubious examination standard. Sixteen candidates had entered who had not passed their medical qualifying exam; four were too young to take an MB[55] and two had taken it and failed.[56] The General Medical Council set up a committee of inquiry, chaired by Sir Walter Foster. On 2 June 1890 it reported that Glasgow's certificate should be removed from the register specifically

[51] Buchanan, George (1831–95). *Dictionary of national biography*, 1st Supplement, 326; Smith, A.L. (1941). *A memoir of the Buchanan family*. Printed privately at the Aberdeen University Press.

[52] Local Government Board (1891). *Miscellaneous correspondence*, Memorandum for conference with Sir Richard Quain, as President of the General Medical Council. 14 March. (Written and signed in George Buchanan's hand), in MH25/86/47244/91.

[53] Local Government Board (1891). *Miscellaneous correspondence*, Letter to Richard Quain, President of the General Medical Council of Medical Education and Registration, 299 Oxford Street. (Signed by Alfred D. Adrian, Assistant Secretary), 25 May, MH25/86/47244/91.

[54] General Medical Council (1890). *Minutes of Council*, **27**, 27 May, 55–60.

[55] In the nineteenth century a Bachelor in Medicine degree (MB) did not qualify its holder to register as a medical practitioner without a licence from a medical corporation.

[56] General Medical Council, op. cit. (note 54).

under the terms of the 'resolution of 1st June 1889'. Glasgow subsequently restructured its diploma course and examinations and, in
order to regain registrable status, it re-examined the candidates of the
1889 examinations. Of the 55 who had previously passed, only four
passed the new exam.[57] The Glasgow case strengthened the General
Medical Council's authority but renewed efforts were needed throughout the 1890s to implement the regulations because each licensing body
continued to interpret the rules individually.[58] The aim of the licensing
authorities was to attract as many candidates to their courses and examinations as possible, increasing their income from fees to a maximum.
They had a vested interest in interpreting the regulations in a way
which would make it as easy as possible for candidates to obtain the
degree.

In 1894 the General Medical Council set up a public health committee
to supervise the implementation of the 1889 regulations. Its first report,
produced in 1895 by its inspector, G. F. Duffey, concluded that despite
the adoption of the regulations, standards still varied widely.[59] The
worst area of discrepancy was the interpretation of the meaning of practical laboratory work and in the completion of outdoor work under the
supervision of a medical officer of health.[60] To counteract the most
serious weaknesses, the General Medical Council issued a new clause in
its Order in 1896 requiring a candidate to show evidence that during a
period of six months, after having obtained a medical licence, he 'had
practically studied the duties of outdoor work under a Medical Officer
of Health'.[61]

By 1898, the new order was still not working effectively. Most
authorities claimed that it was extremely difficult to obtain sufficient
work experience in district health departments for their candidates.[62]
During 1899, therefore, the General Medical Council's Public Health
Committee issued a questionnaire to 170 medical officers of health

---

[57] Ibid. (1890), 27 November, para. 18.

[58] Ibid. (1895). **32**, Appendix 11, 455–743. See Duffey, George (1896). *First report of the Public Health Committee on the inspection of the examinations in sanitary science of the universities and licensing bodies of the United Kingdom.*

[59] Ibid., 455–721.

[60] Ibid., 464ff.

[61] General Medical Council (1898). *Minutes of Council*, **35**, 9 June 1886: 'Every Candidate shall have produced evidence that, during a period of six months after obtaining a registrable qualification, he has practically studied the duties of outdoor work under a Medical Officer of Health'.

[62] Ibid. See Interim report by the Public Health Committee on the interpretation given at different places to the Regulations of the General Medical Council as regards the course of study for the Diploma in Public Health. General Medical Council (1898). *Minutes of Council*, **35**, Appendix 8, 465–73.

throughout the United Kingdom asking their opinions as to how the major obstacles might be overcome.[63]

Responses to the questionnaire provided an important insight into the whole issue of standardizing the DPH. A fundamental division of opinion existed between part- and full-time officers. Part-time officers saw no difficulty in implementing the 1896 rule. Full-time officers, however, pointed out that the General Medical Council had originally intended that outdoor tuition should be conducted by full-time officers only. This was increasingly difficult to achieve because of the lack of co-operation from the local sanitary authorities. The full-time status of a medical officer of health enabled the authority to refuse to allow him to undertake tuition. Some authorities let officers take students on the condition that they did not receive fees for teaching. As a result, there was a shortage of full-time officers for DPH tuition. The instruction of candidates under these circumstances was reduced to informal discussions with sanitary officers and the occasional special inspections of slaughter houses, common-lodging houses, etc., with the medical officer of health. Full-time medical officers of health believed that the six month outdoor tuition period included in the DPH was therefore a 'farce'.[64]

A further contentious issue was the financial burden on candidates. The educational status of the DPH was equivalent to an MD or FRCS. Unlike other postgraduate medical qualifications, it was also an exclusive licence to practise a profession. A majority of full-time medical officers of health believed that fees for outdoor tuition should be set at a level which would discourage candidates who did not intend to use it specifically for entrance to the public health service from taking the degree.[65]

Taken together, the opinions of full-time officers illustrated the central issue regarding the wide variation in standards of the DPH and the need for regulation. By 1891, there were between 200 and 300 candidates taking the DPH every year.[66] Far more candidates were receiving the qualification than there were public health posts to fill. Many were not newly qualified medical students but established general practitioners who were taking the DPH in their spare time. Most were already part-time medical officers of health for their locality, often in small rural districts. In these circumstances the DPH was an insurance policy against the chance that districts would be combined into large

---

[63] General Medical Council, (1899). *Minutes of Council*, **36,** Appendix 21, 759–73.

[64] Ibid., 759–65.

[65] Ibid., 766–7.

[66] General Medical Council (1891). *Minutes of Council*, **28,** Table showing results of professional examinations in 1890 for qualifications in sanitary science, 28.

areas which would then require full-time officers with the compulsory qualifications.[67] Most of the full-time officers who answered the General Medical Council's questionnaire in 1899 believed that this plethora of candidates accounted for the variation of standards amongst the licensing authorities.[68] The General Medical Council's Public Health Committee had reached the heart of the matter concerning state regulation of professional qualifications. Educational standards were directly linked to professional power. Maintaining educational excellence was a means of restricting entrance to the public health profession. Limiting the numbers qualifying also limited the competition for appointments. Specialized labour in preventive medicine became a scarcer commodity and thereby strengthened the bargaining power of the profession over wages and job security. The Committee was acutely aware of the General Medical Council's role when it stated clearly in its report that the numbers of candidates must be reduced through a revision of the rules. The alternative could only be a sacrifice of the standard of tuition, which it believed 'should not be lowered merely to facilitate the obtaining of the Diploma by other practitioners not having that aim [of entering the public health service] in view'.[69]

The General Medical Council's order of 1889 was completely revised by new rules issued in December 1900. These altered the qualifying regulations; changed the rules of practical laboratory instruction and practical work in a public health office; required higher standards of tuition as well as study; and increased fees.[70]

During the 1880s, an uneven standard of excellence in examinations in state medicine resulted from the competition amongst licensing authorities for candidates and their fees. The significance of the DPH as a licence to practise full-time preventive medicine increased its popularity and exacerbated the sacrifice of standards. The aim of the General Medical Council after the Medical Act of 1886 was to ensure that the educational value of the DPH was equivalent to that of the MD and FRCS. This had, as we have seen, led to the unprecedented use of the direct sanctioning power of the Privy Council to institute a state-regulated

[67] Parliamentary Papers, *Local Government (England and Wales) Bill, 1888*. The combination of districts was first encouraged by the 1875 Public Health Act, then later reinforced by the 1888 Local Government Act. See, 'Powers, duties and liabilities of Secretary of State, Board of Trade and Local Government Board transferred to County Councils; section 286 Public Health Act 1875: Power to unite districts for purposes of appointing medical officers of health', *Local Government (England and Wales) Bill* [51 & 52 Vict.] [Bill 138], *Parliamentary Papers*, First Schedule, (1888). 4148.

[68] General Medical Council (1899). *Minutes of Council*, **36**, Appendix, **21**, 768–72.

[69] Ibid., 772.

[70] General Medical Council (1900). *Minutes of Council*, **37**, 29 November, 147–9.

postgraduate examination. Centralized control of the DPH enabled the General Medical Council to monitor its development more closely and eliminate any ambiguity as to the purpose of the qualification. The level of specialization was ensured through the revised rules of 1900 which imposed a stiff penalty, both educationally and financially, upon candidates taking the qualification with no intention of entering the profession.[71]

4. Discontent: professional conflict and the campaign for job security

By the late nineteenth century, the English public health service was made up of a stratified occupational group divided by full- and part-time employment; geographical location (provincial and metropolitan); and between officers who did or did not possess a specialist diploma. The divided occupational structure resulted in conflicting interests and professional goals within the service as a whole. The campaign for job tenure undertaken by the Society of Medical Officers of Health sharply reflected these conflicts.

The Society of Medical Officers of Health came into being in 1889 as the result of the amalgamation of various regional associations and the Metropolitan Association.[72] For the first time, metropolitan and provincial officers combined forces for their mutual benefit and professional strength. The objectives of the new national association were both, in the words of its first secretary: 'academical and . . . political'.[73] Herbert Manley represented the views of many of his provincial colleagues when he suggested that the Society should support and protect medical officers of health from the dangers and difficulties faced in their office.[74] The political nature of this role could have been interpreted, as Manley pointed out, as that of a trade union: 'And as much as others may dislike the title I think there is much to be said in its favour.'[75]

This sentiment was echoed by Alfred Hill, the first president of the new Society, in 1888. He was Medical Officer of Health for Birm-

---

[71] Ibid. (1901). Tables showing results of professional examinations held in 1900, **38**, 4 June, 13–21.

[72] Dudfield, Reginald (1906). History of the Society of Medical Officers of Health. In *Jubilee Number of Public Health* (ed. F.J. Allan), pp. 1–8. Collingridge, London.

[73] Manley, Herbert (1897–98). The Society of Medical Officers of Health: its aims, objects and policy. *Public Health*, **10**, 138–42.

[74] Ibid., 139.

[75] Ibid.

ingham, and Professor of Toxicology and Chemistry at Queen's College. In his presidential address he emphasized that strength lay in unity
and: 'Benevolent socialism or rational communism, which is the root of
most, if not all great and beneficial movements and such union constitutes an indispensable feature of all civilisation and human progress.' [76]
Terms such as 'benevolent socialism' and 'trades unionism' were not
universally appealing to all members of the Society. In its earliest days,
the Metropolitan Association had taken pains to eliminate the term 'combination' from its founding resolution, lest: 'any of the vestries should
suspect anything like a political combination on the part of their medical
officers'. The Association cautiously replaced the term 'combination'
with that of 'mutual assistance'. [77]

Different expectations of the Society emerged in the conflict between
metropolitan and provincial officers during the tenure campaign.
Debates regarding job security were a major issue immediately following
the amalgamation in 1888. In 1888, the Council of the Society resolved to
deplore the fact that the Local Government Bill did not transfer the
power to appoint and dismiss district medical officers of health to the
county medical officer of health. The Council's Resolution, however,
met a mixed response from the general membership of the Society.

At an Ordinary Meeting of the general membership on 20 April 1888,
a group of full-time provincial officers suggested that the Council had
not dealt with the broader inadequacies of the Bill. Specifically, they
wanted the Council to condemn the failure to create large combined districts which would have provided more full-time provincial appointments. [78]

George Wilson, Medical Officer of Health for mid-Warwickshire,
suggested that the Council was not pressurizing legislators into creating a
full-time public health service. He also pointed out that the resolution
should openly condemn the perpetuation of nominal appointments and
believed that unqualified general practitioners holding such posts were
antithetical to the whole purpose of public health administration. Support for Wilson was expressed by a group of provincial officers, who
became leading members of the management of the Society, namely
Francis Bond, Thomas Hime, George Fosboke, John Tathum, and

[76] Hill, Alfred (1888). Presidential address. *Public Health*, **1**, 3–5.
[77] Association of Metropolitan Medical Officers of Health (1856). *Minutes of second meet-ing*, 13 May. See especially the note at the bottom of the page of minutes of the meeting marked with an asterisk. Wellcome Historical Unit, Oxford.
[78] Society of Medical Officers of Health (1888). *Minutes of ordinary meeting of the Society*, 29 April, *loc. cit.* [note 77].

Edward Seaton.[79] Seaton accused Parliament of wholly inadequate appreciation of the issue. He believed that: 'If they wanted a good sanitary service they must have something like prizes in the profession; in districts of only 100 000 . . . there would be none'.[80] The opinions of this caucus of provincial officers did not, however, persuade the majority of the membership, who stood behind the Council's original resolution.

The creation of tenure for appointments in metropolitan districts in 1891 increased pressure within the Society for securing the same terms of employment for provincial officers. By this stage of the tenure campaign the tripartite stratification of the occupation acutely sharpened the conflict. Leading provincial officers expressed deep resentment of the metropolitan-dominated Council of the Society which failed to support their cause. Alfred Bostock Hill (son of the first president) stated openly that: 'one reason why the matter had not come to a satisfactory issue before was that the provincial officers of health had had but little sympathy from their metropolitan brethren, who held office under different circumstances'.[81] Ultimately, Hill warned, the interests of all officers would have to be pursued collectively if the profession was to survive and flourish. The metropolitan officers could not afford to go on 'simply regarding this matter with benevolent neutrality'.[82]

The provincial officers had grounds for being disillusioned with the Society in this regard. After the passing of the Local Government Act in 1888, the Council, under the presidency of William Corfield, petitioned the Local Government Board on behalf of the metropolitan officers concerning their reappointment under the new clauses dealing with the repayment of salaries. They campaigned for compensation for metropolitan officers alone, and made no requests regarding the reappointment of provincial officers. Also, they did not campaign on any of the issues raised during the debates on the Local Government Act by provincial officers during 1888 to 1889.[83]

The Council attempted to redeem the faith of their provincial colleagues by requesting Alexander Wynter-Blyth (the first editor of *Public Health*; and Medical Officer of Health for Marylebone and a barrister-at-law) to investigate the legality of the current tenure held by medical

[79] Ibid.
[80] Ibid.
[81] Hill, Alfred B. (1892–3). Discussion on Dr Page's Paper. *Public Health*, **5**, 18.
[82] Ibid.
[83] See Local Government Board, *General correspondence*, MH25/69/36239/89 and MH25/69/42915/89. (Series of correspondence between C. T. Richie, President of the Local Government Board and W.H. Corfield on behalf of the Council of the Society of Medical Officers of Health.)

officers of health outside the metropolis after 1891. His report merely exemplified the bland neutrality of which the Council had already been accused, but it did emphasize the need to reduce job insecurity by limiting competition through restrictive qualifications. Wynter-Blyth thought the best strategy for job tenure was to make the DPH more expensive to study for and make it harder to pass. The report also stressed the need for solidarity amongst medical officers of health. Collective action was necessary if they were to safeguard salary levels. Oversubscription in the medical profession spilled over into the public health service. Too many newly qualified doctors were chasing too few posts and were prepared to accept low levels of pay, undermining the security of officers already holding appointments and reducing the salary scales as a whole.[84]

The report did not satisfy the full-time provincial officers, but it did bring the part-time officers into the debate. General practitioners amongst the Society's membership felt it was time to defend their position, which was articulated largely by Henry May, Medical Officer of Health for Aston Manor.[85] He noted that full-time appointments only prevented an officer from practising curative medicine. He pointed out that these medical officers of health supplemented their income by combining their office with that of a pubilc analyst, superintendent to a fever hospital, or through a teaching post in hygiene. May suggested that the general practitioner was 'not as bad as he is painted'. He reminded the Council that a great majority of the Society's membership was made up of general practitioners who were part-time officers and warned that they might withdraw their support entirely if they were further alienated by their full-time colleagues.[86]

The full-time officers, however, renewed their campaign throughout the 1890s.[87] During 1893, *Public Health* carried a series of articles by John Thresh, Frederick Adams, and Edward Seaton, which called for the Society to close ranks against part-time general practitioners. Adams insisted that the Society should fight for tenure for full-time officers only. To make part-time appointments permanent would, he claimed, encourage local authorities to expand and perpetuate the system of small districts. He discussed the possibility of banning general practitioners

[84] For Wynter-Blyth's report see Society of Medical Officers of Health (1893). *Minutes of ordinary meeting of the Incorporated Society*, 18 December, loc. cit. [note 77].

[85] May, Henry (1893–94). The status, remuneration and tenure of office of medical officers of health. *Public Health*, **6**, 51–2.

[86] Ibid.

[87] See discussions within the Society of Medical Officers of Health in its *Minutes* throughout 1893 to 1895.

from membership of the Society, but believed that this would be less effective than restricting their entrance to the profession through control of the DPH. This view was also held by John Thresh, who suggested that the supply of medical labour was subject to the same economic laws as 'that of miners and dockers'.[88] Over-subscription devalued the economic and social status of the office. Thresh also agreed with Edward Seaton, who believed that combination of districts and control over the DPH would change the balance of power between the medical officer of health and his employer. Larger districts would result in more jobs for fully qualified officers and would ultimately eliminate general practitioners from the service.[89]

The future of the DPH as a means of market monopoly was discussed amongst the membership during December 1894. Arthur Ransome, Professor of Chemistry at Victoria University and honorary Fellow of the Society, was invited to speak before the Society. He was specifically asked to talk about improvements to the DPH. His paper inspired a vigorous discussion. Leading provincial officers argued for stricter standards regarding bacteriological work and supervision of candidates in outdoor work experience.[90] These were exactly the curricular features the General Medical Council introduced to raise the educational value of the DPH. Ransome responded to the discussion by warning the membership not to make the licence too exclusive, in case it might 'foster a spirit of clique' amongst medical officers of health and alienate their fellow doctors. To this Henry Armstrong, Medical Officer of Health for Newcastle-upon-Tyne, replied that Ransome was out of touch with the situation. It was a 'fact', he suggested, 'that the practitioners of preventive medicine are a distinctly separate caste of their profession'.[91]

[88] Adams, Frederick (1893–94). The status, remuneration and tenure of office of medical officers of health. *Public Health*, **6**, 1–3; Thresh, John. C. (1893–94). Discussion of Dr Adams' paper. *Public Health*, **6**, 3.

[89] Seaton, Edward (1892). Should medical officers of health engage in private practice? Abstract from *Annual report of 1892 for the County of Surrey*. Reprinted in *Public Health* (1893–4) **6**, 5–6. Edward Seaton was son of Edward Cator Seaton (1815–80), who was the epidemiologist appointed by Simon as one of the first inspectors to the Medical Department of the Privy Council. Seaton senior was well known for his dedication to the enforcement of compulsory smallpox vaccination. The younger Seaton followed his father into preventive medicine first as an MOH for Nottingham, then as Medical Officer of Health for Chelsea, and finally the County Medical Officer Health for Surrey in 1891. See *Lancet* (1915). **i**, 516–17.

[90] Ransome, Arthur (1893). The training and qualification of medical officers of health. Read before the Society at an ordinary meeting, 18 December, reprinted in *Public Health* (1893–94). **6**, 242–7.

[91] Armstrong, Henry (1893–94). Discussion of Dr. Ransome's paper. *Public Health*, **6**, 245.

Despite the protestations of provincial full-time officers, the Council continued to pursue a narrow line in its negotiations with the Local Government Board regarding tenure.[92] In 1896, the Council set up a special committee to deal with the tenure campaign, but from the beginning it was accused by Seaton of being single-minded:

> The question appears lately to have been discussed entirely without reference to the essential difference there must be, in the eyes of the whole profession at any rate, between Medical Officers of Health who are making 'public health' their life's work, and officers of health whose main work is that of general practice.[93]

The Tenure Committee did sway in Seaton's direction for a period, but was opposed in the branches, whose voting membership, if not active membership, was largely made up of general practitioners.[94] Alfred Bostock Hill, who had jibed against the metropolitan officers, now re-entered the debate, but this time on behalf of the part-timers, and in him they had powerful support within the management of the Society.[95]

The support that general practitioners received within the Society, however, was not matched by the opinion of the Local Government Board. From the early 1880s, the Board had encouraged, and sometimes coerced, local authorities into appointing full-time officers. In the public records of the department there are numerous cases of dispute between local authorities and the Board regarding this issue.[96] The case of Bishop Auckland, however, set a precedent for dealing with rural districts which refused combination.

Bishop Auckland refused to combine with other districts and also refused to combine appointments within their own district.[97] The district was considered by the Board to be 'an important one and has a population of about 47,000'.[98] In 1883, the Authority applied for repayment of a portion of the salaries of its three medical officers of health, all

[92] See Society of Medical Officers of Health (1895). *Minutes of Council*, 21 March.

[93] Seaton, Edward (1895). Letter to Reginald Dudfield, Secretary of the Society, 19 November. Reprinted in *Public Health* (1895–96). **8**, 163–4.

[94] For analysis of membership and management of the Society see Watkins, op. cit., 100–89 (note 1).

[95] See Society of Medical Officers of Health (1896). *Minutes of Council and minutes of ordinary meeting of the Society*, 16 January and 20 February.

[96] See correspondence of the Local Government Board with local Poor Law unions and sanitary districts: MH12/1421, MH12/1422/2946, MH12/2947, MH12/2629.

[97] See Local Government Board, correspondence (1883). MH12/2946/108/71003/ 80323, 188866; (1884). MH12/2947/108/16139.

[98] Owen, Hugh (1883). Memo to the President of the Board, 9 June. MH12/2946/108/ 74723.

of whom it employed for under £100 per annum.[99] The Board refused. The Local Government Board fought with the Authority throughout the spring and summer of 1883, withholding its approval of the appointments for 1883 to 1884 in an attempt to get the district to appoint a single officer on a sufficient salary to enable him to devote his whole time to the public health office. The Authority pleaded its case with the Board, pointing out that it had tried to form a combination with the adjoining sanitary authorities, who had failed to keep to the agreement. It also offered to increase the individual salaries of the three officers already in post, if the Board would pay a portion of them. But the Board remained adamant and described increased salaries as 'wholly inadequate', confirming its opinion that Bishop Auckland was determined to evade its responsibility. The Board finally refused payment from the grant on the grounds that it was:

. . . not prepared to accept the responsibility of sanctioning a continuance of arrangements which they consider are not calculated to secure the efficient discharge of the duties of Medical Officers of Health, for the purpose of enabling the Sanitary Authority to claim repayment from the Grant.[100]

The annual reports of officers such as those employed in Auckland received by the Board from 'the Country at large' confirmed its opinion that 'such an arrangement is very inexpedient and ought not to be resorted to'.[101] The Board was aware that the Auckland Authority was able to 'appoint one medical officer of health for the whole area at such a salary as would induce him to devote his whole time to their service'.[102] It refused its sanction until Auckland agreed to alter its system.

In negotiations with the Society of Medical Officers of Health, the Board maintained the same stance. The Society followed many diverse strategies to try and obtain the Local Government Board's support for medical officer of health tenure. However, it was finally refused by Gerald Balfour (President of the Board, 1905) because of the implications of an indiscriminate system.[103] He pointed out to a delegation

---

[99] Bruce T. Dundas (clerk to the Rural Sanitary District of Auckland Union) (1883). Letter to the President of the Local Government Board, MH12/ 2946/35315.

[100] Dalton C.M. (assistant secretary at the Local Government Board) (1883). Letter to T. Dundas Bruce, Clerk to the Rural Sanitary Authority of the Auckland Union, 23 July. MH12/2946/108/74723/3446.

[101] Ibid.

[102] Ibid.

[103] Security of tenure for medical officers of health. (Report of the deputation of the Society of Medical Officers of Health to the Local Government Board), (1906–1907). *Public Health*, **19**, 233–9.

from the Society that blanket tenure, which did not discriminate between full- and part-time officers, would give job security to unqualified officers. This would make the task of creating combined districts, to replace small inefficient districts, increasingly difficult for the Board. He believed that this was against the interests of the Board, which wished to be free to remove unqualified men and have them replaced by qualified officers employed full time.[104] Edward Seaton must have felt vindicated.

Job security eluded provincial public health officers for a further 24 years. Part-time public health work was eliminated under the Local Government Act of 1929, which also granted blanket tenure for all medical officers of health subsequently appointed.

5. Conclusion

In the early nineteenth century, public health reform in Britain was led by distinguished individuals: statesmen, philanthropists, and élite members of the medical profession. From the 1870s, a new professionalism emerged in public health practice with the establishment of a national network of medical officers of health. This occupational group established public health administration as its own sphere of expertise, with its own professional standards, aims, and goals. Public health as a process of social reform became diffused into the piecemeal development of a national civil service. Social reformers were replaced by professional administrators of the public health system.

The history of medical officers of health as an occupational group is therefore central to an understanding of public health in the late nineteenth century. The historical stratification of medical officers of health led to intra-professional conflicts and a general failure to consolidate their social and economic position with either their employers, that is to say the Local Sanitary Authorities, or their political masters, namely Parliament and the Local Government Board. Lacking any political force, the professionalizing caucus of the occupational group sought to use standards of expertise to enhance their economic security. This strategy did achieve a limited success. The supply of expertly trained and specially qualified officers was limited through the regulation of the Diploma in Public Health, enhancing the market monopoly of the group over its own labour power. The failure, however, of the professional caucus to control the aims, goals, and practices of the entire

[104] Ibid.

group undermined the overall influence of medical officers of health in the political and economic development of the public health system.

Despite these limitations, the professional strata of medical officers of health developed an ideology of prevention which influenced the discourses on health care by the turn of the century. Discussion of that ideology would require another essay. It was founded, however, on the professional hegemony of medical officers of health and their occupational investment in the expansion of the British public health system.[105]

---

[105] See Porter, Dorothy E. (in press). Enemies of the race: biologism, environmentalism and public health in Edwardian England. *Victorian Studies*; id. and Porter, Roy (1988). The politics of prevention: anti-vaccinationism and public health in nineteenth-century England. *Medical History*, **32**, 231–52; Watkins, op. cit. (note 1), 276–333.

4

The emergence of pioneering public health education programmes in the United States

ARTHUR J. VISELTEAR

> This enterprise, when fully understood, must command the liberal sympathy of those who aim to make their generosity fruitful in substantial and enduring public good.
>
> William Barton Rogers

Schools of public health were established in the United States as a result of a confluence of factors making themselves felt as early as the mid-nineteenth century. Such factors included the changing nature of higher education, the development of commerce and industry, the rise to prominence of the science of bacteriology, and the urbanization of the nation—all coupled with a pervasive spirit of utility and a desire to be, in a word, useful. This chapter will explore each line, leading to the establishment of five public health institutions: the Massachusetts Institute of Technology, the joint programme of Harvard and the Massachusetts Institute of Technology, Yale, University of Michigan, and University of Pennsylvania.

1. Introduction

In 1867, Daniel Coit Gilman, Professor of Physical and Political Geography at Yale's Sheffield Scientific School, published an essay review of seven contemporary publications which treated the subject of scientific education. The publications were prompted by passage of the Morrill Land Grant Act, which had been approved by the United States Congress 2 July, 1862, donating lands to 'the several states and territories' of the United States for the purpose of providing 'Colleges for the Benefit of Agriculture and the Mechanic Arts'. The publications reviewed by Gilman considered the Act itself, the Act's influence on higher education, and the Act's influence on specific institutions: the

University of California, Cornell University, Yale University, and the new Institute of Technology then being planned in Boston.[1]

It was the Civil War that had prompted a national awakening, Gilman wrote. Not only had the nation witnessed the establishment of national banks, a national railroad linking East with West, a national system of weights and measures, national departments devoted to Agriculture and Education, and a National Academy of Sciences, but, with the passage of the new federal Act, 'National Schools of Science'[2] were to receive proper funding and, as a result, the nation would witness and experience an Augustan Age of commerce, advancement, and progress.

Gilman reflected on the new Act's influence on existing institutions of higher learning. These venerable colleges, he concluded, had been devoted to Newman's eternal 'truths in the natural order'. According to this view, knowledge was capable of being its own end. A university education, and again this is Newman:

aims at raising the intellectual tone of society, at cultivating the public mind, at purifying the national taste, at supplying the principles to popular enthusiasm and fixed aims to popular aspirations, at giving enlargement and sobriety to the ideas of the age, at facilitating the exercise of political powers, and refining the intercourse of private life.[3]

Such an education, wrote Newman, would prepare a man 'to fill any post with credit, and to master any subject with facility'. A liberal education was everything; useful knowledge, however, was 'a deal of trash'.[4]

Such views, common in the early nineteenth century, put forth the belief that utility was unimportant. Develop the best educational instrument for the training of the mind (by which was meant classical studies) and, when one's work was finished, the mind would be bright and strong and capable of discharging any labour. Gilman and others believed that this was beautiful theory, but not borne out by results. The nation no longer had the luxury of such theories, as England had determined a decade earlier, when Lord Playfair had undertaken an inquiry into the causes of English inferiority regarding manufacture and found that all of England's continental competitors possessed 'good systems of

[1] Gilman, D.C. (1867). Our national schools of science. *North American Review,* **105**, 495–520. For a brief review of Gilman's life, see Flexner, Abraham (1946). *Daniel Coit Gilman: creator of the American type of university.* Harcourt, Brace and Company, New York.

[2] Gilman, op. cit., 497 (note 1).

[3] Kerr, Clark (1964). *The uses of the university*, p. 3. Cambridge University Press. See Newman, John Henry (1852). Discourse V. Knowledge its own end. In *The idea of a university*. Longmans, Green and Co., London and New York.

[4] Kerr, op. cit., 2 (note 3).

industrial education for the masters and managers of factories and work-shops', whereas England had possessed none.[5] If the United States was not to find itself in the same situation as had England, reform was necessary. The narrow, elementary, and irrelevant curriculum of pres-ent-day universities would have to change. Students, according to A.C. Benson, writing in another time about the same situation, 'were sent out not only without intellectual life, but not even capable of humble useful-ness'.[6] Nowhere in the curriculum was there room for research; nor was sufficient attention devoted to the technical or practical. The older col-leges were sectarian, undemocratic, and dedicated to wealth and privilege. What was needed, in Goethe's words, was more light—the necessary light was soon coming, from science.

Understanding the changed and charged atmosphere in the United States were a group of scientists, financiers, and philanthropists who mortgaged their names and fortunes to the future. Stephen Van Rensse-laer, James Smithson, Abbott Lawrence, Peter Cooper, Joseph Shef-field, Abiel Chandler, Bladina Dudley, and George Peabody had each 'clearly seen the value of training in the mathematical, physical, and natural sciences as a preparation of life', as well as the importance of scientific researches in promoting the development of natural resources.

The pioneer school was founded in 1824 in Troy, New York, by Van Rensselaer. Abbott Lawrence had endowed in 1847 a scientific school at Harvard, and within a few years Yale, Dartmouth, Union, and Colum-bia Universities followed with scientific schools or departments of their own, as did the City of Boston, where an 'Institute of Technology' was soon to be established.[7]

Each new school (in the popular or official phraseology referred to as scientific schools, polytechnics, or technical schools) was fundamentally similar: each had been 'imperfectly endowed' and each had been founded on an 'experimental basis'. Yet each school, according to Gil-man, was 'a very significant indication of the spirit of the age', as each wished to advance knowledge on some other basis than the literature of Greece and Rome; each showed 'the popular craving for what was vaguely termed . . . a *practical* education'; each:

[5] Ashby, Sir Eric (1958). *Technology and the academics: an essay on universities and the scientific revolution.* Macmillan, London. See also Gilman, op. cit., 514–16 (note 1).

[6] Benson, A.C. (1907). Education. In *From a college window*, p. 161. G. P. Putnam and Sons, London.

[7] See Weiner, Charles (1966). Science and higher education. In *Science and society in the United States* (ed. D. D. Van Tassel and M. G. Hall), pp. 163–89. Homewood, Illinois. Sinclair, Bruce (1972). The promise of the future: technical education. In *Nineteenth cen-tury American science: a reappraisal* (ed. G. H. Daniels), pp. 249–72. Evanston, Illinois; and Gilman op. cit. (note 1), 500.

showed that, in some form or other, provision would be made for education in those branches of useful knowledge which tend to exhibit the Creator's works in their true aspects, and likewise in those which are immediately connected with the material advancement and civilization of mankind.[8]

Such was the brief for scientific education, and with the Morrill Act the new schools emerged, not so much to compete with those schools dedicated to language, literature, and history, but to offer an alternative pathway to the future.

What form the new schools took, both in Europe and the United States, is instructive. Gilman recommended that the new schools emerging as a result of the Act should be regional, based on the various needs of the nation. In the agricultural states of the West, agricultural science would be prominent; in California, Nevada, and Pennsylvania, mining interests should receive attention; and in the East, education should be specifically adapted to instruct engineers, mechanics, chemists, and the directors of great manufacturing establishments. The need for buildings and facilities and laboratories of applied research would be met by endowments, tuition, and the funds derived from the Act, but the real need, wrote Gilman, was for 'a corps of instructors, young, manly, thorough, truth-loving, able to teach, speak, and econo-mize'. Such young men would do much to give character and success to a foundation that was still guarded by a 'corps of older men [who never would possess] the spirit of modern inquiry'.[9]

The ultimate object of such an education, Gilman reasoned, was not to have graduates return 'to labor with the hoe or the anvil', but instead to be 'scientifically trained for the higher avocations of life, and especially to take charge of mines, manufactories, the construction of public works, the conduct of topographical and other scientific surveys': in a phrase, educated to be 'leading scientific men'.[10]

The new scientific schools should flourish side by side with the old schools and each, Gilman believed, would be strong in the other's strength: 'The Creator and his laws; man and his development, or, in other words, science and history, alike [affording] abundant discipline for the mind, and appropriate preparation for the active work of life'.[11]

The need for the new pathway was great, and all energies were to be directed towards the great need. As Francis Amasa Walker, to whom we shall soon turn, wrote: ' . . . lands [needed] to be surveyed, roads to be constructed, ships built and navigated, soils of every kind, and under

[8] Gilman, op. cit., 501 (note 1).
[9] Ibid., 517.
[10] Ibid., 519.
[11] Ibid., 520.

every variety of climate, to be cultivated, manufactures . . . established which would [compete] with those of more advanced nations . . . '[12] and science, both basic and applied, as well, to be fostered and understood, propagated, taken to bits, made useful for a growing, progressive, emergent nation.

2. The technical institute versus the university

The older universities were persuaded by the arguments for change. Within half a century, the German universities had become the new model. The democratic, industrial, and scientific revolutions were underway. Newman's gentleman 'at home in any society' would soon be at home in none.[13] With the appointment of a new generation of university presidents—Andrew Dickson White at Cornell, Charles Eliot at Harvard, James Angell at Michigan, and Gilman himself, first at California and then Johns Hopkins University— science had begun to take the place of moral philosophy, research the place of teaching. The universities, according to Abraham Flexner, became 'expressions of their age', which in the latter part of the nineteenth century was vibrant, tumultuous, dynamic, industrial, optimistic.[14]

The sciences entered the university as early as 1727 with the appointment of a mathematician at Harvard. Botany and chemistry appeared at Columbia and Princeton by the end of the eighteenth century. By the 1850s, mathematics, natural philosophy, botany, chemistry, zoology, geology, and mineralogy had found their way into most college curricula. There is not sufficient time to focus on the rise to prominence of American science, to discuss Benjamin Silliman at Yale, for example, or John MacLean, James Dwight Dana, Edward Hitchcock, Ebenezer Emmons, Asa Gray, Joseph Henry, or William Barton Rogers, or to consider the lyceums, museums, popular lectures, or published writings, or to review the rise of civil engineering (developed at West Point in the early 1800s and at Rensselaer in the 1820s);[15] but we should focus our attention on two schools, Harvard and Massachusetts Institute of

[12] Walker was quoting from Francis Wayland, President of Brown University. See Walker, F.A. (1899). Technological and technical education, 1896. In *Discussions in education by Francis A. Walker* (ed. J. P. Munroe), pp. 79–108. H. Holt and Company, New York.

[13] Kerr, op. cit., 3–4 (note 3).

[14] Flexner, Abraham (1930). *Universities: American, English, German.* Oxford University Press, New York.

[15] See Thurston, R.H. (1893). Technical education in the United States: its social, industrial, and economic relations to our progress. *Transactions of the American Society of Mechanical Engineers*, **14**, 855–1013.

Technology, one a classical school at the threshold of modernity and 'Boston Tech', a new school representative of the age.

At both Harvard and Yale, science had made incursions into the curriculum. New professors of chemistry and botany had been appointed in the two schools, and, at Harvard, in 1846, plans were being discussed to establish a graduate school of arts and sciences, eventually to emerge as the Lawrence Scientific School.

Abbott Lawrence, whose fortunes were made as an importer and textile manufacturer, donated $50000 to Harvard.[16] The plans to establish a graduate school were modified and science at Harvard took the form of an undergraduate teaching programme leading to the Bachelor of Science degree, first awarded in 1851; but Lawrence's wish, that the school champion the cause of engineering and the manufacturing sciences, were frustrated when the Board of Overseers appointed as the School's Director, Louis Agassiz, whose principal interests were the natural sciences, especially comparative zoology, rather than the physical sciences.[17]

Science spread elsewhere, to Dartmouth, and Denison Universities, the Universities of Rochester and North Carolina, New York University, and the Universities of Iowa and Missouri. At Michigan, Henry Philip Tappan went a step further, linking the German ideal of research with that of advanced scholarship. This was not 'vocationalism' or applied science, as we shall soon see was to develop, for example, in Boston; rather it was 'true' scholarship, the scholarship of dignity, leisure, and grace.

At Brown, Francis Wayland reinforced Tappan's ideals and recommended that universities throughout the nation experiment, develop electives rather than required courses, and permit their students to enrol in programmes of applied science, agriculture, law, and education. The new universities should be dynamic, temperate, flexible, nondoctrinaire, and adaptive to changing needs.

Carried through to its logical conclusion, the American university accepted the natural and physical sciences as equivalent to the liberal arts; but more than that, as integral to a truly liberal education. This ideal was best expressed by Thomas Henry Huxley in 1883:

That man, I think, has had a liberal education who has been so trained in youth that his body is the ready servant of his will, and does with ease and pleasure all

---

[16] See Love J.L., (1944). *The Lawrence Scientific School in Harvard University, 1847–1906.* Burlington, North Carolina; and Morrison, S.E. (1936). *Three centuries of Harvard, 1636–1936,* pp. 279–80. Harvard University Press, Cambridge, Massachusetts.

[17] For a discussion of Agassiz, see Lurie, Edward (1960). *Louis Agassiz: a life in science.* University of Chicago Press, Chicago.

the work that, as a mechanism, it is capable of; whose intellect is a clear, cold, logic engine, with all its parts of equal strength, and in smooth working order; ready, like a steam engine, to be turned to any kind of work, and spin the gossamers as well as forge the anchors of the mind; whose mind is stored with a knowledge of the great and fundamental truths of Nature and of the laws of her operations; one who, no stunted ascetic, is full of life and fire, but whose passions are trained to come to heel by a vigorous will, the servant of a tender conscience; who has learned to love all beauty, whether of Nature or of art, to hate all vileness, and to respect others as himself. Such an one and no other, I conceive, has had a liberal education; for he is, as completely as a man can be, in harmony with nature. [18]

In Boston, yet another model of science education was developing, this a School of Industrial Science, with a view to aiding 'the development and practical application of science in connection with arts, agriculture, manufactures, and commerce'. The School was the dream of William Barton Rogers, a Professor of Natural Science at the University of Virginia, who had emigrated to Boston with his plan for an Institute of Technology, which began to take shape as a result of a confluence of three discrete but not unrelated events: first, the presence of Rogers himself, an eloquent, erudite, learned man, who represented the unspoken desires of the Commonwealth's emerging and powerful class of 'Manufacturers, Mechanics, Agriculturists, and Other Friends of Enlightened Industry'; secondly, the signing in 1861 of a legislative act granting a charter to the new School and reserving for its use two-thirds of a square of state land in the newly reclaimed Back Bay; and thirdly, a new charter amendment, signed in 1863, providing to the Institute a one-third share of the annual income of the Commonwealth's land grant fund (which had been made possible by the Morrill Act). [19]

The tenets of the School of Industrial Science appear in a document prepared by Rogers in 1864, which embodied the spirit which Rogers wished to infuse in his new institute:

that there is dignity in the mastery of useful knowledge; that science is fundamental to the progress of technology and that together they can contribute significantly to human welfare; that the learning process must be active, for direct experience gives life and meaning to knowledge; and that professional training may profitably be combined with a liberal education in the undergraduate years, to the enrichment of both.

Added to these, was Rogers' principal tenet, that the objectives set

---

[18] Cited by Bibby, Cyril (1960). *T. H. Huxley: scientist, humanist and educator*, p. 44. Horizon Press, New York.

[19] See Prescott, S.C. (1954). *When M.I.T. was 'Boston Tech': 1861–1916*. Technology Press, Cambridge, Massachusetts.

forth were best achieved through 'a special kind of institution, independent and with a clear perception of its central mission'.[20]

As Massachusetts Institute of Technology's President, Richard Maclaurin was to write in 1911, Rogers 'saw what Lowell did, that new times demanded new manners and new men'. The first belief was that science was valuable, that it enhanced 'human comfort and health' and contributed to 'social wealth and power'. As such, the prime motives were those of utility, of being useful, of service to society. As Rogers himself wrote: 'This enterprise, when fully understood, must command the liberal sympathy of those who aim to make their generosity fruitful in substantial and enduring public good'.[21]

It was not without some forethought that Rogers had added the phrase, 'when fully understood'. There were many who did not (or who had chosen not to) understand. Nathaniel Shaler, for example. In 1896, Nathaniel Shaler had already been associated with the Lawrence Scientific School for over 35 years. He had studied geology and zoology under Agassiz, and, after receiving his Bachelor of Science degree in 1862, rapidly made his way up the academic ladder, serving in 1869 as Professor of Paleontology, in 1888 as Professor of Geology, and, between the years 1891 and 1906, as Dean. His courses, especially his introductory geology course, were among the most popular at Harvard; his writings—which considered everything from earthquakes, whales, the moon, climate, hurricanes, floods, sunsets, and mining, to altruism, the silver question, dreams, and race—were thoroughly sound and enlightening; his tenure as Dean enlivening and substantially successful.[22]

Unlike the spokesmen from the Massachusetts Institute of Technology, Shaler had a broad conception of the purpose of studying science, and was more concerned with 'awakening the student's mind than with imparting information'. As the Massachusetts Institute of Technology grew in stature and fame, Shaler could not but look enviously across the Charles River and wonder about the Lawrence's mission in comparison to that of the Massachusetts Institute. Money seemed virtually to flow there, its student body continued to increase, and its future seemed secure and destined for even greater successes.

When the two schools were compared, the Lawrence was certainly anaemic, at sea, less certain of its future. For these and other reasons, Shaler let loose in the *Atlantic Monthly* a broadside attack on the

[20] See *Life and letters of William Barton Rogers, edited by his wife, with the assistance of William T. Sedgwick* (1896), 2 volumes. Houghton Mifflin, Boston.

[21] Ibid.

[22] See *The autobiography of Nathaniel Southgate Shaler, with a supplementary memoir by his wife* (1909). Houghton Mifflin, Boston.

Massachusetts Institute of Technology and other free-standing technological institutes. These schools, he wrote, had prospered based on the
premise that such schools, to which he referred pejoratively as 'trade
schools', were freer, if isolated, 'to go straight forward to their object of
training young men for the highly specialized employments of the arts'.
Training pupils for 'particular tasks', however, invariably led to a 'narrowing of the spirit of education', as Shaler believed 'that the more fit
the youth at graduation for the details of a special employment, the less
likely he is to have the broad foundation on which his subsequent development must to a great extent depend'.[23]

The university had a 'well-affirmed principle' which was to make 'the
enlarged man'; but it was characteristic of all trade work that immediate
ability, rather than the means of continuous growth, commanded the
attention of its managers. Better, wrote Shaler, to 'conjoin' the various
art and science disciplines rather than to have them set apart. Far better
would it be to have 'the influence of contact with able scholars, and of
mingling with fellow students . . . engaged in a great diversity of intellectual occupations'.[24] Only in schools placed within a university, such
as the Lawrence or the Sheffield at Yale, would a technical programme
afford its students all the professional advantages which a separate institution could only hope to provide. Courses here would be interrelated,
intellectual intercourse favoured, a student's learning 'enlarged' and:

Thus, the scholastic life of a young man who intends to be an engineer, a
chemist, or a practical geologist, or who is specially fitting himself to teach
science, [would be] to a great degree spent in a truly academic atmosphere—one
in which knowledge and a capacity for inquiry are valued for their own sake,
and not measured by their use in economic employment.[25]

A response to Shaler's essay appeared in the next issue of the *Atlantic*
written by Francis Amasa Walker, the President of the Massachusetts
Institute of Technology. No man was ever more suited to lead than
Walker; no man ever was more respected or admired. Walker had been a
patriot, scholar, federal bureaucrat, and was selected by Rogers himself as
a man most able to fulfil Rogers' dreams for the Institute.[26] Walker, who
had led cavalry charges in the Civil War, was certainly capable of responding to Shaler's mischievous arguments. He first rebutted the need

[23] Shaler, N.S. (1893). Relations of academic and technical instruction. *Atlantic Monthly*, August, 262.

[24] Ibid., 264.

[25] Ibid., 265.

[26] See Munroe, J.P. (1923). *A life of Francis Amasa Walker*. H. Holt and Company, New York; and Winslow, C-E.A. (1897). Francis Amasa Walker. In *Technique: the book of the class of XCVII*, pp. 33–53. Cambridge, Massachusetts.

for science scholars to be sheltered by a university. Such a need was at variance with the facts, he wrote. Even at the Sheffield Scientific School, a School founded in connection with a university, one which had achieved eminent success, the relationship was less than perfect. Indeed, wrote Walker, the Sheffield had grown up under the 'total neglect' of the Yale Corporation. So little had Yale considered its Science School that, when Batell Chapel was erected in 1873, no provision had been made for giving the Sheffield undergraduate students seats in it. Moreover, the Sheffield's budget was not its own. Requests for facilities and laboratory equipment had to be approved by the University, a situation which in the latter decades of the nineteenth century had proved intolerable. And the same administrative problems were to be found at Columbia's School of Mines and Cornell's Sibley College.[27]

Walker's full assault on Shaler's protective patronage argument was reserved for a discussion of the students. Those pursuing a science education at schools attached to a university, Shaler had written, would be taking their courses with a student body interested in a variety of subjects. Such association Shaler regarded as advantageous, applying to it the felicitous term 'educative companionship'. Walker found the concept ludicrous.

The notion that because a young man is going, two or three years hence, to enter a law school, a medical school, or a divinity school, he therefore contributes some special flavor or savor to his class in chemistry or physics or geology or mathematics today is carrying the doctrine of final cause to an extreme.[28]

Walker continued: 'The fling at technical studies as less "distinguished" than studies which are pursued without a direct object is one heard often', he wrote, 'but those who use [the argument] have not seemed to me to show thereby their own superior liberality of mind'. Young men seeking to qualify for an 'honorable and useful career' could be equally disinterested.

Disinterestedness, in its true meaning, depends not upon the studies pursued, not upon their immediate usefulness or uselessness, but upon the spirit in which the student enters upon and pursues his work. If there be intellectual honesty, if there be zeal in investigation, if there be delight in discovery, if there be fidelity to the truth as it is discerned, nothing more can be asked by the educator of highest aims.[29]

Walker next considered Shaler's argument regarding the favourable

---

[27] Walker, F.A. (1893). The technical school and the university. *Atlantic Monthly*, August, 341.
[28] Ibid., 393
[29] Ibid.

'atmosphere' for learning found at universities in comparison to science schools, implying that the university campus was more conducive to learning that an institute located in a single building. No one who had seen the Massachusetts Institute of Technology would deny this, wrote Walker, but 'the benefits of such environments were easily offset'. The best atmosphere for a student, he argued, was that which a student himself brings with him; the next best atmosphere was that created by 'learned, laborious, and high-minded teachers; the next best that created by a body of devoted fellow-students, all intent upon the work of preparation for life'.[30] Students of technology, as a body, applied themselves to their tasks with 'wonderful energy and enthusiasm'. They would doubtless benefit considerably from a university education, and would bring much to it; but the young men who selected technology schools did not 'greatly care to go to schools where they [were] not respected equally with the best; where all the praise and all the prizes [went] to others; where the stained fingers and rough clothes of the laboratory [marked] them as belonging to a class less distinguished than students of classics or philosophy'. Such prejudices and snobbishness were odious, and the technology students wanted none of it.[31]

Walker concluded with a paean to the Massachusetts Institute of Technology: 'More than one detached school has shown the liberality of sentiment, the comprehensiveness of view, and the high moral courage necessary to place and maintain technical education upon a lofty plane'.[32] The Institute was just one such school, and it is to it that we now turn our full attention.

3. The Massachusetts Institute of Technology

William Rogers and Francis Amasa Walker had a clear, a certain and definite, vision for the Massachusetts Institute of Technology, one from which neither they nor their successors deviated. The commercial and industrial age had dawned, the nation was growing rapidly and the need was great for technically minded and technically trained men and women to maintain the new growth industries of transportation, textiles, steel, mining, agriculture, and construction. Once Walker laid to rest the arguments of Shaler and other sentimentalists, that 'faculties of technology [filled] the minds and [starved] the souls of the young', they never looked back. The Institute prospered and students from 23 states

[30] Ibid., 394.
[31] Ibid.
[32] Ibid.

and eight foreign countries filled, for example, the 1895 entering class of 1200 students.[33] The number of faculty, departments, and course offerings grew as well, and by the end of the century, students were matriculating in many different areas of study: civil engineering, mechanical engineering, mining engineering and metallurgy, architecture, chemistry, electrical engineering, biology, physics, chemical engineering, sanitary engineering, geology, naval architecture, and general studies (which included economics, political science, German, French, history, and English).[34] Rogers had laid down a few simple but far-reaching principles, as we have seen, the foremost of which was the importance of being useful, or, in Rogers' words, 'efficiency in the science of society'.

Commenting in 1911, Richard Maclaurin, the fourth President of the Massachusetts Institute of Technology, quoted from Goethe: 'How can man learn to know himself? Never by thinking, but by doing'.[35] The Institute was a place for doing, for action; it was also a place 'not for boys to play, but for men to work', as Walker was fond of reiterating to each entering class of 'Tech Men'.[36] When students visited the Institute from the English High School in Boston, one of its principal feeder schools, as C-E.A. Winslow had done in 1894, they were shown the workshops and laboratories first, shown the library next, and then interviewed by the directors of the various programmes. After Winslow's lengthy interview session with William T. Sedgwick, Sedgwick commented: 'Well Winslow, I think you can be a *useful* man'.[37] The powerful educational engine at the Massachusetts Institute of Technology was driven by a dedicated and distinguished faculty, each of whom infused in their students a burning ambition to excel and a desire to make their 'generosity fruitful' by contributing substantially to the 'public good'.

This spirit of usefulness pervaded the Institute. It was apparent in each course, in each speech of its administrators, in each message of its alumni, in each lecture of its faculty. It was apparent in the physical science courses, the engineering courses, even the general studies courses; but, in no course was it more apparent than in those taught by

[33] Massachusetts Institute of Technology (1895). *Annual report of the President and Treasurer*, 9–10.

[34] Prescott, op. cit., 158 (note 19).

[35] Maclaurin, R.C. (1911). Some factors in the Institute's success. In *Technology and industrial efficiency: a series of papers presented at the Congress of Technology, opened in Boston, Mass., April 10, 1911, in celebration of the fiftieth anniversary of the granting of a Charter to the Massachusetts Institute of Technology*, pp. 1–7. McGraw-Hill Co., New York.

[36] Munroe, op. cit., 248 (note 26).

[37] *American Journal of Public Health* (1942). Sedgwick Memorial Medal for 1942 awarded to Dr C–E.A. Winslow, **32**, 1416–7.

Sedgwick, who seemed the very embodiment of the concept, despite the fact that his early scholarly career had been dedicated not to applied but to basic research.

Sedgwick graduated from the Sheffield Scientific School at Yale University in 1877, spent two years at the Medical College there, where he served as a teaching assistant to Russell Chittenden, but for the most part was bored by the primarily didactic nature of the programme taught by community physicians who were too busy to keep up with the scientific literature or to encourage young students to higher aspirations.[38]

Such an educational programme Sedgwick found profoundly unattractive, and he abandoned it, having the good fortune to be recommended and accepted for a Fellowship in Biology at the Johns Hopkins University. It was at the Hopkins that Sedgwick experienced the uncommon vitality of scholarly research, for here had Daniel Coit Gilman assembled Sylvester in mathematics, Gildersleave in the classics, Rowland in physics, Remsen in chemistry, and Martin in biology.

Biology was from the start one of the principal features of the Hopkins. Indeed, Gilman had invited Thomas Henry Huxley to deliver the address at the formal opening in 1876 of the Johns Hopkins University. In this famous address, Huxley discussed elementary education, admissions policy, primary and secondary schools, courses of study leading to higher degrees, the Johns Hopkins Hospital, and the object and essentials of medical education, the new science, and the need for research. He stated:

The future of the world lies in the hands of those who are able to carry the interpretation of nature a step further than their predecessors; so certain is it that the highest function of a university is to seek out those men, cherish them, and give their ability to serve their kind full play . . . My own conviction is that the best investigators are usually those who have also the responsibilities of instruction, gaining thus the incitement of colleagues, the encouragement of pupils, and the observation of the public.[39]

Such principles were embodied not in the practice of medicine, but only in a career which led to teaching and research. Sedgwick soon came under the influence of Newell Martin, serving as fellow and instructor in Martin's laboratories and eventually receiving in 1881 the degree Doctor

---

[38] See Jordan, E.O., Whipple, G.C., and Winslow C–E.A. (1924). *A pioneer of public health: William Thompson Sedgwick*. Yale University Press, New Haven. Information about the Sheffield Scientific School may be found in Chittenden, R.H. (1928). *History of the Sheffield Scientific School of Yale University, 1846–1922*, 2 volumes. Yale University Press, New Haven.

[39] Huxley, T.H. (1877). Address on university education. In *American addresses, with a lecture on the study of biology*, pp. 97–127. Appleton and Company, New York.

of Philosophy for a dissertation entitled: 'The influence of quinine in the reflex excitability of the spinal cord.' For the next two years, Sedgwick served as Associate in Biology and received shortly thereafter a call from the Massachusetts Institute of Technology, in 1883, to take up the duties of an Assistant Professor of Biology in a department which had previously been named 'Natural History'.

Sedgwick's was one of the first academic posts in the United States to be so designated. Fresh from studies with Martin, Sedgwick intended to have biology take its rightful place with the physical sciences. He wanted biology, comparative anatomy, histology, and physiology, to serve as a pre-medical course of instruction, which he had missed at the Sheffield, and which at that time had eluded most college students intent upon a career in medicine.

Despite so logical a position, Sedgwick was unable to attract many students to the field of biology. Only a few students from the Massachusetts Institute of Technology went on to medical school and, try as he may, he could not convince students of the potential of this field of study. Students at the Institute were interested, it seems, more in applied than basic science, and Sedgwick was forced to adapt his work to more practical areas, for example, by offering courses in bacteriology to students enrolled in the civil engineering programme and by lecturing to high school teachers, enrolled as external students, about the new science.

Biological studies at the Institute, then, expediently and properly followed another line, into bacteriology and microbiology, and for very good reason. The 1870s and 1880s witnessed the important work of Pasteur and Koch. The germ of tuberculosis had been discovered in 1882, and the aetiological agents causing cholera, tetanus, diphtheria, and typhoid fever were discovered very soon thereafter. Those working in this nascent field, Major G. M. Sternberg of the United States Army, T. J. Burrill, Professor of Botany at the University of Illinois, and H. J. Detmers of the Department of Agriculture, together with Sedgwick, perhaps the only persons in the nation engaged in the study of the new science of bacteriology, recognized almost immediately the significance of its applications to sanitary science.

Concurrent to these discoveries, state officials in Massachusetts had turned their attention toward the sanitary condition of the water supplies and rivers of the Commonwealth of Massachusetts.[40] Members of

---

[40] See Whipple, G.C. (1917). *State sanitation: a review of the work of the Massachusetts State Board of Health.* Cambridge, Massachusetts; and Rosenkrantz, B.G. (1972). *Public health and the state: changing views in Massachusetts, 1842–1936.* Harvard University Press, Cambridge, Massachusetts.

the faculty of the Institute had already been asked to prepare, on behalf of the State Board of Health, chemical and biological studies of the water supply. In 1888, Sedgwick had been placed in charge of the research programme of the Lawrence Experiment Station and in 1890, issued a major report of the Station's biological research on sewage and filtration.[41] In subsequent years, Sedgwick also investigated the typhoid fever epidemics which had occurred in the Merrimack Valley, especially in Lowell and Lawrence, employing both epidemiological methodology, and bacteriological and chemical analysis, and, as well, investigated another typhoid fever outbreak, in Springfield, due to infected milk.[42]

Francis Amasa Walker commented on the potential of these new studies and consultations in his 1888 annual report:

The great advances recently made in this line of investigation [sanitary bacteriology], and the almost limitless possibilities of the future in this respect, have not only caused the minds of many of our students to turn in that direction, but have created a demand from outside for skilled bacteriologists, which up to this time the Institute has not been able fully to meet.[43]

Bacteriological studies at the Massachusetts Institute of Technology were soon applied to the study of brewing, controlling the fermentative processes occurring in milk, butter, and cheese, in canning and food preservation, in tanning, tobacco curing, and in the manufacture of various acids and dyes. In addition, of course, bacteriology was also applied to public health, to determining and preserving 'the purity of public supplies (such as air, water, milk, and ice) as well as the more urgent and difficult problems of drainage and sewerage'. As Winslow wrote in 1906, about his own experiences at the Institute:

A whole field of novel sciences has grown up, bound together by the fact that all bear on a single biological problem—the adaptation of the human mechanism to its environment, and in particular in relation to certain microparasites. Taken together they form what is practically a new profession, founded on its own special basis of pure knowledge—the profession of sanitary science.[44]

Within a few years of his arrival, then, the chief aim of Sedgwick's

[41] Sedgwick, W.T. (1890). *A report of the biological work of the Lawrence Experiment Station.*

[42] See especially Sedgwick, W.T. (1892). *Investigation of recent epidemics of typhoid fever in Massachusetts.* Representative Board of Health of Massachusetts, Boston, Massachusetts; Sedgwick, W.T. (1894). *On an epidemic of typhoid fever in Marlborough apparently due to infected skimmed milk.* (privately printed) Boston, Massachusetts.

[43] Massachusetts Institute of Technology (1888). *Annual report of the President and Treasurer,* p. 67.

[44] Winslow, C–E.A. (1906). The teaching of biology and sanitary science in the Massachusetts Institute of Technology. *Technology Quarterly,* **19**, 416–25.

emergent Department of Biology, which in subsequent years was renamed the Department of Biology and Public Health, became primarily 'to furnish recruits for the great sanitary campaign'; and it was from his Department of Biology and the collateral Department of Sanitary Engineering that such recruits emerged, to take their place, as laboratory workers and engineers, alongside physicians. The engineers and the laboratory workers, he believed, could also serve as planners, evaluators, and administrators, as it was no longer necessary for those medically trained to be the chief executive. After all, he reasoned, the physician, in the course of his medical training, found very little in the medical syllabus that was concerned with public health.

Sedgwick eventually concluded that sanitary science, or public health, based on the new science, should stand alone as a professional discipline. Public health, he believed, should no longer be merely a 'subsidiary function' of the practice of medicine. Medicine might very well be the 'mother of sanitary science' but it was now time for a proud parent to understand that its child had attained majority.[45] Moreover, the two fields had become unrelated, distinctly detached from one another. Medicine, for example, was interested in disease; sanitary science in health.

Curative and preventive medicine had already been separated in schools of medicine, and in a speech before the American Public Health Association, Sedgwick pointed to this dichotomy of interests:

It is today absurd for the average well-trained medical student to think of becoming an expert in such branches of hygiene as water supply, sewage, heating and ventilation, street building, street cleaning and watering, garbage collection and disposal, gas and other forms of light supply, ice supply, milk supply, the abatement of nuisances, etc. These belong rather to the sanitary engineer, sanitary chemist, and sanitary biologist; to sanitation rather than hygiene.[46]

Here, then, was a call to a new profession, one which Sedgwick and his colleagues in the Massachusetts Institute of Technology were ready to advance and develop. Sedgwick reasoned as follows. The physician was already in place, but was primarily trained to diagnose and cure disease. Physicians understood the new science, but their interests and responsibilities were not similar to the interests of those in sanitary science. Indeed, there were really three professional interests to be addressed: the physician, the laboratorian, and the engineer.

Winslow addressed these divergent careers in his 1906 paper. Public

---

[45] Ibid., 419–20.
[46] Sedgwick, W.T. (1905). The readjustment of education and research in hygiene and sanitation. *Public Health Papers and Reports*, **31**, 115–20.

health was concerned with the control of contagious diseases, which included diagnosis, laboratory examination, isolation, disinfection, and serum therapy. Health departments were usually staffed by two types of experts, those, for example, who were clinically trained physicians, who could diagnose disease, administer antitoxin and inspect schools, and those who were trained in laboratory diagnosis, who did not need a medical training but rather one instead in chemistry, histology, and bacteriology. This latter group, who would be best trained in scientific departments or scientific schools and not in medical schools, were responsible for preparing vaccines and serums, preparing cultures, testing disinfectants, and determining infectious agents in milk, ice, water supplies, or food. They were the trained laboratory specialists, those who applied pure science to the work of public hygiene, and who had already attained professional status and recognition as evidenced in the newly established Laboratory Section of the American Public Health Association.[47]

The third group were the sanitary engineers, the men who '[dealt] directly with the inanimate environment and remodelled it in accordance with the advice of the physician and the laboratory expert'. Winslow added that the sanitary engineer had risen to a supreme importance, especially with 'the aggregation of masses of people in great cities', making the problem of healthful conditions at once more difficult and more imperative. 'The city [was] an organism which [demanded] as the first essential for its life a supply of pure water, food, and air, and the removal of its waste products', he wrote. There was a need also for engineering experts in ventilation, heating, housing, and industrial hygiene, such recruits as would be trained in the Department of Sanitary Engineering in the Massachusetts Institute of Technology.[48]

Thus the focus of the new public health was in biology and sanitary engineering. Sedgwick's Department of Biology would develop the laboratory expert, who in some cases of special aptitude would later become a health officer or administrator. For such training, a student, as had Winslow and his colleagues, enrolled in a rigorous and demanding programme which included courses in general chemistry and bacteriology, advanced courses in the chemistry and bacteriology of air, water, food, and clinical and microscopical examination of foods and drugs, the principles of sanitary science and municipal sanitation, vital statistics, and the study of parasitology as applied to the laboratory diagnosis of the infectious diseases. Winslow also was required to take courses

---

[47] Winslow, op. cit., 421 (note 44).
[48] Ibid.

in the bacteriology of sewage and water, geology, mineralogy, social welfare, three mathematics courses, and courses in German, English literature, social welfare, and history.[49]

Collateral to the programme in biology was the Institute's Department of Sanitary Engineering, organized on the triple base of engineering, chemistry, and biology. Students who enrolled in this department were trained as civil engineers, in surveying, railroad and highway engineering, stereotomy, applied mechanics, structures, and hydraulics. Following these courses, the students were taught the rudiments of chemistry and biology, 'since sanitary engineers were to an extent also chemists in order that they [should know how to] plan and interpret sanitary analyses'. Similarly, the sanitary engineer '[would have to] be to some extent a biologist, acquainted with the significance of bacteriology and the laws which [governed] the causation of disease'.[50]

Advanced course work was also available for students at the Institute's Sanitary Research Laboratory and Sewage Experiment Station. Founded in 1902 after an anonymous donor had made available $5000, the Sanitary Research Laboratory was to determine how best to improve methods of sewage disposal, 'especially those adapted to large cities', and established also for the following purposes:

(1) keeping up with the investigations of the best men in all countries;
(2) using this knowledge in the work of the Institute;
(3) original experiment;
(4) distributing all over our country in such words that they who [are responsible for city health and sewage] may read the results of the work; and
(5) inciting the students to make plain and simple statements of the results of their studies.[51]

The Sanitary Research Laboratory began operations in July 1903, under the direction of Sedgwick, with Winslow, then an Instructor in Sanitary Bacteriology at the Institute, Biologist-in-Charge, and E.B. Phelps, also of the Institute and soon to be associated as Chemist at the Lawrence Experiment Station of the State Board of Health, as Research Chemist and Bacteriologist. Appearing in the volumes of published papers emanating from the Laboratory were research papers which considered Boston sewage, microscopic enumeration of bacteria in sewage

[49] Massachusetts Institute of Technology, Office of the Registrar. *Class of 1898*, Vol. 35, pp. 348–9.
[50] Winslow, op. cit.,421–2 (note 44).
[51] Massachusetts Institute of Technology (1905). *Contributions from the Sanitary Research Laboratory and Sewage Experiment Station*. Boston, **1**, 5.

effluent, septic tanks, sand and contact beds, and trickling filters. Graduate students from other programmes collaborated on research projects, as did personnel from the United States Geological Survey and other State agencies.[52]

The success of Sedgwick's programme was readily apparent. In 1906, when Winslow completed his review of the teaching programme at the Institute, he had found that 12 graduates of the Massachusetts Institute of Technology held positions with the State Board of Health: five as engineers, five as chemists, and two as biologists, including the Biologist of the Lawrence Experiment Station. In Ohio, the engineering department of the State Board of Health was composed entirely of graduates of the Institute. The State Boards of Health of New York and Minnesota had appointed new chief engineers, each of whom was an alumnus . The Chief Engineer of the State Water Commission of Pennsylvania and his first assistant were alumni, as were the chemists and biologists of boards in New Jersey, Maryland, Louisiana, Vermont, Rhode Island, Connecticut, and Iowa. A graduate of the Massachusetts Institute of Technology even had been hired by the United States Geological Survey to study water and stream pollution problems.

Similarly, the Institute furnished health officers, bacteriologists, and chemists for many municipal departments, and Winslow cited as examples Richmond, Boston, Cleveland, Pittsburgh, New Orleans, Albany, as well as many smaller municipalities in New York and New Jersey.[53]

The battle had been joined. The expected results were already being tabulated. Death rates and morbidity rates had fallen and would more than likely continue to fall, as the nation built more sewage systems and waste disposal plants, and as the Massachusetts Institute of Technology and similar schools or programmes trained more laboratorians and sanitary engineers to staff and administer state and local health departments. As Winslow wrote, somewhat exultantly:

This is the field for [the Institute's] graduates in sanitary science. The Biological Department continues to offer a fundamental scientific training to those entering upon the study and practice of medicine. It prepares men and women for the teaching of natural science in the school, the high school, and the college. It furnishes specialists in the increasing applications of biology to the development of the arts and industries. Its chief function, however, is to train recruits for the new crusade against disease; and this function is limited only by the number of volunteers and by the facilities necessary for their equipment.[54]

[52] See the published papers appearing in ibid., Vols 1–9.
[53] Winslow, op. cit., 423–4 (note 44).
[54] Ibid., 425.

Regarding the primary sanitary expert to which Winslow had made reference, the physician in public health work, the Institute had much to offer; but very few takers. Sedgwick had slanted the biology course toward sanitary science and, with a few minor modifications, easily developed a two-year course of study for physicians. He lamented the fact that so few of the nation's medical schools had made the attempt to educate their students to serve as sanitary experts, especially at a time when such experts were sorely needed. He believed that the general impression, that a medical degree qualified someone for public health work, was wrong and should be set right. As Winslow wrote regarding this problem: 'The ordinary physician [was] no better fitted for this side of public health work than the ordinary civil engineer or the ordinary systematic biologist [was] for theirs'.[55] Despite the opportunity for training graduate physicians at the Massachusetts Institute of Technology, by 1921, the year of Sedgwick's death, only a handful had matriculated from Sedgwick's department, a situation which was also to prove true for Yale, as we shall soon see.

4. The Harvard–Massachusetts Institute of Technology School for Health Officers and the Department of Public Health, Yale University

The story I shall now relate moves in two directions, one towards Harvard and Milton Rosenau and George Whipple, and the other towards Yale and Charles-Edward Amory Winslow. The problem of public health education for physicians had troubled Sedgwick for over 40 years. If the public health campaign was to succeed, the trained physician would have to take his proper place in the scheme of things. Early in his career, Sedgwick had recognized that public health administration was bound to medicine. Both fields were distinct, but if real success was to be realized, the roles of the non-medically trained laboratorian and sanitary engineer would have to be co-ordinated. In 1914, the potential for this ideal was fulfilled, for it was on 11 June of that year that the first Certificate of Public Health (CPH) was conferred on students matriculating from the School for Health Officers of Harvard University and the Massachusetts Institute of Technology. The origins of this school may be traced to 1912, when Harvard's Professor Whipple met with Harvard's President Lowell at the Colonial Club, the latter asking the former to think of ways to develop a co-ordinated plan which would

[55] Ibid., 423.

link Whipple's Department of Sanitary Engineering with the Massachusetts Institute of Technology, leading to a course of study for health officers. Meetings followed with the Institute's President Maclaurin, Professor Sedgwick, and Harvard's Professor Milton Rosenau, the latter having served since 1909 as Chairman of Harvard's Department of Preventive Medicine and Hygiene. In May 1913, the plans took further form when the Board of Overseers of Harvard University appointed Sedgwick, Rosenau, and Whipple as members of the new School's Administrative Board, with similar action being taken by the Executive Committee of the Massachusetts Institute of Technology shortly thereafter (July 1913). Sedgwick served as the Board's first Chairman, Rosenau as Director, and Whipple as Secretary and Treasurer.[56] The object of the School, as stated by Rosenau, was:

To prepare young men for public health work and especially to fit them to occupy administrative positions as health officers, or members of boards of health, or sanitary agents, district health inspectors or technical experts of health organization . . . [The School intends to] provide the scientific groundwork in the sanitary sciences which underlies efficient health administration. The country needs leaders in every community fitted to guide and instruct the people in the art of hygienic living; qualified to direct the expenditure of energy, time and money in public health work into fruitful channels; and able to initiate plans to meet novel conditions as they arise.[57]

Admission requirements were very strict, as the Board believed it imperative to pick only men of considerable technical ability. Although the medical degree was not a 'prerequisite' for the degree, candidates were advised to become medically qualified before specializing in public health work. The principal reason for this was the fact that preferment for positions and advancement to higher administrative positions appeared to come more readily to those who already possessed the MD degree.[58] Nonetheless, those who had matriculated BS from the Massachusetts Institute of Technology in biology and public health, and from other recognized institutions, would be admitted on their records, as were Masters of Civil Engineering of Harvard or similar degree recipients in Sanitary Engineering from the Institute. These later candidates, however, were to be required to devote at least a year in preparation before being accepted as candidates for the CPH. In addition, other

[56] See Curran, J.A. (1970). *Founders of the Harvard School of Public Health, with biographical notes, 1909–1946*, pp. 9–21. Josiah Macy Jr. Foundation, New York.

[57] Rosenau, M.J. (1915). Courses and degrees in public health work. *Journal of the American Medical Association*, **64**, 794–6.

[58] School for Health Officers (1915). *Catalogue and announcement, 1915–16*, p. 7. Boston, Massachusetts.

graduates of technical or scientific schools or colleges would be admitted provided their collegiate courses included course work in physics, chemistry, biology, French, and German; but such students would be required to spend two or more years in preparation before being declared eligible for candidacy for the CPH.

In addition to the CPH, the School for Health Officers also offered the Doctor of Public Health degree (Dr.P.H.). As with the CPH, candidates were admitted without the MD degree, such as those who wished to specialize in sanitary engineering, sanitary architecture, sanitary biology, sanitary chemistry, demography, or other branches of public health work. The programme for this category of students was to extend over four years, including the submission of an acceptable thesis 'embodying the results of original research'. For the MD, those who already possessed a knowledge of sanitary engineering, vital statistics, and preventive medicine, the course was for no less than one year (although Rosenau had himself believed that it would be impossible to accomplish all the requirements in such a short period of time), and also included the presentation of an acceptable thesis containing results of original research. An additional requirement was for each candidate to prepare a sanitary survey of a city, a requirement Rosenau considered of great importance in the education of future health officers.[59]

The faculty of the combined programme was impressive. Over 70 courses were interwoven, by Whipple and his associates in sanitary engineering and in demography at Harvard in Cambridge; by Sedgwick, Prescott, Dewey, and others at Boston; by Rosenau, Theobald Smith, and Richard Strong at the Harvard School of Tropical Medicine; and by Ernst and others at the Harvard Medical School. The courses included everything we would expect to find in an advanced public health programme (preventive medicine and sanitary science, personal hygiene, public health administration, sanitary biology, sanitary chemistry, special pathology, communicable diseases, sanitary engineering, and demography), and, as well, special courses and lectures in infant mortality, social service work, mental hygiene, oral prophylaxis, the prevention of ear, nose and throat disease, hygiene of the eyes, industrial hygiene and medicine, eugenics, genetics, and sanitary law.[60]

But more needed to be done. Physicians entered the programme, but not in the numbers expected. Sedgwick wished to press further ahead, and perhaps beyond, the advanced School for Health Officers.

[59] Rosenau, M.J. (1924). The sanitary survey as an instrument of instruction in medical schools. *Methods and problems in medical education*, pp. 7–11. Division of medical education, The Rockefeller Foundation, New York.

[60] See note 58, 14–16.

Moreover, he was troubled by the administrative plan of the School. Neither the Massachusetts Institute of Technology nor Harvard wished to give the School complete autonomy. The degrees the students received, for example, were unique to the School, as neither the Institute nor Harvard would agree to joint degrees, which meant that neither institution was willing to legitimize the School's students with parental blessings. For these and other reasons, including Sedgwick's primal loyalty to the Institute, something which transcended even his loyalty to his science and the field of public health, Sedgwick developed a new plan. His proposal, set forth in an 8 December, 1916 memorandum to President Maclaurin, was for a new Institute of Public Health in the Massachusetts Institute of Technology.[61]

The plan was bold, unusual, and comprehensive. An Institute would be created, subdivided into four principal divisions:

(1) a Division for Health Officers;
(2) a Division of Testing and Research;
(3) a Division of Publicity and Education; and
(4) a Division of Library and Museum.

The *Division for Health Officers* was derivative of programmes of the Harvard–Massachusetts Institute of Technology School, as the *new* Institute would be designed for medical and other advanced science graduates, college graduates, special students, and technicians, and would award the CPH, the Doctor of Public Health, and the Sanitary Inspector's Certificate. The *Division of Testing and Research*, which would be 'the central nucleus' of the whole establishment, would have the following subdivisions: (1) Laboratories; (2) Sanitary Engineering; (3) Vital and Social Statistics; (4) Personal Hygiene (and Applied Physiology); (5) Epidemiology; (6) Industrial Hygiene; and (7) Sanitary Law. The laboratories would be devoted to work in economics, bacteriology, pathology, biochemistry, diagnosis, and the production of sera and vaccines, while the sanitary engineering subdivision would deal with water supply, sewage, water purification, sewage purification, garbage collection and disposal, street cleaning, and the mechanical aspects of ventilation. The *Division of Publicity and Education* would be 'in the hands of a carefully selected man', one experienced in public health promotion by means of 'lectures, posters, leaflets, booklets, advertisements, lantern slides, moving pictures, textbooks, school books, and manuscripts'. The *Division of Library and Museum* would be under the direction of a

[61] Sedgwick to Maclaurin, 8 December (1916). Massachusetts Institute of Technology (Ac 13), 530.

competent librarian/curator, who would assemble a suitable library and museum containing not only the regular books and periodicals germane to the subject, but the very numerous reports of state and local Boards of Health, the publications of the United States Public Health Service, historical documents, 'apparatus historical or otherwise important', and stock cultures of microbes of all sorts, together with models and diagrams suitable for reference or for use in the conduct of practical Board of Health work.

Sedgwick's plan was expensive—$40 000 would be necessary each year for salaries for faculty, staff, apparatus, and supplies. In addition, a building would be necessary, and the land alone was likely to cost more than $200 000; if the plan were to be undertaken $1 000 000 would need to be raised.

Sedgwick concluded his report with the revealing comment:

Perhaps I ought to emphasize more than I have done my profound conviction that the need for an institution of this kind is today of the gravest and the time the most opportune. Never before in the history of the human race has so much interest been felt as it is felt today in personal and public health; never before has the scientific knowledge available been so abundant or so easily applied; never before have communities and individuals stood as ready as they are today to make fundamental reform in their Boards of Health and the work which these Boards may do.

The opportunity for rapid work in every direction is unparalleled, and the promise so inspiring that I find it difficult to write with the necessary reserve.[62]

Nothing came of Sedgwick's bold venture and he found it necessary to reign in his characteristic enthusiasm. As told so well by Elizabeth Fee, the monies necessary to implement such a plan went neither to Massachusetts Institute of Technology, nor Harvard University, nor the Universities of Pennsylvania, Michigan, or Columbia, but instead to the Johns Hopkins University, about which we shall learn more in Chapter 5.[63]

What now of Yale and Winslow, Sedgwick's most dedicated pupil and disciple? The Yale programme had two antecedents, one dating from 1907, in the form of Irving Fisher, Professor of Political Economy at Yale, and the other in the form of a bequest from the family of Anna M.R. Lauder, arriving in the hands of the Yale Secretary in 1914. In 1907, Fisher drafted a proposal which was sent to a colleague, Dr

---

[62] Ibid.
[63] See Fee, Elizabeth (1983). Competition for the first school of hygiene and public health. *Bulletin of the History of Medicine*, **57**, 339–63; and Fee, Elizabeth (1987). *Disease and discovery: a history of the Johns Hopkins School of Hygiene and Public Health, 1916–1939*. The Johns Hopkins University Press, Baltimore, Maryland.

George Blumer, Professor of Medicine at Yale. With a minor reorganization of courses already being offered in the Sheffield Scientific School and the graduate and medical schools, Fisher believed that an outstanding public health programme could be developed. The medical school already offered courses in hygiene and bacteriology, the economics department had several members 'particularly interested in the sociological applications of preventive medicine', and the Scientific School had 'already made a reputation for itself in sanitary engineering and dietetics'.[64]

Together with Blumer and a third colleague, the physiological chemist Lafayette Mendel, Fisher prepared an outline for a new department which they believed could be called either 'Public Health and Public Service' or 'Hygiene and Philanthropy'. Students matriculating in the proposed department would have to meet the strict prerequisites of the graduate school and be expected to take a total of 41 courses, including courses in anthropology, bacteriology, law, natural and physical sciences, 'public hygiene' (which comprised vital statistics, sanitary administration, quarantine, and occupational health), tropical medicine, 'economics and labor history', 'poverty and crime', and 'practical philanthropy'. The graduates of such a programme would receive a diploma of some sort and were expected to enter any number of public health and welfare positions in charity and voluntary associations or settlement houses, or become public health officers or public health nurses.

The plan never got off the ground, as the faculty of the medical school considered it unwieldy, desultory, and unfocused. The clinical and scientific aspects were not unified and the students, many of whom would enter with different backgrounds, were expected to seek mutually exclusive goals. Better, wrote Yandell Henderson, if the programme deleted the roles of the Sheffield Scientific and Graduate Schools, and be redesigned for medical students only, who would take, concurrent to their medical school courses, an additional comprehensive course in 'Sanitary Science'. If this revised plan were accepted, medical students at the completion of their course of studies would receive both the MD degree and a second degree, the Diploma in Public Health, the latter a degree awarded then only in Great Britain and Canada.

The plan set forth by Fisher and his colleagues and the revised plan advanced by Henderson were both ruled 'inoperable' by the Yale Corporation and never implemented. So, whereas public health pro-

---

[64] For a discussion of early Yale public health, see Viseltear, A.J. (1982). C–E.A. Winslow and the early years of public health at Yale, 1915–1925. *Yale Journal of Biology and Medicine*, **55**, 137–51.

grammes had already been established at the Massachusetts Institute of Technology, Harvard, Pennsylvania, and Michigan, Yale demurred and remained oblivious to both its own resources and the opportunities in this new discipline until 1914 when, as a result of an intense fund-raising effort planned to coincide with the Centennial of the School of Medicine, Yale University received a substantial endowment of $500 000 from the Lauder family for the specific purpose of establishing a chair in public health.[65]

There were restrictions on the bequest. The professorship, for example, was to be offered to a physician experienced in public health and sanitary affairs, someone capable of dealing effectively with the public and astute in politics. Especially necessary as a stated objective was that the department lead the drive to revise existing public health laws and redesign the administrative public health programme of the State.

Many suggestions were forthcoming from public health and medical leaders, including Biggs, Sedgwick, Rosenau, Jordan, Park, and Westbrook. Recommended were Joseph Goldberger, Wade Hampton Frost, John Anderson, George McCoy (all of the United States Public Health Service) and other prominent sanitary engineers, bacteriologists, and health officers. The choice ultimately fell on a non-physician, Charles Edward-Amory Winslow, whose own career had served as a paradigm for the non-medically trained public health expert.

Winslow was (forever it seems) one of 'Sedgwick's Boys'.[66] He received his BS from the Massachusetts Institute of Technology in 1898, his MS a year later, and for the next 10 years was a member of Sedgwick's department and the Biologist at the Sanitary Research Station. Winslow next went to Chicago as a half-term replacement for Professor E.O. Jordan, and in 1910 was called to City College, New York, as an Associate Professor of Biology, while concurrently appointed Curator of Public Health at the American Museum of Natural History. Shortly thereafter he was hired by Hermann Biggs to serve as Director of Publicity in the New York State Department of Health, and, in 1915,

---

[65] Ibid., 139.

[66] For information about Winslow, see: Fulton, J.F. (1957). C.–E.A. Winslow, leader in public health. *Science*, **125**, 1236; Hiscock, I.V. (1957). Charles-Edward Amory Winslow, 1877–1957. *Journal of Bacteriology*, **73**, 295–6; Editorial (1957). Charles-Edward Amory Winslow, 1877–1957. *American Journal of Public Health*, **47**, 153–67; Viseltear, A.J. (1980). Charles-Edward Amory Winslow. In *Dictionary of American biography*, pp. 701–3. Scribner Company, New York; Acheson, Roy M. (1970). The epidemiology of Charles-Edward Amory Winslow. *American Journal of Epidemiology*, **91**, 1–18. The papers of C–E.A. Winslow have been deposited in the Contemporary Medical Care and Health Policy Collection, Manuscripts and Archives, Yale University Library.

received the call to Yale to serve as Anna M. Lauder Professor and Chairman of the Department of Public Health at Yale.

Why Winslow was ultimately selected is conjecture, as no document exists which precisely answers this question. There are, however, a number of explanations, including the very strong recommendations written on his behalf by Biggs, Sedgwick, and Henry Fairfield Osborn; the latter Director of the American Museum. Sedgwick had indoctrinated Winslow in the sciences basic to public health and Biggs had tutored Winslow to appreciate and reckon with those external forces of sloth, ennui, and greed which retarded and occasionally engulfed public health goals. Reviewing Winslow's recommendations and publications, Blumer doubtless recognized that Winslow's potential, as scientist, administrator, and emergent statesman, was best suited to set the agenda for the new department.

Unlike the Massachusetts Institute of Technology, the Department of Public Health at Yale was to be situated within the medical school. It was neither a school of public health nor an institute, and this administrative peculiarity may serve as another explanation as to why Winslow had been selected. Winslow understood the administrative structure of Yale University and his objectives for Yale's new department were compatible with the programmes of the University's three major scientific components, the Graduate School, the Scientific School, and the School of Medicine. When Blumer and Winslow met to negotiate the position, Winslow expressed the opinion that public health at Yale should not duplicate educational programmes already in place elsewhere. Instead, Winslow decided to focus his attention on 'the education of undergraduate medical students along the lines of preventive medicine'.[67]

Winslow then seemed to be in a perfect location to enlighten the medical students about public health and the great potential for serving the public good if they proceeded into public health careers. He not only intended to spread the 'preventive spirit' in his courses, but to capture a handful of the 'right sort' for the public health campaign.

However, despite the fact that Winslow's department was assigned 150 hours for course and field work by the curriculum committee, despite his ability to effect close working relationships with and co-operation from medical school colleagues, including the Dean, despite his ability to effect relationships with the other University departments and programmes, and despite the fact that Winslow's courses in the

---

[67] See Winslow, C–E.A. (1928). Department of Public Health, Yale University. In *Methods and problems of medical education*, 10th series, pp. 31–41. Division of medical education, The Rockefeller Foundation, New York.

1920s and 1930s included contemporary medical care topics and seminars, Winslow was singularly unsuccessful in convincing medical students to go on in public health. His courses and lectures undoubtedly 'broadened their vision', but his primary responsibility became, as had been true of Sedgwick, to instruct public health students studying for the CPH, the Ph.D., and the Dr.P.H.

The phrase, 'broadening vision', in the case of Yale medical students, is worthy of another paragraph. One of Winslow's greatest talents was diplomacy. As Yale began to revise its curriculum, reducing the number of hours reserved for didactic lectures, in a word 'streamlining' the curriculum by salvaging over 1500 hours, a policy which resulted in the reduction of Winslow's own curriculum by 45 hours, Winslow sought to influence medical education in another direction, toward the realm of social medicine. The Dean of the School of Medicine, Milton Winternitz, wished to give Yale a personality, to set it apart from other front-rank schools. One way to achieve this goal was to develop a new educational plan of instruction, whereby students would be encouraged to enroll in elective courses, be required to pass only two comprehensive examinations (instead of countless course examinations) and engage in independent research leading to an MD thesis, all the while advancing at their own pace through the curriculum.[68]

A second means of setting Yale apart was a plan for a new collaborative research and training institute, the Institute of Human Relations.[69] Winternitz believed that medicine had become atomized, narrow, and provincial. Physicians had become specialists, turning ever inward, unaware of the society around them, unappreciative of the social, cultural, political, economic, legal, even theological aspects of health and disease. The School needed more light. Together with the Deans of the law and graduate schools, Winternitz developed a programme whereby medical students would be educated together with students of the Schools of Law, Nursing, and Divinity, and take courses offered in the Departments of Psychology, Industrial Relations, Sociology, and Social Work. From such a programme would emerge a new physician, one tuned into a broader, more realistic world of the patient seen as a whole person.

[68] See Viseltear, A.J. (1986). The Yale plan of medical education: the early years. *Yale Journal of Biology and Medicine*, **59**, 627–48; Acheson, Roy M. and Payne, A. M–M. (1967). Preventive medicine at the Yale School of Medicine, 1950–1965. *Milbank Memorial Fund Quarterly*, **65**, 287–301.

[69] See Viseltear, A.J. (1984). Milton C. Winternitz and the Yale Institute of Human Relations: a brief chapter in the history of social medicine. *Yale Journal of Biology and Medicine*, **57**, 869–89.

This plan ultimately failed. As more and more advances were being made in the basic and clinical sciences, the belief that the Institute of Human Relations would solve societal problems, problems of unemployment, poverty, welfare, and poor nutrition, was seen by many as misguided. Winslow had played a valuable role in helping Winternitz conceptualize the Institute of Human Relations and in helping Winternitz to hone his arguments to further advance social medicine; but, in the end, mere geographical proximity had not worked its magic. The fact that core faculty representing cognate disciplines were located in a single building had not necessarily meant that outstanding collaborative research would be achieved. The Institute of Human Relations failed because medicine had once again become reductionist and the medical school curriculum, at Yale and elsewhere, soon reflected a return to its original mission and traditional concerns: the patient and not the community; sickness and not health; cure and not prevention—all goals at variance with the ethos of public health.

5. Public Health in the Universities of Michigan and Pennsylvania

Let us leave Yale and turn momentarily to Michigan and Pennsylvania. As we have seen, the period immediately prior to the Civil War had been a period of major industrial growth. New jobs were created and science schools established (thanks to the Morrill Land Act) to provide society with technologically trained leaders. Cities grew in size as immigrants and others gravitated to find employment and a better life. The major epidemics of the mid-nineteenth century revealed the need for a protective arm in the form of benevolent public health to guard against societal diseases: cholera, typhoid, and tuberculosis. Nascent health departments emerged in the mid-1800s, in Louisiana (1855), and in the States of Massachusetts (1869), California (1870), Virginia and Minnesota (1872). Impressed by the success being achieved in Massachusetts and elsewhere, Dr H. B. Baker framed a bill which, enacted in 1873, established the Michigan State Board of Health.[70]

Bacteriology developed early at Michigan. Two years before Sedgwick had arrived at the Massachusetts Institute of Technology, the Board of Regents of the University of Michigan established a School of Political Science. Among the courses listed in the Bulletin was one in

[70] Sundwall, John (1956). The division of hygiene and public health. In *The University of Michigan, an encyclopedic survey in nine parts*, (ed. W.A. Donnelly), Part VIII, pp. 1149–57. University of Michigan Press, Ann Arbor.

Sanitary Science taught by Dr V.C. Vaughan, then an Assistant Professor of Physiological Chemistry. Vaughan's one-term elective course, offered in October 1881, embraced 12 main topics, including ferments and germs, physiological fermentation, disease germs, filth diseases, antiseptics and disinfectants, quarantine, and vaccination. In 1884 Vaughan proposed a new course, to be offered under the aegis of the Department of Chemistry. Called at first 'Sanitary Examinations', the course, which dealt with the analysis of water, foods, and drugs, was eventually redesignated as 'Methods of Hygiene'.[71]

In 1883, Vaughan was appointed to the Michigan State Board of Health and investigated numerous outbreaks of water- and food-borne disease. He realized that the State Board needed its own laboratory to assist in scientific examinations, and decided that the best location for such a laboratory would be the University. The Board of Regents were eventually persuaded by his arguments and established a Laboratory of Hygiene in which original clinical, microscopical, and biological investigations were to be carried out. Attention was to be given to the analysis of water, the adulteration of food, and the practical investigation of other problems of sanitary science. Primarily, however, the Laboratory of Hygiene was established owing to a rash of outbreaks of food poisoning, especially as a result of milk and cheese adulteration. The outbreaks had been so severe that the State's cheese industry had been threatened with extinction. In the same way that Sedgwick, as a member of the Massachusetts State Board of Health, had mobilized resources to contain the typhoid outbreaks occurring in towns and cities along Massachusetts' rivers and streams, Vaughan, a member of Michigan's State Board, tackled the problems of the cheese industry. After numerous studies, Vaughan eventually determined that the conditions in the processing plants were primitive. No one, he wrote, had thought at the time to clean the udders of cows; nor had anyone thought it necessary to require that the milker wash his hands or draw the milk in clean receptacles. Vaughan drew up rules of inspection, enlisted the co-operation of the principal players, and the epidemics were contained.

Recognizing the economic benefits of the State Board's scientific endeavours, the Michigan Business Men's Association backed the Board and petitioned the University Board of Regents to appropriate sufficient funds to establish at the University a Hygienic Laboratory, with the following objectives: (1) research into the causation of disease; (2) examination of food and drink and other materials which might be sent to the

[71] Novy, F.G. The Department of Bacteriology and Serology and the Hygienic Laboratory, in Donnelly, op. cit. (note 70), 821–6.

Laboratory by physicians and health officers; and (3) instruction of students in bacteriology. Reminiscing about these events in a letter written in 1926 to Winslow, Vaughan admitted that the petition never had the 'full-hearted support' of the University authorities; but the request could not be ignored owing to the strong support of the State's commercial interests. Eventually, $100 000 was appropriated by the State Legislature and, in 1887, the new Laboratory of Hygiene officially dedicated. Vaughan was appointed Professor of Hygiene and Physiological Chemistry and Director, and Frederick Novy, a man of uncommon ability, appointed Instructor in Hygiene and Physiological Chemistry.[72]

Michigan's Hygienic Laboratory developed quickly. Vaughan and Novy went abroad to work in Koch's laboratory in 1888. New apparatus and equipment were purchased, and a course of instruction prepared on a host of topics, including bacteriology and sanitary science.

More systematic professional public health education was established in May 1911 when the Regents gave the medical faculty permission to 'provide for a course of two years' instruction, leading to the Doctor of Public Health (DPH)'. The Regents believed that there was 'a great demand, and a growing one', for health officials who should know not only medicine, but the principles of heating, ventilation, plumbing, sewage and garbage disposal, and about water supplies and methods of purification of water. The requirements for admission to the DPH (Doctor of Public Health) were for candidates to have both a BS and an MD, conferred by the University of Michigan, or from a 'medical school of equivalent standing'. The course was to extend for two years, half to be given by the medical school and half by the Department of Engineering.[73]

The Regents also established the degree of Master of Science in Public Health, designed as a one-year course of study for post-baccalaureate candidates who possessed the MD degree. The students were not only required to complete satisfactorily their course work, but each was 'to carry out a piece of original investigation of sufficient value, and . . . present a thesis on the same'.[74] By 1916, the 'and' an MD degree was changed and 'or' an MD degree substituted, doubtless owing to the fact that Vaughan had experienced the same difficulty as had Sedgwick, Rosenau, and Winslow.[75] Laboratory workers and sanitary engineers were needed for the great sanitary campaign, as were physicians trained in sanitary science; but if the physicians remained uninterested then the

[72] Vaughan to Winslow, 3 February (1926). Yale University, Winslow MSS I/30/777.
[73] Sundwall, op. cit., 1152 (note 70).
[74] Ibid.
[75] Ibid.

schools would have to inure themselves to the inevitable and devote their attention in another direction: the non-medically trained sanitarian. As Winslow had determined at Yale, however, all was not lost because one could still attempt to capture for public health the medical students; and, if not capture, at least make cognizant of the preventive spirit.

In the early 1920s, Vaughan was to teach at Michigan, as Winslow had done at Yale, the principles of hygiene and public health to hundreds of medical students.[76] Whether or not any of them proceeded to careers in public health is uncertain. Medical students at Michigan, as was true for Yale, had simply not accepted the argument of service for the public good.

The same was to hold true at Pennsylvania. Public health education at Pennsylvania dates from the period following the Civil War. The war had brought to the nation's consciousness, as the great waves of epidemics had done, the need for hygienic practices, in military camps and hospitals as well as in urban centres.[77] In the early 1870s, a chair in hygiene had been awarded to Henry Hartshorne, who, in 1877, was succeeded briefly by Horace Binney Hare and Joseph Richardson. Additional faculty were appointed (N. Arthur Randolph, Seneca Egbert, and especially Samuel Dixon, about whom we shall learn more below),[78] but it was not until 1889, based on a bequest by Henry C. Lea, that a building was established to house the Department of Hygiene. This was soon to be an Institute, if William Pepper, Provost of the University and one of the nation's leading medical statesmen and academic administrators, had anything to say about the matter. Building upon Lea's original bequest, and adding his own personal subscription of $10 000, Pepper personally negotiated the services of John S. Billings, who assumed the directorship of the new Institute in 1892.[79] Billings, army surgeon, librarian, organizational genius, and hospital planner, was quite a catch, but remained at the Institute only until 1896.

When Billings arrived at the Institute, instruction in hygiene had been a part of the medical curriculum for over 20 years. Given new life by the

---

[76] Ibid. For information about V. C. Vaughan, see Vaughan, W.T. (1930). *Victor Clarence Vaughan. Journal of Laboratory and Clinical Medicine*, **15**, 817–20.

[77] Corner, G.W. (1965). *Two centuries of medicine: a history of the School of Medicine, University of Pennsylvania*, pp. 128–9. University of Pennsylvania Press, Philadelphia. See also William Pepper's review of the 12–14 May, 1886 meeting of the Pennsylvania Sanitary Convention in *The Sanitarian* (1886), **17**, 111–7.

[78] See University of Pennsylvania, *Minutes of the Board of Trustees*, 6 February (1877), (11/380); 6 April (1877), (11/383); 7 December (1886), (12/285); 4 December (1888), (12/431).

[79] Ibid., 5 November (1889), (12/501) and 5 May (1891) (12/593). See also Corner, op. cit., 180–1 (note 77).

science of bacteriology, a laboratory of hygiene had been established as early as 1888, under the directorship of Samuel Dixon.

Dixon had begun his adult professional career as an attorney, but owing to a weak constitution, found law too strenuous and decided to become a medical scientist. He received his MD degree in 1886 and proceeded immediately to Europe, to study bacteriology in London and at Pettenkofer's Institute of Hygiene in Munich. In 1888, he was appointed Professor of Hygiene and director of a laboratory devoted to bacteriological research. Dixon's Pennsylvania career as bacteriological researcher, however, came to an abrupt end when Pepper began his negotiations with Billings. The Pennsylvania archives contain many letters revealing Dixon's concern, embarrassment, and then anger, and when Pepper offered the chair to Billings, few were surprised when Dixon resigned his clinical professorship.[80] Dixon went on to do substantial research at the Academy of Natural Sciences where he eventually rose through all the staff ranks to assume the Academy's Presidency. George Corner tells us that Dixon not only had a 'creditable career' in science, but a distinguished one in public service, serving as a member of Philadelphia's school board (from which post he improved hygienic conditions in the public schools), and as health commissioner of Pennsylvania (placing the state's public health activities on a firm scientific basis).[81]

Once established at the Institute, Billings named as his assistant Alexander Abbott, a graduate of the University of Maryland and a student of William Welch at the Hopkins. Abbott had studied abroad, with both Pettenkofer and Koch, and returned in 1889 to Hopkins, where Welch put him in charge of a research laboratory modelled after Koch's laboratory. Abbott did not have time to establish himself at Hopkins, as Billings (who interestingly was the man responsible for bringing Welch to Hopkins) hired Abbott for the assistantship at Pennsylvania.

Billings and Abbott began instruction in hygiene and bacteriology in 1892. Corner tells us that the first class of 11 students was equally divided between the two subjects. Ten of the 11 were physicians, including Charles Harrison Frazier, who later became Professor of Surgery and Dean of the Medical School. Enrolment increased slightly, with more and more students seeking instruction in bacteriology, whereas the number of students enrolled in Billings' course in hygiene dwindled. Disappointed by his inability to attract students, Billings resigned in 1896, to take on yet another new task, negotiating the

---

[80] Corner, op. cit., 181–3 (note 77). See also Dixon to Pepper [Provost], 31 December (1889) and 1 January (1890). General Archives, University of Pennsylvania.

[81] Corner, op. cit., 181–2 (note 77).

merger of the Lenox and Astor Libraries into the New York Public Library.[82]

With both Dixon and Billings removed from the scene, Abbott, primarily a bacteriologist interested in infectious diseases, had difficulty developing the Institute for 'effective community service'. Despite his success in having his laboratory serve as the public health laboratory for a handful of municipalities located throughout the state, no one was surprised when the Provost, as early as 1910, but not consummated until 1914, led the Institute back into the medical school and departmental status. From this new locus, it appears that Abbott intended to follow the same academic path as had Sedgwick, Rosenau, Winslow, and Vaughan, and with the same lack of immediate success.

Abbott first attempted to reach the physicians and requested that his department, now a department of the medical school, be permitted to mount a programme leading to the degree Doctor of Public Health. Recognizing the need for non-medically trained sanitarians, Abbott also requested that he be permitted to admit for study non-medically trained students, such as engineers, who would be eligible for the designation, 'Certified Sanitarian'.[83] Both requests were approved, one with a slight alteration. Instead of the title 'Doctor of Public Health', the Regents recommended a redesignation to 'Doctor of Hygiene', a degree actually awarded retroactively in 1912 to three physicians who had completed the course two years earlier.[84] (The degree Doctor of Public Health was not restored until 1920, as a result of the recommendations derived from the conference on the standardization of degrees in public health, held in New Haven on 28 February, 1919.)[85]

It is not clear when Abbott became disillusioned with the medical school, but he soon came to realize that a proper public health programme needed more degrees of freedom than permitted by the medical school and began to petition the Regents to redesignate his department a department of the University. In these petitions, Abbott pointed out that very few physicians had enrolled in his programme and that students with an interest in public health, such as civil and sanitary engineers, students of architecture, and 'teachers or workers in domestic science',

---

[82] Ibid., 182.

[83] Abbott to Smith [Provost], 15 December (1911), University of Pennsylvania Archives, 'Hygiene and public health, 1911'.

[84] Robins [Secretary] to Abbott, 10 January (1912), ibid., 1912.

[85] See American Public Health Association, *Standardization of public health training. Report of the Committee of Sixteen of the American Public Health Association*. Boston, Massachusetts, April (1921); and University of Pennsylvania, *Courses leading to degrees in public hygiene, session 1919–20.* University of Pennsylvania Archives, 'Hygiene, 1919'.

had no intention or interest in gaining admittance to the medical school, from which administrative body the public health degrees were awarded.

In 1914, Abbott wrote to Provost Edgar Fahs Smith that he wished the Laboratory of Hygiene to be independent of the medical school. The Laboratory, he wrote, needed the goodwill and co-operation of the medical school, but—as the Laboratory also had co-operative arrangements with the School of Biology (zoology and entomology), the Towne Scientific School, the Departments of Architecture and Civil Engineering, the Wharton School (Statistics), the Veterinary School, the Department of Physical Culture, and with many branches of municipal government (the Bureau of Public Health, the Hospital for Contagious Diseases, and the Department of Public Works)—Smith should understand that 'Public Hygiene, in its modern development, [was] in fact a social question more than a strictly medical one, and should be encouraged to so develop'.[86]

Abbott's request was denied and, as had Winslow in 1915 at Yale, he petitioned the Provost to permit his department to accept into a public health degree programme students who did not meet the requirements for entrance to the medical school. Such students as enrolled in his department would be awarded either one of two degrees, 'Certified Sanitarian' or 'Bachelor of Public Hygiene'. It was Abbott's wish that a programme so designated, distinct but related to the medical school, and effecting co-operative relationships with other university-wide and municipal departments and affiliations, would attract outside funding, such as was then being discussed by the Rockefeller Foundation prior to its 1916 decision to establish a fully equipped school of hygiene and public health at Johns Hopkins.

The programme Abbott envisioned was as comprehensive as the Institute programme set forth by Sedgwick in 1916 at the Massachusetts Institute of Technology and the programme at the Harvard-Massachusetts Institute of Technology School for Health Officers. For example, in the 1919–20 Bulletin,[87] 16 subjects were listed comprising the course of study:

A.   Sanitary Engineering
  1.   Municipal Water Supplies and Water Works
  2.   Sewage and Sewage Disposal
  3.   Disposal of Municipal Refuse and Street Cleaning

---

[86] Abbott to Smith [Provost], 10 December (1914), University of Pennsylvania Archives, 'Hygiene, 1914'.

[87] *Courses leading to degrees*, op. cit. (note 85).

B.   Sanitary Engineering of Buildings
    1.   Heating
    2.   Ventilation
    3.   Drainage
C.   Inspection of Meat, Milk, and Other Animal Products
    1.   Milk Hygiene
    2.   Meat Hygiene
D.   Practical Hygiene
    I.   Clinical and Physical Methods as Applied to:
        1.   Atmosphere
        2.   Water
        3.   Sewage
        4.   Disposal of refuse, cremation of garbage, etc.
        5.   Soils and building sites
        6.   Foods
        7.   Clothing
    II.   Sanitary Bacteriology
E.   Protozoology
F.   Arthropods
G.   Helminthology and General Medical Zoology
H.   Pathology of Tropical Diseases
I.   Personal and Military Hygiene
J.   Sanitary Legislation
K.   Medical Inspection of Schools
L.   Vital Statistics
M.   Industrial Hygiene
N.   Public Hygiene and Epidemiology
O.   Field Work
P.   Sanitary Surveys

As had colleagues in other schools, Abbott lamented the fact that, whereas his programme had attracted fairly large numbers of students from various disciplines, including the Schools of Education and Architecture, very few students had enrolled from the medical school, and probably few ever would.[88]

6. Conclusion

We have now discussed the early years of five schools, the Massachusetts Institute of Technology alone, and then in collaboration with

---

[88]   Abbott to Smith (note 86).

Harvard, and Yale, Michigan, and Pennsylvania, and have reached that time when we must ravel the threads of our discussion and set forth some conclusions.

I have maintained that the schools examined emerged from a confluence of factors manifested in the nineteenth century. Such factors included the development of commercial enterprise; the need for technically trained students to advance the manufacturing sciences; the development of schools dedicated to applied science, fostered by the passage of the Morrill Land Grant Act, which provided funds for that purpose; the urbanization of the nation and the need to resolve problems attendant thereto; the water-borne epidemics of typhoid and cholera and other epidemics which threatened lives and commercial interests, leading to the sanitary awakening; the need for skilled public health professionals, abundantly made clear by emergent problems not only in the urban city, but in Civil War military camps and hospitals; the emergence of state boards of health; the rise to prominence of the sciences of bacteriology and immunology: all of which may be coupled with a pervasive spirit of utility—a desire to correct society's ills—by developing a cadre of professionally trained and thereby eminently useful sanitarians.

In each school examined, evidence of these factors was apparent. The Massachusetts Institute of Technology, for example, was established for the primary purpose of providing students with a technical course of study. Once established, its educational policy never varied, and even served as a model for numerous similar institutions. Graduates of the Massachusetts Institute helped develop industries, generally added to the national welfare by the application of scientific methods to the 'great practical problems of the day', and, thanks to Sedgwick and those whom he trained, helped to conserve the health of all citizens.[89] As William Barton Rogers had written, 'the value of science [is] in its great modern applications to the practical arts of life, to human comfort, and health, and to social wealth and power'.[90] To meet these ends, Sedgwick, from his strategic post at the Massachusetts Institute, applied his science in many arenas, in the State Board of Health, the Lawrence Sanitary Station, the Massachusetts Institute's Sanitary Research Laboratory and Sewage Experiment Station, as teacher and mentor to a battalion of sanitarians and engineers, and as national consultant[91] and sanitary statesman.

[89] Maclaurin, op. cit., p. v (note 35).
[90] Ibid., 4–5.
[91] See Leighton, M.O. (1907). *Pollution of Illinois and Mississippi rivers by Chicago sewage*. Government Printing Office, Washington, DC.

Sedgwick carried his ideas forward into the productive but short-lived combined Harvard–Massachusetts Institute of Technology School for Health Officers, where the resources of both institutions were united into a coherent programme for both medically and non-medically trained students wishing to take their place as leading players in the public health crusade. The School more than fulfilled its great potential, but suffered from its uncertain administrative arrangements and its inability, owing to its organizational setting, to award its own degrees. Both institutions refused to make modifications in the original charter and the School maintained itself only until 1921.[92]

Recognizing the combined School's anomalous situation and based on a fierce pride and loyalty for his own institution, Sedgwick in 1916 attempted to develop at the Massachusetts Institute of Technology an Institute of Hygiene. Comprehensive and bold in design, the plan lacked only financial support, support such as went from the Rockefeller Foundation to Johns Hopkins.

At Yale, a new department of public health was established in 1915 with Winslow, Sedgwick's disciple, as Chairman. Winslow believed that from this administrative arrangement a viable public health teaching and research programme could be developed; and it was. Winslow reached into the medical school and established cooperative relationships with the departments of bacteriology, pathology, and psychiatry, and the Child Study Center; he extended these relationships to the departments of engineering and the Sheffield Scientific and Law Schools; thanks to the strong support of his Dean, Milton Winternitz, he strengthened his department by consolidating it with the graduate school departments of bacteriology and pathology; and with the Provost's approval, Winslow was able to admit to his programme qualified non-physicians for studies leading to the CPH, Dr.P.H., and Ph.D. degrees.

Unsuccessful in reaching the physician, as Sedgwick had been, Winslow focused on two special groups of clientele: non-medically trained students and medical students. The first group was to receive degrees and take their place as laboratory workers and sanitary engineers, as leaders in the public health campaign; the second group, those whom he especially hoped to capture for the profession, he settled for simply pervading with the preventive spirit.

Vaughan, at Michigan, followed a path very similar to Sedgwick's. Serving on the State Board, Vaughan revealed the importance to health,

---

[92] Curran, op. cit., 19 (note 56).

and commerce, of public health science. With strong support from the State Board of Health and commercial interests, but surprisingly not from the Governor or the University's Board of Regents, a Laboratory of Hygiene was established in 1887, in the same year that the Marine Hospital Hygienic Laboratory was established[93] and five years before the University of Pennsylvania's Hygienic Laboratory.

With the able assistance of Novy, Vaughan developed courses in sanitary science and bacteriology and made substantial contributions to the literature of both applied and basic research. Vaughan, as had Sedgwick, found it difficult to reach the physicians and requested that the administration permit him to admit non-physicians to his programme. And, as necessity dictated, he, like Winslow, found that his primary objective had become to educate laboratorians and sanitary engineers and to offer courses in sanitary science to the medical students.

At Pennsylvania, Abbott made similar inroads into state-wide, but primarily local, public health, developing his Institute for 'effective community service'; but he too failed in his desire to reach the physicians. Abbott's Laboratory, like Winslow's Department, was administratively a part of the medical school; but whereas Winslow had been singularly successful in maintaining a visible and effective medical school teaching programme, while achieving for his programme graduate school status, Abbott found himself confined by the medical school, until that time when they relented and permitted him to admit to his programme students who had not first qualified for admission to the medical school. Once established, Abbott's programme was as comprehensive a programme as existed in any of the schools I have studied.

A final point concerns the medical students and physicians. Why was it so difficult, even from the proximity of departmental status, to bring them into the public health campaign? Why had the programmes sought so desperately for school or university rather than departmental status? Why were there not more physicians of high quality finding their way into the field? Answers to such questions are not easy to find; but some help may be forthcoming from a questionnaire prepared in the early 1920s by E.O. Jordan, Professor of Bacteriology at Chicago, and one of Sedgwick's former students.

Jordan had distributed questionnaires to medical students of four different universities. Questions were designed to determine why students had decided on a medical career rather than on one in public health. He

---

[93] See Harden, V.A. (1986). *Inventing the N.I.H.: federal biomedical research policy, 1887–1937.* The Johns Hopkins University Press, Baltimore, Maryland.

received 461 replies. Of these, 103 students stated that they had, at one time or another, considered public health while the remaining 358 stated that they never had taken the possibility seriously. Most cited as reasons for this lack of interest their insufficient knowledge of the field; some replying that they knew absolutely nothing about public health work. Some believed medicine more suited to their personality, interests, and curiosity; while others expressed their hostility to public health because it was thought to be wrapped-up in local and state politics and considered to stifle initiative. Some addressed the issue of remuneration, believing it so slight in public health that it would not make up for the many arduous years of study necessary to enter the field.[94]

Each of the schools considered the problems, some with the characteristic shrug of resignation or the belief that perhaps medical schools were admitting the wrong type of students; others, Winslow, for example, by identifying the problem as one based on the way we, in the United States, had decided to organize, finance, and deliver health services. As long as a financial barrier existed between those who needed and those who provided medical care, then medicine, as Winslow was to say in 1926, would never be truly preventive and public health never fully realize its potential.[95]

As expressed at the 1922 conference on 'The future of public health in the United States and the education of sanitarians', the hope was that professional standards would be raised, that medical students would become more informed about the nature and opportunities of public health work as more medical schools adopted quality programmes in public health, that physicians trained in the techniques of public health would be drawn into public health work, and that vigorous and systematic education campaigns would be mounted to influence the public, state legislatures, and the medical profession.[96]

The early schools and programmes, which began their institutional history based on utility, science, and optimism, reached maturity in the 1920s. They closed ranks, consolidated achievements, and began to identify new avenues for expansion. One such avenue lay in the direction of clinical medicine, toward maternal and child health, occupational

---

[94] See *Report of a conference, the future of public health in the United States and the education of sanitarians, March 14 and 15 (1922)*. Public Health Bulletin, No. 124, 19–21. Washington, D.C.

[95] See Winslow, C–E.A. (1920). The untilled fields of public health. *Modern Medicine*, **2**, 183–91; and Winslow, C–E.A. (1926). Public health at the crossroads. *American Journal of Public Health*, **16**, 1075–85.

[96] *Report*, op. cit., 21–5. (note 94).

medicine, clinical epidemiology,[97] tropical medicine, and preventive medicine;[98] another in the potentially dynamic field of medical care.[99]

How the schools adapted themselves to these new missions and how their responsibilities succeeded or failed, were modified or abandoned, will be discussed in Chapters 5 and 7.

[97] See Viseltear, A.J. (1982). John R. Paul and the definition of preventive medicine. *Yale Journal of Biology and Medicine*, **55**, 167–72.

[98] See Leavitt, J.W. (1980). Public health and preventive medicine. In *The education of American physicians* (ed. R.L. Numbers), pp. 250–72. University of California Press, Berkeley.

[99] See Viseltear, A.J. (1973). The emergence of the medical care section of the American Public Health Association, 1926–1948. *American Journal of Public Health*, **63**, 986–1007; and Viseltear, A.J. (1973). Compulsory health insurance and the definition of public health. In *Compulsory health insurance: the continuing American debate* (ed. R.L. Numbers), pp. 25–54. Greenwood Press, Westport, Connecticut.

5

Designing schools of public health for the United States

ELIZABETH FEE

1. Introduction

In the late nineteenth century, public health in the United States was institutionalized in city and state health departments, but there were few formal requirements for public health positions, no established career structures, and little job security for health officials. Most public health positions were part-time appointments at nominal salary; many who devoted effort to public health did so on a largely voluntary basis. As Arthur Viseltear has explained, some of the better medical, engineering, and technical schools offered courses in public health, preventive medicine, and sanitary engineering but there was no standardized system of training and little agreement about the forms of knowledge necessary for public health practice. Most public health officers in the north and east had medical degrees, but some were engineers and others were lawyers, chemists, or biologists.

Public health programmes, when organized at all, were organized locally: as Robert Wiebe has argued, the United States in the nineteenth century was a society of 'island communities' with considerable economic and political autonomy.[1] The first public health organizations had been those of the rapidly growing port cities of the eastern seaboard in the late eighteenth century. By 1860, public health activities were just beginning to move beyond the confines of local city politics, and in the 1870s and 1880s, most of the states created their own boards of health.[2]

---

[1] Wiebe, Robert H. (1967). *The search for order, 1877–1920*. Hill and Wang, New York.

[2] The first state board of health, largely an organization on paper, was created in Louisiana in 1855. The first working state health board was formed in Massachusetts in 1869, followed by California (1870), the District of Columbia (1871), Virginia and Minnesota (1872), Maryland (1874) and Alabama (1875). Paterson, R. G. (1939). *Historical directory of State Health Departments in the United States of America*. Public Health Association, Columbus, Ohio.

The impact of these state boards of health should not, however, be overemphasized; by 1900, only three states (Massachusetts, Rhode Island, and Florida) spent more than 2 cents per capita for public health services.[3]

The development of public health departments, especially in the cities, had been prompted by the industrial transformation of the late nineteenth century. The populations moving from the land to the rapidly growing cities competed for living space with the flow of immigrants from Western, Southern, and Eastern Europe; families crowded into tenement housing, back alleys, and damp basement apartments, supplied with communal privies and polluted water sources. City streets were heaped with garbage, including dead and decaying animals, and the waste products of small manufactories; factories produced their own noise, smells, smoke, and industrial wastes to add to the dirt and confusion of the new industrial order. Children died young of diarrhoeal and respiratory diseases, diphtheria, whooping cough, smallpox, and typhoid fever. Tuberculosis and other infectious diseases killed young adults and further impoverished families already struggling for survival. City health departments, especially in the eastern port cities, faced overwhelming social and health problems.[4]

An increasing number of voluntary reform groups were organized to address social and sanitary reforms. In 1872, the American Public Health Association was started by a small group of social reformers in New York City; other municipal associations were also active in attempting to improve the conditions of the poor or in campaigning for specific

[3] Abbott, S. W. (1900). *The past and present conditions of public hygiene and state medicine in the United States.* Wright and Potter, Boston.

[4] Blake, John (1959). *Public health in the town of Boston, 1630–1822,* Harvard University Press, Cambridge, Massachusetts; Rosenkrantz, Barbara (1972). *Public health and the state: changing views in Massachusetts, 1842–1936.* Harvard University Press, Cambridge, Massachusetts; Duffy, John (1968). *A history of public health in New York City, 1625–1866.* Russell Sage Foundation, New York; Duffy, John (1974). *A history of public health in New York City, 1866–1966.* Russell Sage Foundation, New York; Galishoff, Stuart (1975). *Safeguarding the public health: Newark, 1895–1918.* Greenwood Press, Westport, Connecticut; Leavitt, Judith Walzer (1982). *The healthiest city: Milwaukee and the politics of health reform.* Princeton University Press, Princeton, New Jersey; Winslow, C–E.A. (1929). *The life of Hermann M. Biggs: physician and statesman of the public health.* Lea and Febiger, Philadelphia, Pennsylvania; Jordan, E.O., Whipple, G.C., and Winslow, C–E.A. (1924). *A pioneer of public health: William Thompson Sedgwick.* Yale University Press, New Haven; Cassedy, James H. (1962). *Charles V. Chapin and the public health movement.* Harvard University Press, Cambridge, Massachusetts; Rosenberg, Charles E. and Carroll S. (1968). Pietism and the origins of the American public health movement. *Journal of the History of Medicine and Allied Sciences,* **23**, 16–35; Shryock, Richard H. (1937). The early American public health movement. *American Journal of Public Health,* **27**, 965–71.

social reforms.[5] Progressive reform organizations aided, pushed, and provoked city governments to act on some of the most obvious threats to cleanliness, order, and health in the urban environment.[6]

Gradually, the functions of city health departments, especially in the North and East, expanded. In addition to divisions of street cleaning, sanitary engineering, and vital statistics, they started bacteriological laboratories, divisions of tuberculosis and venereal disease control, and divisions of child and maternal health. The heads of these divisions held full-time posts, supported by a growing corps of public health nurses, sanitary inspectors, and statistical clerks. The main difficulty of most city health departments was to find personnel trained and competent to do the job, while resisting pressures to make political appointments of unqualified people. These official activities of the municipal health departments were supplemented by the energetic efforts of voluntary agencies dedicated to specific reforms.

The northern industrial cities thus displayed the social and health problems brought by rapid industrial growth, but they also generated the progressive reform movements to address the most obvious problems. By contrast to the Northeast, the Southern states after the Civil War resembled an underdeveloped country within the United States. In the Southern states, levels of literacy, agricultural production, and economic efficiency were all low due to a legacy of slavery. The integration of the South into a growing industrial economy required far-reaching social and cultural changes. In this context, Northern industrialists began investing in education as well as in cotton mills and railroads, and John D. Rockefeller, on the suggestion of Frederick Gates, created the General Education Board to support 'the general organization of rural communities for economic, social and educational purposes'.[7]

Charles Wardell Stiles convinced the Secretary of the General Education Board that the real cause of misery and lack of productivity in the

[5] Smith, Stephen (1921). The history of public health, 1871–1921. In *A half century of public health* (ed. Mazyck P. Ravenel), pp. 1–12. American Public Health Association, New York. Ravenel, Mazyck P. The American Public Health Association: past, present, future, in Ravenel, op. cit., 13–55.

[6] The American Red Cross had been formed in 1882, the National Tuberculosis Association in 1904, the American Social Hygiene Association in 1905, the National Committee for Mental Hygiene in 1909, and the American Society for the Control of Cancer in 1919. See Smillie, Wilson G. (1955). *Public health: its promise for the future*, pp. 450–8. Macmillan, New York; Rosenkrantz, Barbara (1974). Cart before horse: theory, practice and professional image in American public health. *Journal of the History of Medicine and Allied Sciences*, **29**, 57.

[7] Fosdick, Raymond B. (1962). *Adventure in giving: the story of the General Education Board*, pp. 57–8. Harper and Row, New York and Evanston, Illinois.

South was hookworm, the 'germ of laziness'.[8] In 1909, Rockefeller agreed to provide $1 million to create the Rockefeller Sanitary Commission for the Eradication of Hookworm Disease, with Wickliffe Rose, originally a philosophy professor in Tennessee, as Director. Rose worked to establish an effective and permanent public health organization in the Southern states.[9] At the end of five years of intensive effort, his campaign had greatly expanded the role of public health agencies. In 1914, the organizational experience gained in the Southern states would enable the Rockefeller Foundation to extend the hookworm control programme to the Caribbean, Central America, and Latin America. A major problem faced by the Rockefeller Foundation's efforts in the Southern states had been to find adequately trained and competent public health workers; the leaders of the hookworm campaign found, by bitter experience, that they could not depend on the competence and efficiency of part-time public health officers, nor could they depend on the support or co-operation of most private medical practitioners. As a result of his experiences in the South, Wickliffe Rose decided that a new profession of public health must be created, with full-time public health workers who had been specifically trained for the job, and whose loyalties would be committed to public health rather than to clinical medicine.

2. Toward a new profession of public health

Public health had been defined in terms of its aims and goals—to reduce disease and maintain the health of the population—rather than by any specific body of knowledge. Many different disciplines contributed to public health work: physicians diagnosed contagious diseases; sanitary engineers built water and sewage systems; vital statisticians provided quantitative measures of births and deaths; lawyers wrote sanitary codes and regulations; public health nurses provided care and advice to the sick in their homes; sanitary inspectors visited factories and markets to enforce compliance with public health ordinances; and administrators tried to organize everyone within the limits of their budgets.

Physicians claimed to make a special contribution to public health, but so did other groups including chemists, nurses, engineers, lawyers,

[8] For a detailed account of the Rockefeller Sanitary Commission, see Ettling, John (1981). *The germ of laziness: Rockefeller philanthropy and public health in the new South*. Harvard University Press, Cambridge, Massachusetts.

[9] Rose, Wickliffe (1910). *First annual report of the Administrative Secretary of the Rockefeller Sanitary Commission*, p. 4, as cited in Fosdick, Raymond B. (1952). *The story of the Rockefeller Foundation*, p. 33. Harper & Brothers, New York.

bacteriologists, and statisticians. The attempt to create a new profession of public health meant that these diverse and often competing interests would have to be brought together with a single vision, a common philosophy, and a unified educational program. If each group had different specific skills, they would have to learn to work together in practice. To create a more unified profession, their different professional identities would have to be integrated in the interests of a larger goal. Programmes of education and training and of licensing would have to be shaped to their different levels of educational experience and scientific knowledge.

By the second decade of the twentieth century, non-medical public health officers were beginning to protest the increasing dominance of public health by medical men. By this time, the sanitary engineers were the only professional group strong enough to challenge the physicians' assumption that the future of public health should be theirs. Civil and sanitary engineers had created relatively clean city water supplies and adequate sewerage systems. With the benefit of hindsight, we can say that the sanitary engineers, through their work in improving water supplies and sewerage systems, surely deserve much of the credit for the decline of infectious disease mortality and morbidity in the late nineteenth century.[10] Professional competition between the sanitary engineers and the physicians became intense in the early years of the twentieth century as physicians reinforced their dominance in public health departments, and as sanitary engineers vociferously complained about the increasing 'medical monopoly' of public health.[11]

Physicians, sanitary engineers, and public health leaders, such as

[10] It is difficult to be confident about mortality rates in the United States before 1900, when the death registration areas began regular reporting. The evidence seems, however, to suggest that mortality rates between 1850 and 1880 remained relatively constant, with wide annual variations depending on the presence of epidemics. In the 1880s, the mortality rates began to decline, and continued this decline, with minor fluctuations, throughout the period from 1890 to 1915. The major component of the decline was in infant mortality, especially mortality rates from the infectious diseases and infant diarrhoea. This pattern is consistent with the thesis that the extension of municipal water systems and the filtration of water supplies played a major role in the decline in mortality. The pasteurization of milk was probably also an important contributing factor. On the estimation of mortality rates for the period, see Meeker, Edward (1972). The improving health of the United States, 1850–1915. *Explorations in Economic History*, **9**, 353–73; Haines, Michael R. (1979). The use of model life tables to estimate mortality for the United States in the late nineteenth century. *Demography*, **16**, 289–312; Hoffman, Frederick L. (1906–1907). The general death rate of large American cities, 1871–1904. *Publications of the American Statistical Association*, **10**, 1–75. For a general discussion of the social impact of infectious diseases, see Duffy, John (1971). Social impact of disease in the late nineteenth century. *Bulletin of the New York Academy of Medicine*, **47**, 797–811.

[11] Knowles, Morris (1913). Public health service not a medical monopoly. *American Journal of Public Health*, **3**, 111–22.

William Sedgwick, trained as a biologist, and Wickliffe Rose, originally a professor of philosophy, agreed on one unifying idea: the new profession of public health should be based on a scientific education. The discoveries of Louis Pasteur, Robert Koch, and other bacteriologists in the 1870s and 1880s had been rapidly integrated into public health practice in the United States; as Sedgwick aptly expressed the impact of bacteriological discoveries: 'Before 1880 we knew nothing; after 1890 we knew it all; it was a glorious ten years'.[12]

The new bacteriology became an ideological marker separating the 'old' public health, mainly the province of untrained amateurs, from the 'new' public health, which would belong to those trained in the techniques of science and laboratory research. The new emphasis on scientific knowledge would also provide a means of insulating public health practice from political pressures by making appointments more dependent on knowledge and training than on personal and political loyalties. At the same time, scientific training would differentiate public health professionals from the broader enthusiasms of voluntary reformers; in public health, the social reform impulse would be tempered by scientific knowledge and expertise. Public health leaders were committed to the idea that health activities should be planned along scientific lines by a scientifically trained élite, and not left either to the good intentions of voluntary reform groups or to changing political pressures and special interests.

Some of the more progressive state governments, such as New York, were already by 1913 passing legislation to require minimal levels of scientific training for those appointed to public health positions. Such legislation was, however, in advance of the educational system: there were few real opportunities for education in public health and most public health workers were necessarily trained on the job. Where the federal and state governments were slow to act, the private foundations, and especially the Rockefeller Foundation, took the lead in organizing public health programs and professional public health education.

One critical event in shaping the future structure of the public health profession was a conference held in New York on 16 October 1914. This conference, held in the offices of the General Education Board of the Rockefeller Foundation, would have a dramatic impact: the decisions taken on that occasion would lay the basis for the future development of professional public health education. The public health leaders and Foundation representatives involved set themselves the task of defining the necessary knowledge base for public health practice and

---

[12] As cited in Jordan, Whipple, Winslow, op. cit., 57 (note 4).

designing the educational system needed to train a new profession. William Henry Welch and Wickliffe Rose refined these ideas, each inserting his own favoured emphasis, in their two versions of the famous Welch- -Rose report of 1915—the central reference point for the design of schools of public health.

The creation of public health as a profession in the United States— however incomplete the process—was thus part of a deliberate plan and strategy. By examining the specific decisions taken, we can better understand the subsequent development of education in public health and, with the benefit of hindsight, evaluate the results of this early planning. At the time, there were several possibilities for organizing professional education in public health. One option was to regard public health as a unique amalgam of the biomedical, engineering, and social sciences, requiring specialized training in each of these fields. Some suggested that public health be treated as a combination of sanitary engineering and bacteriology, so that the contributions of engineers and physicians could both be honoured. Others regarded public health as mainly a problem of social reform and social organization, in which social and political scientists should take a leading role. Yet others thought that public health should be a specialized branch of medicine, drawing on physicians' knowledge of disease processes, diagnosis, and therapy.

The question of the relationship of public health to other disciplines and professional groups was simultaneously the question of the content and methods of the field. Should public health identify closely with bacteriology and the successes of the germ theory of disease, or should it seek a broader definition, trying to understand the influence of social, economic, and environmental conditions on the health of individuals? Were the social sciences of fundamental importance to understanding the definition, patterns, and distribution of health and disease, or were they a side issue qualifying the serious business of biological research? If public health constituted the study of disease in society, how much attention should be devoted to disease and how much to society?

The most fundamental issues in the design of public health education were the tensions between public health and clinical medicine, and between the social and biological approaches to health. A series of other related issues also structured the debates about public health education. The first concerned the relative importance of advanced education for the few versus minimal training for the majority of public health practitioners. Those wanting training efforts to be directed at practising public health officers urged the creation of short courses, correspondence courses, and extension courses rather than lengthy full-time degree programmes, so that people already working in the field would have access to some specialized education.

The second issue, related to the first, was whether educational programmes should concentrate on research and research methods—the means of developing new knowledge—or on the more practical skills needed in running a health department, planning an immunization campaign, or establishing a new clinic. Those advocating a research-oriented education argued that the demands of practice were constantly changing so that education in specific methods would soon be outdated; research training provided the basic scientific principles that could be applied to any problems arising in the future. Those advocating more practically oriented programmes argued that the most urgent task was to implement existing public health knowledge rather than to devote resources to new research. They cited the British model of education in public health, described by Roy Acheson in Chapter 2, which they saw as being oriented toward administrative skills, and with licensure dependent on a combination of course work and practical training. Those advocating a research-oriented education referred to the German research institutes of hygiene as their model. In the debates about the form of education in public health in America, the term 'public health' usually referred to the English administrative model, while 'hygiene' implied the German emphasis on research.

A third related issue in education in public health was the relative importance to be given to mass education for the general public. Most agreed in principle that public education in the broadest sense was important in improving the public's health, but they differed in the real priority they gave to popular education. Those most interested in promoting research tended to give a lower order of importance to popular health education than did the advocates of practical training programmes. These issues were not, however, synonymous, and some laboratory researchers were ardent advocates of popular education.

3. Wickliffe Rose and the Rockefeller Sanitary Commission

Wickliffe Rose, the architect and organizer of the Rockefeller Sanitary Commission's campaign against hookworm, was described by Abraham Flexner as 'a thoroughly intellectual type' and as 'a great general and strategist'. Rose indeed thought of the world as a battlefield in the conquest of disease.[13] The general, however, needed an army: officers

[13] Flexner, Abraham (1960). *I remember: an autobiography*, p. 134. Simon and Schuster, New York; Fosdick, Raymond (1958). *Chronicle of a generation: an autobiography*, p. 255. Harper & Brothers, New York.

and soldiers trained in the most effective and efficient methods of fighting disease, possessed with zeal for the battle, and properly equipped for the seriousness of the task. Rose knew that he did not want to rely upon part-time health officers, or on physicians whose main income came from private practice.

In the hookworm campaign, Rose had attempted to work through local health officials in each community. He had discovered that public health was strictly a part-time avocation for these men, and that their primary interest was in medical practice. He had early come to the conclusion that a new profession was needed, composed of men who would devote their whole careers to the control of disease. Rose insisted, as had Edwin Chadwick before him, that there must be two separate professions: medicine, for curing disease on an individual level, and public health, for preventing and controlling disease on a population level.

4. Abraham Flexner and the General Education Board

As the first step in the implementation of his plan, Rose turned to the General Education Board and to Abraham Flexner, whose 'Flexner Report' of 1910 had been central to the reorganization of American medical education.[14] Flexner was not very interested in public health, but he knew a great deal about medical education, and the General Education Board held general responsibility for all Rockefeller education programmes. At the time, Flexner was struggling to get medical school professors to give all their time to teaching and research and not be permitted to earn income from private practice—a principle that some accepted and others violently opposed. To Rose, the need for full-time health officers appeared in a similar light: real progress would depend on the separation of public health work from the competing loyalties of medical practice. In December 1913, Rose asked the General Education Board to consider ways of training men for public health service.[15]

Abraham Flexner immediately began to explore the existing facilities for training health officers. He soon discovered that Wickliffe Rose's concern about professional training was widely shared. Hermann Biggs, the energetic Commissioner of Health in New York State, was especially bitter about the lack of properly trained men for health

---

[14] Flexner, Abraham (1910). *Medical education in the United States and Canada*, Bulletin no.4. Carnegie Foundation for the Advancement of Teaching, New York. For Flexner's interest in preventive medicine see Brieger, Gert H. (1985). The Flexner Report: revised or revisited? *Medical Heritage*, January/February, 25–34.

[15] Archives of the Rockefeller Foundation (1913). *Minutes of the Executive Committee of the International Health Commission*, 19 December, record group 1.1, series 200.

department work.[16] In 1913, Biggs had manoeuvered a bill through the New York State legislature to allow the State Board of Health to set minimum qualifications for local health officers.[17] This bill had no immediate effect, for there were no applicants with any special training in public health, and no training programme available in the state. Massachusetts, Pennsylvania, and Maryland had similar legislation, but again, it was ineffective without a supply of trained men to fill the available positions. The legal framework remained meaningless until provision could be made for educating the new professionals.

Existing training courses in public health were insufficient to meet the demand. Alexander Abbott, who had studied with Welch, Pettenkofer, and Koch, was graduating a small number of students from his public health programme at the University of Pennsylvania.[18] Edwin Jordan at Chicago had a modest programme for public health training, and E.P. Lyon had been trying to start a programme in Minnesota. William W. Ford reported from Baltimore:

Even with the most favourable interpretation of our facilities . . . it must be admitted that the subject of Hygiene or Public Health is in its infancy at Johns Hopkins, and that we would not be justified in maintaining for a moment that we have the opportunities for properly training men for a career in Public Health.[19]

As noted in Chapter 4, the most developed model for public health training was the School for Health Officers run jointly by Harvard University and the Massachusetts Institute of Technology. By combining existing courses in Harvard and the Massachusetts Institute of Technology with a number of new offerings, the School for Health Officers had produced an impressive catalogue of courses in communicable diseases, sanitary engineering, preventive medicine, personal hygiene, demography, public health administration, sanitary biology, and sanitary chemistry. Two or three years of academic work were required for

[16] Hermann Biggs was perhaps the first great public health administrator in the United States. Biggs was extremely successful as a private medical practitioner and had formed relationships with the politically powerful in New York City; he used his influence—and the wealth he had gained from private practice—to further the cause of public health in New York.

[17] On Biggs' efforts in reorganizing the New York State Department of Health, see Winslow, C–E.A. (1929). *The life of Hermann M. Biggs: physician and statesman of the public health*, pp. 251–88. Lea and Febiger, Philadelphia, Pennsylvania.

[18] University of Pennsylvania (1909). *Courses in public health, 1909–1910*. University of Pennsylvania, Philadelphia. This catalogue gives a complete listing of courses leading to the diploma in public health; Abbott to Flexner, 20 January (1914), Archives of the Rockefeller Foundation, (RFA), loc.cit. (note 15).

[19] Ford to Flexner, 16 January (1914), RFA, loc.cit. (note 15).

a certificate in public health.[20] The Harvard–Massachusetts Institute of Technology School graduated a small number of highly trained health officers each year: five received certificates in 1914.[21] Some of those trained were medical men, but most were scientists and engineers. The School's Director, Milton J. Rosenau, had written the classic text, *Preventive medicine and hygiene*.[22]

As soon as Rosenau heard of the General Education Board's interest in the training of health officers, he wrote to Flexner proposing that 'such a project might well be entrusted to Harvard University'.[23] At the same time, Charles-Edward A. Winslow suggested a school in New York. Thinking of the immediate practical needs of the New York State Health Department, Winslow visualized a school that would concentrate on training public health nurses, sanitary inspectors, and health officers for small towns: the rank-and-file of the profession, not just the highly trained élite. He argued forcibly that the laws recently passed in New York State called for many hundreds of trained men and women to work in areas such as industrial hygiene, infant mortality, and school inspections.[24]

On 28 May, 1914, Wickliffe Rose presented his own report on 'Training for Public Health Service' to the General Education Board.[25] Rose argued that the public health officer of the future would not be a practising physician but would follow an 'independent career'. Opportunities for professional employment already existed; a properly equipped school would find an immediate market for its graduates. Rose suggested that the General Education Board begin formulating a concrete plan to establish, on an experimental basis, one or two schools 'at such places as Boston or New York'.[26] Abraham Flexner agreed to organize a planning conference for the following October.

At this juncture, Columbia University submitted a proposal for a

---

[20] Rosenau, Milton J. (1915). Courses and degrees in public health work. *Journal of the American Medical Association*, **64**, 794–6. See also, Catalogue and announcement, (1913). *Circular of the School for Health Officers*, **1**, 1–41.

[21] Curran, Jean Alonzo (1970). *Founders of the Harvard School of Public Health, with biographical notes, 1909–1946*, p. 7. The Josiah Macy Jr. Foundation, New York.

[22] Rosenau, Milton J. (1913). *Preventive medicine and hygiene*. D. Appleton and Company, New York and London.

[23] Rosenau, Milton J. (1914). Memorandum, and letter to Abraham Flexner, 9 January, RFA, loc.cit. (note 15).

[24] When Winslow later became Professor of Public Health at Yale University, he would be mainly concerned with educating medical students and physicians; he would continue, however, to be actively involved in training public health nurses.

[25] Rose, Wickliffe (1914). First report to the General Education Board: training for public health service. 28 May, RFA, loc.cit. (note 15).

[26] Ibid., 3.

school of public health in New York. The Columbia plan, submitted by
Edwin Seligman, Professor of Political Science, called for a combination
of medical, engineering, and social science courses, leading to a Doctor
of Science degree. Abraham Flexner now had to add a representative
from Columbia to his invitation list for the October conference. Nicho-
las Murray Butler, the President of Columbia University, suggested
Seligman. Instead of inviting Seligman, or even one of the other distinguished Columbia faculty such as Hans Zinsser, Professor of Bacteriology, or Mary Adelaide Nutting, Professor of Nursing, Flexner asked
Daniel Jackson, a junior faculty member from the Engineering Department, to represent Columbia. Protesting, Butler asked that Seligman be
invited to the conference, but Flexner was adamant, and Jackson, who
had neither an MD nor a Ph.D., received the invitation. In vain, Seligman warned that 'the broader social side was in danger of not being adequately represented'.[27]

The Columbia plan placed unusual emphasis on the importance of the
social and political sciences and insisted that public health was a social
and political problem, as well as a medical and engineering one. In the
discussions that followed, three competing conceptions of public health
emerged: the engineering or environmental approach, the socio-political, and the biomedical. In the end, the biomedical conception was to
dominate, with socio-political and environmental concerns relegated to
a very subsidiary role, just as Seligman had feared.

Yale University was also planning a programme in public health.
Yale had been given an endowment to establish a chair of public health,
and had asked Flexner for advice in selecting a candidate; Flexner suggested that the university postpone all plans until after the October conference.

As Flexner drew up his plans for the conference, Wickliffe Rose was
clarifying his own idea of the necessary organization of training in public health. By 7 October, 1914, Rose already had the outlines of a plan to
place schools of public health in strategic centres across the United
States.[28] He sent Flexner a long list of men and organizations to be consulted, including, in addition to medical school representatives, the
United States Public Health Service, the medical departments of the
army and navy, state, city, and county health officers, food control
officials, registrars of vital statistics, life insurance companies, industrial
health managers, and sanitary engineers. Most of the men on Rose's list
were never contacted; Flexner was not very interested in the opinions

[27] Seligman to Flexner, 10 October (1914), RFA, loc.cit. (note 15).
[28] Rose to Flexner, 10 July (1914), RFA, loc.cit. (note 15).

and concerns of practising health officers, except those at the very highest level.

By contrast to Flexner, Hermann Biggs, like Winslow and Rose, wanted public health training to be closely tied to the practical needs of local communities. Biggs argued the need for short courses given in many different universities, supplemented by extension and correspondence courses, so that at least minimal training could be provided for the health officials of small towns and rural areas. In Biggs's view, the provision of graduate training for higher level health officials was less urgent.[29]

By the time of the conference in October 1914, Flexner thus had a variety of plans and proposals: Harvard and Columbia both wanted to establish schools, Biggs wanted a network of courses at different universities, Rose wanted a series of schools to be set up across the country, and both Abbott of Pennsylvania and Whipple of Harvard argued that no new schools would be needed if their existing facilities were expanded.

5. The General Education Board conference: 16 October 1914

On 16 October, the General Education Board conference brought together eleven public health representatives and nine Rockefeller trustees and officers. The public health men were Alexander C. Abbott, Professor of Bacteriology at the University of Pennsylvania; Hermann M. Biggs, Health Commissioner of New York State; Frederick Cleveland, Director of the New York City Bureau of Municipal Research; Daniel D. Jackson, Assistant Professor of Engineering at Columbia; Edwin Jordan, Professor of Bacteriology at the University of Chicago; William H. Park, Director of the New York City Public Health Laboratory; Milton J. Rosenau, Professor of Preventive Medicine at Harvard; Theobald Smith of the Rockefeller Institute for Medical Research; William H. Welch, Professor of Pathology and Dean of the Johns Hopkins School of Medicine; George C. Whipple, Professor of Sanitary Engineering at Harvard; and Charles-Edward A. Winslow of the New York State Health Department.

Flexner began the meeting with a relatively safe question: what were the different types of public health officers for whom training was required? Biggs said there were three classes of health officers: executives, technical experts, and field workers. The 'health officials of the

[29] Biggs to Flexner, 15 October (1914), RFA, loc.cit. (note 15).

first class', men with executive authority, included state and district health officers, and city commissioners of health. In the 'second class' were the technical experts: the bacteriologists, statisticians, engineers, chemists, and epidemiologists who would conduct research and implement health department programmes. Third were the 'subordinates' or 'actual field workers', the local health officers, factory and food inspectors, and public health nurses. This latter and most numerous group were the 'foot-soldiers' in Rose's war against disease.[30]

How, then, should these three classes be trained? Should the first class have broad, general training and the second class specialized training? William H. Welch argued the importance of basic scientific principles: 'Train them in the fundamental principles. The rest, of course, requires specialized training, but it almost takes care of itself, and is easily supplied'.[31]

But who should be trained? The single most difficult question was whether public health officials ought to be medical men. Was it reasonable to suppose that physicians would be willing to abandon their independence to become salaried employees? One consequence of the Flexner reforms in medical education had been a decline in the number of practising physicians and a rapid increase in their incomes; it was hardly the most propitious moment to expect an influx of medical men into public health, when, as Frederick T. Gates pointed out, 'the attractions of practice are becoming so extraordinary'.[32] Indeed, one effect of the General Education Board's previous intervention into medical education was to undercut the possibility of creating a new cadre of salaried medical men in public health.

Welch refused to see the situation that had thus been created; he insisted that public health would be as attractive to medical men as the inducements of private practice.[33] Many physicians, he thought, would be eager for graduate training in public health, and would see it as a 'splendid opportunity'. Welch at that moment showed himself a poor prophet, for the majority of physicians in the United States were to demonstrate little enthusiasm for specialist public health education.[34]

Welch proposed that a qualified health officer should have a medical degree, hospital internship, and two additional years of special training

---

[30] *Transcript of General Education Board meeting*, (1914). 16 October, p. 21, RFA, loc.cit. (note 15).

[31] William H. Welch, ibid., 30 (note 30).

[32] Frederick T. Gates, ibid., 47 (note 30).

[33] William H. Welch, ibid., 47 (note 30).

[34] Williams, Greer (1976). Schools of public health—their doing and undoing. *Milbank Memorial Fund Quarterly*, **54**, 489–527.

in a public health school. Frederick Gates and Hermann Biggs argued against the requirement of a medical degree: Biggs preferred men 'reasonably qualified to do the work' rather than to wait forever for an 'unattainable' ideal.[35] Gates suggested that many medical men failed to establish successful practices; perhaps the failures in private practice might become students of public health? The idea of public health as a refuge for failed physicians hardly augured well for the new profession, but many at the conference felt that public health officers needed medical qualifications. Even Theobald Smith, who argued that physicians were 'absolutely colour-blind to the preventive point of view', thought that the health officer needed an MD so that he could 'stand on a level with the medical man'.[36] Abbott explained that the health officer would be dependent upon the co-operation of the medical profession in his community; a non-physician would find it doubly difficult to gain the respect and attention of local physicians.[37]

At this time, the increased activity of state and city health departments in the identification and control of infectious diseases often brought health officers into conflict with private practitioners; many practising physicians regarded public health with deep suspicion as a form of governmental encroachment on their freedom. When public health took on the battle against specific diseases, it threatened the territory of medicine; lacking strong state authority, public health officials had to cultivate the goodwill of the doctors. As John Duffy has argued, this had the effect of making public health officers 'cautious to the point of timidity' in the period between 1906 and the 1930s, so reluctant were they to undertake any programmes that might disturb the interests of their medical colleagues.[38]

The men at the 1914 conference, unable clearly to define the relationship between medicine and public health, were swayed by Welch's benign assurance that no real conflict existed. Welch, however, was much too optimistic; the issue, in different forms, would continue to plague the development of public health as a profession. In the United States, and in Britain, as Dorothy Porter describes in Chapter 3, the interests of private medical practitioners and those of public health officers often conflicted; from the point of view of the physicians, public health officers interfered with the doctor–patient relationship, trespassed

[35] Biggs, *Transcript of General Education Board meeting*, (1914). 16 October, 48, loc.cit. (note 15).

[36] Theobald Smith, ibid., 85 (note 30).

[37] Abbott to Flexner, 10 October (1914), RFA, loc.cit. (note 15).

[38] Duffy, John (1979). The American medical profession and public health: from support to ambivalence. *Bulletin of the History of Medicine*, **53**, 1–22.

on their autonomy, and threatened to provide patients with free services—such as immunizations—for which private physicians might
otherwise be paid.

This question of the larger relationship of public health and medicine
was closely connected to the decision about the structural relationship
between public health and medical education. Welch had initially
spoken of public health as a department of a medical school, Rosenau
envisioned a completely separate school, and Biggs wanted a system of
public health training independent of any existing institutions. Biggs
and Winslow, colleagues in New York State, argued that association
with a single university would severely limit the possibilities for field
training, hamper the school's ability to influence legislatures and appropriations, and make it impossible to standardize educational and professional qualifications.[39]

Wickliffe Rose now laid out an elaborate and carefully articulated
plan. He argued the need for a national scientific school of public health,
well endowed for research. This school should be affiliated with a
university, but have its own independent identity, not simply be one
department of a medical school. It must have its own building, grounds,
endowment, and a faculty who would give their whole time to teaching
and research. It should be located in a port city, 'with its immigration
element' but be within reach of opportunities for rural health work.[40]
This school would select its students from across the country and place
its graduates in strategic positions throughout the United States.

The central school was, however, only the beginning of the plan; it
would be linked to smaller schools of public health to be established in
every state. These simpler state schools would focus on teaching rather
than on research, be linked to state health departments and medical
schools, give short courses for public health officers in the field, and
provide extension services for rural health education. Both central and
state schools would teach public health education methods and seek to
extend popular health information to the entire population.

Rose's plan brought together most of the elements of the initial discussion; his description of the central school in a port city might have
applied to Boston, New York, Philadelphia, or Baltimore. Biggs called
the plan 'admirable'; Theobald Smith found it 'magnificent'; and Welch
pronounced it 'stirring and inspiring'. Wallace Buttrick, President of the
General Education Board, then suggested that Welch and Rose together
work out a plan for the new school that could be mailed to all partici-

---

[39] *Transcript of General Education Board meeting*, (1914). 16 October, 67–8, RFA, loc.cit.
(note 15).
[40] Rose, ibid., 71–80 (note 39).

pants for criticism and suggestions. Welch agreed, if Rosenau and Biggs would join them. Flexner left the arrangements to Welch, and the meeting adjourned.

After the meeting, Boston and New York both laid claim to the new school. From Harvard, Whipple wrote that he had been gratified to see how closely the ideal school, outlined by Rose, corresponded to their efforts: 'It makes us feel all the more certain that we are on the right track'.[41] Edwin Seligman produced a more detailed plan for a 'School of Sanitary Science and Public Health' at Columbia University.[42] In addition to the two-year course of study for graduates of medicine and engineering, this plan called for a certificate in public health for nurses, sanitary inspectors, and local health officers. With his proposal, Seligman enclosed a letter from E. H. Lewinski-Corwin arguing for the conception of public health as a social science. According to Lewinski-Corwin, most public health issues were not medical or technical problems, but questions of political economy:

Congestion of population in cities, the condition of tenement houses, the elimination of slums, recreation centers, alcoholism, prostitution, the standard of living, social insurance, the saving of human wear and tear in industry, the elimination of the insane and feeble minded and many other similar problems affect the public health as much as the sewerage system, food inspection, and the quarantine of measles.[43]

On this argument, social science and political economy should be at the centre of the public health curriculum, together with 'the principles of administration and efficiency'. But this social conception of public health was to receive little attention, as the emphasis on biomedical sciences came to dominate the social and environmental approaches to public health.

6. The Welch and Rose Reports: May 1915

While Harvard and Columbia were making their appeals to Abraham Flexner, Wickliffe Rose and William Henry Welch were supposed to be meeting in Baltimore, to outline the proposal for a new school of public health. Welch had first promised to write a draft proposal in October, in time for a second conference.[44] By March, Welch was still saying that

---

[41] Whipple to Flexner, 22 October (1914), RFA, loc.cit. (note 15).
[42] Seligman to Flexner, 23 December (1914), RFA, loc.cit. (note 15).
[43] Lewinski-Corwin to Seligman, 15 September (1914), RFA, loc.cit. (note 15).
[44] Rose to Flexner, 27 October (1914), RFA, loc.cit. (note 15).

he would soon have the report ready.[45] By April, Rose was becoming increasingly anxious: the next General Education Board meeting was set for May 27, and Welch had still not written the report. By May 12, Rose had become still more anxious: where was the report? By this time, Rose had produced his own memorandum, entitled 'School of Public Health': he only wanted Welch to add his ideas to the draft. At the very last moment, Welch produced a document retitled, 'Institute of Hygiene', which was then presented at the General Education Board meeting as the 'Welch–Rose report'. By delaying until the last possible moment, Welch had avoided another conference; even Rose did not have time to review the report before its official presentation.

There are thus two quite distinct versions of what has come to be known as the Welch–Rose report: the first, written by Rose, and the second, rewritten by Welch. The longer Rose version was his plan for a national system of public health training, with a central school of public health as the focal point of a network of state schools. The central school would create 'thoroughly trained and inspired leaders to mould public opinion and train the army of workers in the state's public health service'.[46] It would develop a new 'science of hygiene' and establish public health service as 'a distinct profession'. Rose clearly differentiated medicine from public health and asserted that 'the science of protection is quite distinct from the science of cure'.[47]

Although the central school would be essential for creating this new science of hygiene, Rose's main focus was on the state schools and extension courses. Here, his model was the agricultural extension courses and farm demonstration programmes used by the Rockefeller Foundation to modernize agricultural production in the Southern states.[48] The Smith–Lever Act of 1914 had placed these programmes under the management of state agricultural colleges, and Rose wanted to reproduce this pattern in public health: 'This lesson which has been learned by the teachers of agriculture through a long period of costly experimentation we shall adopt bodily in our system of public health education'.[49]

The main conception of these programmes had been that real change in agricultural methods depended less on scientific research than on

---

[45] Rose to Flexner, 17 March (1915), RFA, loc.cit. (note 15).

[46] Rose, Wickliffe (1915). School of public health, p. 10, RFA, loc.cit. (note 15).

[47] Ibid., 11 (note 46).

[48] For a description of these programmes, see Fosdick, *Adventure in giving: the story of the General Education Board,* op.cit. (note 7); and Flexner, Abraham (1915). *The General Education Board, 1902–1914,* pp. 18–70. General Education Board, New York.

[49] Rose, op.cit., 8 (note 46).

persuading the farming population to put new knowledge into practice: agricultural extension workers travelled from farm to farm urging individual farmers to try new crop techniques and organizing their children into clubs concerned with raising pigs, cattle, and poultry. In the same way, public health teachers would take instruction to 'workers in the field' and would teach by practical demonstration. According to Rose, the central school would take the whole country as its 'field of operations', sending out 'an army of workers' to demonstrate the best methods of public health, and bringing back practical experience to be 'assembled and capitalized' in research at the centre of operations. In line with this conception, Rose emphasized three of the more practical departments in the curriculum: epidemiology, public health nursing, and public health administration.

The orientation of Welch's version of the 'Welch–Rose report' was quite different. The change in title was significant: the substitution of 'institute' for 'school' implied a focus on research rather than teaching; the substitution of 'hygiene' for 'public health' meant an emphasis on science rather than on practice.[50] Welch wanted an 'Institute of Hygiene': a centre for scientific research and the production of knowledge, not the command headquarters for an army of practical workers as envisioned by Rose.

In his introductory pages, Welch contrasted public health and hygiene in England and Germany by explaining that in Germany, hygiene was taught as a scientific subject in the universities, while in England, emphasis was placed on practical public health administration.[51] Although Welch said that the ideal American plan would give due weight to both the scientific and the practical aspects of public health, he made obvious his own conviction that scientific research must take priority over practice. In fact, Welch's version of the report essentially ignored Rose's proposed system of state schools, practical demonstrations, and extension courses. Enthusiastic paragraphs about the need for public health nurses and special inspectors disappeared; Welch combined Rose's three departments of epidemiology, public health nursing, and public health administration into a single 'Division of General

[50] The word 'hygiene' had traditionally been broadly defined as the promotion of health; Welch, however, gave the term a new and specific meaning, by using it to refer to the German research tradition in health, epitomized by the German 'institutes of hygiene'.

[51] Welch based this summary on a report prepared for him by William W. Ford of Johns Hopkins Medical School: The present status and the future of hygiene or public health in America. March (1915). William Henry Welch papers, The Alan Mason Chesney Archives, The Johns Hopkins University, Box 118.

Hygiene and Preventive Medicine'.[52] Welch insisted that the school's main purpose would be to cultivate and advance 'the science of hygiene in its various branches' and not to meet the immediate needs of the public health service: 'It would be a misfortune if this broader conception of the fundamental agency required for the advancement of hygienic knowledge and hygienic education should be obscured through efforts directed solely toward meeting in the readiest way existing emergencies in public health services'.[53]

In describing the institutional relationships of the new 'school' or 'institute' the differences between the Welch and Rose reports might appear minor, but they were to be highly significant in choosing its location. Rose argued that the school of public health must not be a department of a medical school: 'the two have divergent aims and must stand apart'.[54] Nevertheless, the school of public health had to be close to a medical school 'in the interest of economy and efficiency' so that basic medical courses would not have to be duplicated. Welch dropped Rose's phrase about the divergent aims of medicine and public health, and substituted the milder expression that the institute of hygiene should have 'an independent existence'. He then added a short paragraph stating that the institute must have access to the facilities of 'a good general teaching hospital' for study and training in preventive medicine.[55] This was a critical point as the location of the new school would be largely decided by evaluating the medical schools and teaching hospitals of Boston, New York, and Baltimore.

On 27 May, 1915, the Welch version of the Welch–Rose report was presented and accepted by the General Education Board, and the report mailed to the original conference members for their comments and criticisms. Most of the responses were highly favourable; the Harvard men supported it but seemed not to see its potential implications. Indeed, Whipple viewed the report as an endorsement of the Harvard–Massachusetts Institute of Technology School: 'The ideal of our School for Health Officers, which is much broader than its name implies, is very well set forth in the report of Dr. Welch and Dr. Rose'.[56]

The New York men were more alarmed. Charles-Edward A. Winslow complained that the report was closer to the German than the English conception of public health, and should have emphasized practical field work; he also wanted the title changed to the 'institute of public

---

[52] Welch (1915). Institute of Hygiene, 27 May, 11, RFA, loc.cit. (note 15).
[53] Ibid., 8 (note 52).
[54] Rose (1915). School of Public Health, May, 12, RFA, loc.cit. (note 15).
[55] Welch (1915). 27 May, 8, op.cit. (note 52).
[56] Whipple to Flexner, 12 June (1915), RFA, loc.cit. (note 15).

health and hygiene'.[57] William H. Park wanted part-time men from city health departments, school health departments, and industrial plants to participate in teaching.[58] Frederick A. Cleveland urged that emphasis be shifted 'to make administration the big idea and statistics the ancillary one'.[59] Edwin Seligman wanted the new centre to be called a 'school' rather than an 'institute' and complained pointedly about the emphasis given to the medical side of public health:

Nothing is said of the need of studying the substantial forces in our economic and social environment and the various plans for social and economic reform which frequently have a great influence on the health of the community. Again, such a matter as accident and sickness insurance, which usually occupies about half of any European book on social medicine, is not mentioned in the outline.[60]

Seligman agreed that connection with a medical school would be important, but argued for equal emphasis on the relation to a school of engineering and to other university departments: the majority of students would come, he thought, from departments of chemistry, biology, engineering, and from the social and political sciences, rather than from medical schools. Abraham Flexner responded that the medical school relation was essential: public health officers had to deal with the prevention and management of *disease*, and had therefore to gain their experience and understanding 'in the laboratories and hospital of a medical school'.[61] By this reply, Flexner demonstrated either his distaste for, or ignorance of, the conception of public health held by the social and sanitary reformers; Flexner's was a 'disease model' of public health practice. Flexner discounted Seligman's emphasis on social science as simply a self-interested position; he wrote to Rose that Seligman was 'doubtless conscious of the fact that, on the medical school side, the position of Columbia is . . . vulnerable'.[62] As Seligman was professor of political science, he had a 'tendency to underrate the importance of the medical school'. Rose answered mildly that Seligman was not underrating the importance of the medical school so much as wanting more emphasis on other departments, especially sociology. 'We did recognize this relation and it could be expanded in much more detail'.[63]

Rose did not share Flexner's adamant commitment to the medical

[57] Winslow to Flexner, 14 June (1915), RFA, loc. cit. (note 15).
[58] Park to Flexner, 3 July (1915), RFA, loc. cit. (note 15).
[59] Cleveland to Flexner, 11 June (1915), RFA, loc. cit. (note 15).
[60] Seligman to Flexner, 10 August (1915), 4, RFA, loc. cit. (note 15).
[61] Flexner to Seligman, 13 September (1915), RFA, loc. cit. (note 15).
[62] Flexner to Rose, 13 September (1915), RFA, loc. cit. (note 15).
[63] Rose to Flexner, 16 September (1915), RFA, loc. cit. (note 15).

model of public health, but it was Flexner who was to push forward the
plans for education in public health. In June 1915, Flexner wrote a
memorandum to the Rockefeller Foundation proposing that a director
and location be chosen for the 'Institute of Hygiene'. The director could
then make detailed plans of organization.[64] By this time, Flexner had
probably already settled on his choice of Baltimore as location, and on
William Henry Welch as Director of the Institute. However, Jerome D.
Greene, Secretary of the Rockefeller Foundation, thought the choice
narrowed down to Boston and New York, 'with the chances very much
in favour of New York, in view of the large opportunities here for both
municipal and rural practice'.[65] Hurriedly, Flexner replied that it would
be 'unfortunate' to restrict narrowly the number of possible locations
before having examined 'all fairly possible situations' and 'unfortunate
to gravitate towards any one place prematurely'. He added on a disin-
genuous note that 'the factors are so many and so complicated that I
have myself no idea as to what the ultimate decision should be'.[66]

7. Choice of location: the site visits

In September 1915, Wickliffe Rose proposed to Flexner and Greene that
they visit Boston, New York, Philadelphia, Baltimore, Washington,
DC, Chicago, and St. Louis, thus examining, as Flexner had suggested,
'all fairly possible situations'.[67] Boston was the first on the list; only four
cities would in fact be visited—as the tour stopped at Baltimore. For the
first three days, Flexner directed the interviews at Harvard: instead of
dealing with issues specific to public health, these focused on the administrative relationships between the medical school and its affiliated hospitals. Flexner continually emphasized the fact that Harvard did not
control the hospitals it used for teaching.[68]

The need for medical schools to control hospital appointments was
one of Flexner's most cherished themes, an important, although little
discussed, part of the 'Flexnerian reforms' in medical education. However, in the context of planning a school of public health, Flexner's

---

[64] Flexner, A. (1915). Memorandum on the subject of public health, 13 June, RFA,
loc.cit. (note 15).

[65] Greene to Flexner, 29 June (1915), RFA, loc.cit., (note 15).

[66] Flexner to Greene, 1 July (1915), RFA, loc.cit., (note 15).

[67] Rose to Flexner, 16 June (1915), RFA, loc.cit., (note 15).

[68] For the historical context of the struggle for control of hospital appointments, see
Rosenberg, Charles E. (1979). Inward vision and outward glance: the shaping of the
American hospital, 1880–1914. *Bulletin of the History of Medicine*, **53**, 346–91.

obsession with the administrative control of hospitals seemed out of place. Flexner ignored Harvard's experienced public health teachers and researchers, considerable scientific talent, plentiful opportunities for field work, and progressive and co-operative city health department. He paid little attention to the School for Health Officers and, to add insult to injury, even failed to call on William T. Sedgwick, founder of the School, a leading light in public health circles, and the main proponent of a separate educational track for public health.

On his return from Boston, Flexner apologized to Sedgwick for his 'unintentional and inadvertent' failure to invite him to the conference on public health.[69] Sedgwick replied graciously but went on to criticize the Welch–Rose report.[70] He urged that the new centre for public health training be called 'An American Institute of Public Health,' and that it be given a less German, more American and democratic orientation. It should have 'an almost absolute independence' to avoid being submerged by the medical school and should articulate with federal, state, and municipal organizations to 'keep in vital contact with the traditions, customs and spirit of American Democracy'.[71] Sedgwick insisted that the new profession of public health be 'coordinate, but not subordinate' to medicine and that the medical and engineering sides of public health be equally represented. Flexner's interests, however, were entirely medical and he continued to display a thinly veiled impatience with the environmental approach to public health. Flexner made his apologies to Sedgwick and then continued to ignore his views.

The visit of Flexner, Rose, and Greene to the University of Pennsylvania was brief. Alexander Abbott seemed to have little idea of how to establish the proposed school of public health. When asked how the school would be organized, for example, he simply replied, 'I have not thought it out definitely'.[72] Pennsylvania had few resources in comparison to Harvard, but Abbott had modest ambitions. He declared that he already had ample facilities, and would just like an increase in staff: not the kind of inspiring vision that members of the General Education Board expected.

The third visit, to Columbia University, was more extensive. Columbia had an excellent programme in public health nursing run by Mary Adelaide Nutting, and New York City had a progressive and co-operative city health department, led by Haven Emerson. On the other

---

[69] Flexner to Sedgwick, 6 November (1915), RFA, loc.cit. (note 15).

[70] Sedgwick to Flexner, 8 November (1915), RFA, loc.cit. (note 15).

[71] Sedgwick to Flexner, 26 November (1915), 4, RFA, loc.cit. (note 15).

[72] Conference held at the University of Pennsylvania, 8 November (1915), 19, RFA, loc.cit. (note 15).

hand, the medical school provided no basis for optimism. The medical professors, meeting at the Century Club, appeared to have little comprehension of public health work or of its possible implications. Most strongly asserted that public health officers should be medical men, but beyond this, had few suggestions. It became clear that Columbia's strength lay in engineering, nursing, the social and political sciences, and in the opportunities for practical field work: all issues that in Flexner's mind were much less important than the quality of the medical school and hospitals.

The last site visit was to Baltimore and the Johns Hopkins University, which epitomized Flexner's ideal of medical education as he had amply demonstrated in the Flexner report of 1910.[73] Both the medical school and the hospital were heavily committed to the research ideal. As at Columbia, the medical school faculty had almost total power over the running of the medical institutions, but Flexner explained the difference: 'they have a tremendous organization, a thoroughly homogeneous one, sympathetic to their authorities to start with. They have not got a lot of old fogies here'.[74] At Hopkins, the medical school and the hospital were in theory independent corporations, but in fact, they had interlocking boards of trustees and tended to act as a single unit. Flexner was reassured that there would be no difficulty in using the hospital for research and training or in opening special hospital departments if needed.

Welch emphasized the advantages of Baltimore: property was cheap, the city was close to the southern states for practical public health work, and also close to the United States Public Health Service in Washington. Co-operative relationships with federal and state health departments could easily be developed. Welch promised the school could be flexible in taking students with or without a medical degree. Theodore Janeway of the medical school was equally optimistic. Baltimore, he claimed, had many diseases not available in New York: amoebic dysentery, pellagra, and hookworm from the South, and tropical diseases from Cuba and the West Indies.[75] J. Whitridge Williams, the Professor of Obstetrics and Gynaecology, summed up the advantages of Baltimore: 'If this school comes here the best thing we have to offer you is Dr. Welch. I feel sure that Dr. Welch with very little urging will take it on his shoulders to develop it . . . Another thing we have 100 000 darkies here with all their diseases, and their mortality twice as high as the whites,

[73] Flexner, op.cit. (note 14).

[74] Meeting at Johns Hopkins Hospital to consider the establishment of a school of hygiene in connection with the Johns Hopkins University, 18 January (1916), 23, RFA, loc.cit. (note 15).

[75] Ibid., 84.

and three times as much tuberculosis, and four or five times as much syphilis'.[76]

The visitors were evidently persuaded; within a week, they had submitted their report to the General Education Board with Baltimore as the heavy favourite.[77] Harvard, Columbia, and Pennsylvania were criticized because of the independence of their medical schools and hospitals, and especially the fact that medical professors tended to be locally prominent practitioners rather than academic researchers. The resources of the Johns Hopkins University in engineering, the sciences, and sociology were declared to be 'modestly developed' although 'modern in spirit'. The City Department of Health was 'far inferior to that of Boston, New York, or Philadelphia' although 'the attitude of the authorities assures the University a free hand in utilizing its resources and possibilities, whatever they are'.

The real advantage of Hopkins was its medical school, with a small faculty 'animated by high ideals and very efficiently led'. In summary, the report concluded: 'The general resources of the University and of the community are inferior—in some respects much inferior—to those found in New York, Boston and Philadelphia; the Medical School fulfills the requisite conditions in the highest degree anywhere obtainable'.[78]

The decision in favour of Baltimore produced considerable bitterness between Hopkins and Harvard. Abraham Flexner has been accused of rank favouritism for Hopkins, of hating Harvard, of being 'Welch's matchmaker', and of dogmatic conviction that Hopkins was the only medical school worthy of respect.[79] Certainly, Charles W. Eliot, President of Harvard, was infuriated by the decision. He wrote to Flexner:

The personality and career of Dr. Welch are the sole argument for putting the Institute in Baltimore—and he is almost sixty-six years old, and will have no similar successor. This is the first time that a proposed act of a Rockefeller Board has seemed to me to be without justification or reasonable explanation.[80]

Flexner replied that the Welch–Rose report—as rewritten by Welch— had earlier been endorsed by the Harvard men, and had pointed to the department of medicine as the single most important factor in locating the Institute of Hygiene. 'Viewed from this angle the personality and

---

[76] Ibid., 184.

[77] Institute of Public Health: final report of the General Education Board, 26 January (1916), RFA, loc.cit. (note 15).

[78] Ibid., 9–10.

[79] Williams, op.cit. (note 34).

[80] Eliot to Flexner, 1 February (1916). See also Eliot to Flexner, 18 February (1916), RFA, loc.cit. (note 15).

present activities of Dr Welch, helpful as they might be at the outset, are not so essential as the character of the medical school organization, a thing which will surely endure'.[81]

The question remains: why did Wickliffe Rose and Jerome Greene agree that the organization of the medical school should be the determining factor in locating a school of public health? Why did they give such importance to the management of hospitals, when these institutions were irrelevant to most public health activities? Why did Rose sign Welch's version of the report at the last moment and agree formally to present it to the Foundation, thus allowing his own vision of a comprehensive system of public health education to be eclipsed by Welch's narrower focus on a single institute of research?

From Jerome Greene's letters, it is clear that Wickliffe Rose had the deciding voice in giving the new school of public health to Welch and to Baltimore. Flexner had his mind set on Johns Hopkins; Greene favoured Harvard; Rose was not only the most impartial of the three, but also the one who best knew from experience the practical side of public health. Rose had decided on Baltimore. It seems paradoxical, but Rose had emphasized the quality of the medical school precisely because he believed that the aims of public health contradicted the interests of the majority of the medical profession. Rose was entirely serious in his ambition to eliminate disease from the earth; he hoped, and believed, that in controlling infectious diseases, he would eventually put much of the medical profession out of business. As he saw the situation in the South: 'A physician has to make a living but that depends on the prevalence of disease. Insofar as this function (prevention) is successful it diminishes the prevalence of disease and therefore diminishes his work and his income'.[82]

In the southern states, Rose had found that the medical profession often constituted the main obstacle to public health programmes. Even in New York, physicians had attacked the City Health Department for infringing upon their professional rights; the Rockefeller Foundation had wanted to fund public health activities but had retreated in the face

[81] Flexner to Eliot, 11 February (1916). There can be little doubt that Flexner was biased toward his old college, Johns Hopkins, and toward his old family friend, William Henry Welch. In his autobiography, Flexner recalled the site visits and decision in the following terms: 'Someone in each of these centers had more or less vague ideas, but one man alone possessed the requisite knowledge and vision. I reported to Rose that it was immaterial where the school was located; it mattered only who directed it. The only possible director, in my opinion, was Dr. Welch; the school might be placed wherever he wished'. Flexner, op.cit., 197 (note 13).

[82] Conference at Columbia University, November 13 and 15 (1915), 77, RFA, loc.cit. (note 15).

of strong medical opposition.[83] Many physicians saw the Rockefeller activities in public health as an assault on their interests as small (medical) businessmen and as an effort to invade their markets. Rose understood this point of view and openly declared his ultimate aim to undercut the practice of medicine through the prevention of disease.

To Rose, therefore, the medical practitioners represented, in theory and often in practice, the potential opposition to the new profession of public health. For this reason, the influence of powerful local practitioners on the faculty of the medical schools at Harvard, Columbia, and Pennsylvania might threaten the survival of a new school of public health. Johns Hopkins was different: there, the medical professors were full-time men, committed to research and teaching rather than to private practice.[84] These men would not be economically challenged by public health activities. They might be sympathetic to the new school or indifferent, but in any case, they were unlikely to destroy the fledgling institution by overt or covert opposition.

In April 1916, the Executive Committee of the General Education Board accepted the site visit report of Flexner, Rose, and Greene. Welch was to be Director of the Institute, with William Howell, Professor of Physiology in the Medical School, to undertake its 'executive management'. Welch and Howell formally presented a detailed plan of organization to the Board of Trustees of the Rockefeller Foundation.[85] On 12 June, 1916, the Executive Committee of the Rockefeller Foundation approved the plan, appropriating $267 000 for the initial operation of the new school at Johns Hopkins University. They gave the school a name representing a compromise between those who had wanted a 'school of public health' on the English model and those who favoured an 'institute of hygiene' on the German model.[86] The new school thus gained its unwieldy title: 'The School of Hygiene and Public Health' —implying

---

[83] Ibid., 45.

[84] Johns Hopkins was the first medical school to move toward the full-time system for both clinical and pre-clinical departments. By 1916, the full-time system had been instituted for three of the major clinical departments: medicine, surgery, and pediatrics. See Turner, Thomas (1974). *Heritage of excellence: The Johns Hopkins Medical Institutions, 1914–1947*, especially pp. 3–22. The Johns Hopkins University Press, Baltimore, Maryland; Chesney, Alan M. (1963). *The Johns Hopkins Hospital and The Johns Hopkins University School of Medicine*, Vol. 3. The Johns Hopkins University Press, Baltimore, Maryland.

[85] Welch, W.H. and Howell, W. (n.d.) Suggestions regarding organization of an institute or school of hygiene. William Henry Welch Papers. The Alan Mason Chesney Archives, The Johns Hopkins University, Box 118, 1.

[86] Britain did not have schools of public health as such, but as shown in Chapters 2 and 8, it did have a national system of public health training, one that was pragmatic, and oriented to the demands of practice, in contrast to the German emphasis on research.

that it would be both an institute for basic scientific research and, at the same time, a school for practical public health training.

8. William Henry Welch and the Hopkins School

When William Henry Welch won the competition to start the first of the central research and training institutes supported by Rockefeller Foundation dollars, he gained the ability to put his own ideas of public health education into practice.[87] At Hopkins, the alignment of the conceptual frameworks and methodologies of scientific medicine and public health were assured, as was the orientation toward research rather than practical training. Welch was now able to implement his own version of the Welch–Rose plan. However, he still needed money for a building and an endowment, and for this, he needed the support of the International Health Board of the Rockefeller Foundation. Throughout the initial years of organizing the school, Welch continually pushed his idea of a research institute of hygiene, while the Rockefeller Foundation urged that more attention be paid to public health administration, applied public health, short training courses, and popular health education.

The resulting structure of the school represented a negotiated agreement between Welch and the Rockefeller Foundation. Welch agreed to offer short training courses for International Health Board officers and other carefully selected student groups; he allowed somewhat more curriculum time for public health administration and made limited excursions into the field of health education for the general population. When the Rockefeller Foundation provided extra funding in 1932, the school worked with the city health department to establish the Eastern Health District, an area that served as a 'population laboratory' for research and the practical training of students in field surveys and administrative methods. On the whole, however, the school continued to be strongly oriented toward laboratory research and the biomedical model of public health. Welch had indeed obtained the institute of hygiene he had planned ever since, as a young man, he had visited the research institutes in Germany. In terms of research productivity, the School of Hygiene and Public Health would be very successful: the faculty and students

---

[87] Welch's original model of a research institute in hygiene had been Pettenkofer's Institute of Hygiene in Munich, which had deeply impressed him when, as a young man, he had visited several of the leading German medical research laboratories. In 1901, Welch had become one of the seven founding trustees of the Rockefeller Institute, the first American institute to be devoted to biomedical research on the German model. Its director was Simon Flexner, originally one of Welch's students, and Welch probably had

turned out research publications at a rapid rate. In terms of training public health workers, the school produced a small and élite group of graduates who were often more interested in research and teaching than in the practical activities of public health departments.

This would not have been problematic had the rest of the Rose plan for public health education been instituted: if, for example, state schools of public health had been training large numbers of public health workers in the practical methods of public health. The state schools, however, were built more slowly, much later, and in fewer numbers than needed; the correspondence and extension courses needed to train large numbers of public health workers would come many decades later, or not at all. Perhaps Rose could have used the Hopkins school as the starting point for designing a comprehensive national system of public health education for the United States, but Rose was soon to be distracted from the national scene by his appointment as Director General of the International Health Division of the Rockefeller Foundation, with responsibility for public health activities around the world.

9. New schools of public health

Once the Hopkins school had defined the Welch model of public health, other schools tended to pattern themselves in the same image. Even the pioneering Harvard–Massachusetts Institute of Technology School for Health Officers, which had preceded the Hopkins school (see Chapter 4, Section 4), was reformulated into a structure similar to the one at Hopkins. In an important symbolic move, the school cut its ties with the Massachusetts Institute of Technology and sanitary engineering, and went over to the medical campus at Harvard University. The new Harvard School of Public Health, opened in 1922 with an endowment from the Rockefeller Foundation, was located beside the Harvard Medical School, and the Dean of the Medical School, David L. Edsall, was also made Dean of the School of Public Health.

The argument for an intimate relationship between the medical and public health schools was that the medical school would thus be imbued with the spirit of public health. This turned out to be a naïve hope: Harvard Medical School continued, as did Johns Hopkins, to demonstrate a distinct lack of interest in public health. The perspective of medicine was not, after all, determined by administrative arrangements, but was the synthesis of more fundamental political and economic forces, scientific

the Rockefeller Institute in mind as an example of the kind of research institute he intended to establish at Johns Hopkins.

advances, and technological change. The cutting edge of medicine followed technical possibilities in diagnosis, therapeutics, and surgery;
high technology medicine was both exciting and lucrative. The growing
economic power and resources of academic medicine contrasted with
the relative and sustained poverty of public health. In such a context,
bringing medical and public health education together was rather like
merging a large corporation with a small one; public health tended to
become submerged in the powerful interests of academic medicine and
clinical research.[88]

Both the Hopkins and Harvard schools were identified with strong
medical schools and with the 'medical model' of public health; both
were clearly oriented towards research, with a relatively small and élite
postgraduate student body, and both were similarly organized into
departments and disciplines.[89] Both schools trained a small number of
American students (especially relative to the demand for public health
officers) and tended to offer an élite route into high-level public health
positions—the kind of educational mission consistent with the traditions
of two private universities that prided themselves on their academic
standards, highly qualified faculty, selective admissions policies, and
institutional commitment to research.

Within the next few years, several major universities in the United
States established or reorganized their public health programmes. The
specific formal organization of these programmes differed: Yale University developed a department of public health within the School of Medicine; Columbia University established the De Lamar Institute of Public
Health, and the University of Michigan created a division of hygiene
and public health.[90] While these programmes had individual differences,
the basic model of the content and methods of public health education
would be similar to that instituted at Hopkins and Harvard.

10. Public health, the Depression, and the Social Security Act

A major stimulus to the development of public health practice came in
response to the Depression, the New Deal, and the Social Security Act

---

[88] The history of the Harvard school has been described by Curran, op.cit., 7 (note
21).

[89] There were differences in emphasis: Hopkins was especially noted for epidemiology
and nutrition research, whereas Harvard was stronger in industrial and child hygiene.

[90] See Chapter 4 in this volume; Sundwall, John (1956). The division of hygiene and
public health. In *The University of Michigan. An encyclopedic survey in nine parts* (ed. W.A.
Donnelly), Part 8, pp. 1149–59. University of Michigan, Ann Arbor; Viseltear, Arthur J.
(1986). The Yale plan of medical education: the early years. *Yale Journal of Biology and*

of 1935. The Social Security Act expanded financing of the Public Health Service and provided federal grants to states to assist them in developing their public health services. Federal and state expenditures for public health actually doubled in the decade of the Depression.

Federal law required each state to establish minimum qualifications for health personnel employed through federal assistance, and recommended at least one year of postgraduate education in an approved school of public health. For the first time, the federal government provided funds, administered through the states, for public health training. Overall, the states budgeted for more than 1500 public health trainees, and the existing training programmes were filled to capacity. As a result of the growing demand for education in public health, several state universities began new schools or divisions of public health and existing schools of public health expanded their enrolments.

In 1936, the American Public Health Association reported that 10 schools offered public health degrees or certificates requiring at least one year of residence; of these, the largest were Johns Hopkins, Harvard, Columbia, and Michigan.[91] By 1938, more than 4000 people, including about 1000 doctors, had received some public health training with funds provided by the federal government through the states. The economic difficulties of maintaining a private practice during the Depression had pushed some physicians into public health; others were attracted by the new availability of fellowships or by increased social awareness of the plight of the poor and of their need for public health services. In 1939, the federal government allocated over $21 million for public health programmes: $8 million for maternal and child health, $9 million for general public health work, and $4 million for venereal disease control.

11. Evaluation of schools of public health

In 1938, the Rockefeller Foundation decided to evaluate the status and future of public health education.[92] The Scientific Directors of the International Health Division selected Thomas Parran, the Surgeon General,

Medicine, **59**, 627–48; Viseltear, Arthur J. (1982). C–E.A. Winslow and the early years of public health at Yale, 1915–1925. *Yale Journal of Biology and Medicine*, **55**, 137–51; Acheson, Roy M. and Payne, Anthony M–M. (1967). Preventive medicine at the Yale School of Medicine, 1950–1965. *Milbank Memorial Fund Quarterly*, **65**, 287–301.

[91] Leathers, W.S. and others (1937). Report of Committee on Professional Education of the American Public Health Association. Public health degrees and certificates granted in 1936. *American Journal of Public Health*, **27**, 1267–72.

[92] Fosdick, op.cit., 42–3 (note 7).

and Livingston Farrand, recently retired as president of Cornell University, to study the schools of public health in the United States and Canada.[93]

Parran and Farrand estimated that about 300 public health physicians and between 2000 and 4000 public health nurses would be required each year to staff the public health services. The demand for other kinds of public health personnel—sanitary engineers, statisticians, epidemiologists, etc.—was also increasing dramatically. They noted that 10 universities offered degrees in public health: California at Berkeley, Columbia, Harvard, Hopkins, Michigan, Massachusetts Institute of Technology, Minnesota, Pennsylvania, Wayne State in Detroit, and Yale. The numbers of graduates per year (in 1939) ranged from 75 at Hopkins to 1 at Wayne State, with a total of 199 graduates. Of these, 63 per cent were physicians. There were also 20 universities and colleges offering programmes in public health nursing, together graduating about 500 students each year. Twelve engineering colleges offering degrees in public health engineering together graduated about 80 students per year.[94] Some of those schools, especially the nursing schools, offered only undergraduate degrees; a total of 24 schools and universities offered postgraduate courses in public health. In whatever manner the numbers of graduates were estimated, they were clearly not sufficient to meet the projected needs for trained personnel.

In addition, most of the public health officers already employed by health departments needed further training to satisfy the new federal requirements. A Public Health Service survey of health departments had found that one-half of the physicians, one-third of the nurses, and two-thirds of the sanitary officers had no public health training whatsoever and were seriously under-educated by the new professional standards.

Again, legislation was in advance of the capacities of the educational system. The national need for public health graduates far exceeded the numbers being trained by existing schools. Federal training funds were now allotted to California, Michigan, Minnesota, Vanderbilt, and North Carolina to develop short courses for the rapid training of public health personnel. These short courses were recognized as an emergency measure until the schools were able to develop more adequate post-

---

[93] Livingston Farrand had previously worked for the International Health Board as Director of the tuberculosis programme in France during the First World War; he had been Chairman of the Central Committee of the American Red Cross, Treasurer of the American Public Health Association, and also President of the University of Colorado. He was President of Cornell University from 1921 to 1937.

[94] Parran, Thomas and Farrand, Livingston (1939). Report to the Rockefeller Foundation on the education of public health personnel. 28 October, RFA, loc.cit. (note 15).

graduate educational programmes. The University of Michigan, the University of Minnesota, Columbia University, Yale University, and Vanderbilt University were all expanding their graduate programmes in an effort to meet the demand. The University of Michigan, for example, had registered 176 full-time professional public health students in 1939; of these, 25 per cent were medical, 25 per cent engineering, and 50 per cent other disciplines including health education, statistics, and the laboratory sciences.[95] In addition, Michigan was training 186 public health nurses.

In their report to the Rockefeller Foundation, Parran and Farrand recommended increased support for Hopkins, Harvard, and Toronto, as the leading schools in the United States and Canada, to sustain research in public health disciplines, especially bacteriology, biostatistics, epidemiology, and public health administration. To help solve the national need for increased public health training, they recommended that regional training schools be supported in the West, the Mid-west, and the South. They suggested that the University of California at Berkeley, the University of Michigan, and Vanderbilt University seemed probable choices for the development of a second tier of public health education: they urged that new regional schools be oriented to practical training more than to research.[96] In essence, the Parran-Farrand report was recommending a limited version of the original Rose report on public health training: schools of public health in each major region of the country (rather than each state), with emphasis to be placed on training larger numbers of public health personnel.

12. International expansion

Wickliffe Rose, in the meantime, had turned his attention to international public health. As Director-General of the International Health Board, he was now in a position to expand his conception of education in public health from a plan for the United States to a plan for world public health. He started by extending the hookworm control programmes, begun in the southern states, to other countries, beginning with British Guiana, Trinidad, Grenada, St. Vincent, St. Lucia, Antigua, Panama, Costa Rica, Guatemala, and Egypt. Rose next expanded the focus of the International Health Board to include malaria and yellow fever, and developed major new programmes in China, Latin America, and Central America.

[95] Ibid., 69.
[96] Ibid., 89.

In each country, the International Health Board offered Rockefeller Foundation Fellowships to experienced public health officers, both medical and non-medical, and to new medical graduates; the Rockefeller Fellows came to the United States for public health training and then returned home to participate in, and often to lead, their national health programmes. Eventually, the International Health Board intended to establish schools of public health in these countries, staffed by faculty who had been trained in the United States. In other words, the original 'Rose plan' for public health training was to be implemented on an international level.

The project of developing international schools of public health relied heavily on what the Rockefeller Foundation referred to as the 'West Points of Public Health', a reference to the leading military academy in the United States. For the United States and, to a large extent, for all countries under United States influence, these were the Johns Hopkins School of Hygiene and Public Health and the Harvard School of Public Health. For Britain and its Empire, this role would be filled by the London School of Hygiene and Tropical Medicine, founded in 1924 and funded by the Rockefeller Foundation; for Canada and the British West Indies, the University of Toronto School of Hygiene was funded in 1924. In China, the Peking Union Medical College, opened in 1919, provided an élite form of medical and public health training in a country otherwise somewhat isolated from United States influence. The first of the Latin American schools was established in São Paulo, Brazil, with assistance from the Rockefeller Foundation. Later, schools in India, Japan, and the Philippines provided centres for professional health training on the western model. Thus, a network of training centres was established in Europe, Latin America, and Asia, with faculty and students rotating among these centres on Rockefeller Fellowships, teaching exchanges, and research projects. As Raymond Fosdick described it:

Rose and his successors as head of the International Health Board undertook the implementation of a bold and creative plan literally to girdle the globe with schools and institutes of public health, including public health nursing . . . The schools and institutes were located in Prague, Warsaw, London, Toronto, Copenhagen, Budapest, Oslo, Belgrade, Zagreb, Madrid, Cluj, Ankara, Sofia, Rome, Tokyo, Athens, Bucharest, Stockholm, Calcutta, Manila, São Paulo, and the University of Michigan . . . A migration of public health personnel back and forth across national boundary lines would be an enriching experience by which the new ideas and techniques of one area could become the common property of all.[97]

[97] Fosdick, op.cit. (note 7).

13. Medicine and public health: the unhappy marriage

The relationship between the emerging profession of public health and the well-established profession of medicine would continue to be problematic and controversial. The increased activities of health departments in the control of infectious diseases brought them into repeated conflicts with private practitioners; as soon as public health had left the confines of sanitary engineering and took on the battle against specific diseases, it had begun to challenge the boundaries of medical autonomy. As John Duffy has noted, the medical profession moved from a position of strong support for public health activities in the late nineteenth century to a cautious and suspicious ambivalence, and often, outright hostility in the early decades of the twentieth century.[98]

The Flexner reforms in medical education had been only a symptom of the larger transformation occurring in medical knowledge and practice in the early twentieth century.[99] As medical practice became dependent on developing scientific knowledge and technology, it was institutionalized in hospital settings.[100] Hospitals became dependent on physicians and physicians in turn became dependent on access to hospital facilities. As physicians became ever more interested in the technical possibilities of scientific medicine and abandoned general practice for specialist training, they became even less interested in community and preventive activities. As the standards of education and criteria for admission to the profession became more controlled and demanding, the numbers of practitioners fell and their incomes rose. Medical practice was an intellectually and financially rewarding field. Few physicians were attracted to public health with its relatively low incomes, political pressures, and comparative lack of individual autonomy.

Schools of public health had been established with the expectation that young physicians would take advanced training in public health after graduating from medical school. But young medical graduates showed themselves more drawn to the glamour, excitement, and rewards of curative medicine and surgery. The schools of public health at Johns Hopkins, Harvard, Yale, and Columbia all reported the same problems: most of their applicants for training in public health were either experienced older men who had worked in public health positions

---

[98] Duffy, John (1979). The American medical profession and public health: from support to ambivalence. *Bulletin of the History of Medicine*, **53**, 1–22.

[99] Brown, E. Richard (1979). *Rockefeller medicine men*. University of California Press, Berkeley; Starr, Paul (1982). *The social transformation of American medicine*. Basic Books, New York.

[100] Rosenberg, Charles (1987). *The care of strangers: the rise of America's hospital system*. Basic Books, New York.

without specialist qualifications, or young scientists interested in bacteriology, epidemiology, and other public health disciplines, but who lacked the medical degree now regarded as an essential qualification for public health leadership.[101] Important positions in public health were often offered to physicians without specialist training in preference to non-physicians with doctorate degrees in public health; the demand for physicians was such that they rarely needed public health training as a professional job requirement. As a result, the incentives for physicians to take specialized degrees in public health were further reduced, and schools of public health admitted the ever larger numbers of nurses, engineers, statisticians, and biologists who enthusiastically sought public health training. This structural problem in the relationship between medicine and public health, already clear by 1920, was never entirely resolved. Public health in the United States would continue to be open to many professional groups and disciplines, while maintaining a special and privileged status for those with medical qualifications.

The relationship of public health to medicine was a continuing preoccupation of those organizing and implementing the expansion of public health education. The fond hope that schools of public health allied to medical schools would serve to permeate those medical institutions with the spirit of preventive medicine proved illusory. After 20 years of public health teaching, public health and medicine still seemed far apart and often moving in opposite directions. The situation in the United States in 1939 suggested a thriving and expanding public health movement, supported by new federal and state health programmes, but developing in general isolation from the medical profession as a whole.

The officers of the Rockefeller Foundation, who were pouring money into education in medicine as well as in public health, continued to be optimistic that eventually the two would form a closer and more harmonious relationship. Indeed, they often asserted that, with the increasing success of medical science in curing disease, the emphasis within medicine would gradually shift from cure to prevention. The industrial and mechanical metaphors in which they conceptualized medicine transformed this dream into good business sense:

A railway spends more money on train and track inspection than on wreck crews. The average automobile owner is on the watch for signs of motor trouble and does not wait until there is trouble. The factory manager looks solicitously after his machines and does not wait until there is a breakdown. The

---

[101] Viseltear, op.cit. (note 90); Fee, Elizabeth (1987). *Disease and discovery: a history of the Johns Hopkins School of Hygiene and Public Health, 1916–1939.* The Johns Hopkins University Press, Baltimore, Maryland.

human body, which is vastly more complex than any machine, is in need of vigilant care and frequent examination. Yet for the most part it is neglected until pain and disability sound an unmistakable alarm. Then the doctor is called in and too often expected to do the impossible. He is thought of as a wreck crew rather than as a train and track inspector.[102]

In the United States, repeated attempts were made to bring preventive and curative medicine closer together by creating new educational programmes in preventive medicine in medical schools, often with the aid of schools of public health. These attempts to change the nature of medical education were mainly remarkable for the recurrent enthusiasm of the efforts and the consistent failure of the results. Reviewing the organizational relationships and co-operative efforts between schools of public health and schools of medicine, Russell Nelson, President of the Johns Hopkins Hospital, in 1974 noted: 'It is a sad story of unfulfilled expectations, numerous failures, frequent tensions, and some bad feelings'.[103] Rejecting the idea that schools of medicine and public health should be combined or that medical schools should 'take over' public health, Nelson added that 'Medical schools are already too large and complex to manage their present, and future, responsibilities, let alone take on others . . . In short, medical schools don't want to take over public health; the idea, it seems to me, appeals only to some administrators and armchair critics'.[104]

Waller S. Leathers, Dean of the School of Medicine at Vanderbilt University, noted that in most United States medical schools, the teaching of preventive medicine was 'of a desultory, uninteresting and poorly organized type'.[105] Departments of preventive medicine were usually small and relatively weak, with low budgets and few faculty positions. In part, this was the consequence of a political problem: preventive medicine, to the extent that it was equated in many physicians' minds with 'socialized medicine', seemed to represent a potential economic threat; medical schools were, in general, more willing to express vague support for the concept of preventive medicine than to provide active advocacy or strong financial commitment to the idea. The continuing efforts by some proponents of preventive medicine to dissociate it from

---

[102] Vincent, George E. (1921). *The Rockefeller Foundation: a review for 1920*, p.4. The Rockefeller Foundation, New York.

[103] Nelson, Russell A. (1974). Organizational relationships of schools of public health with schools of medicine. In *Schools of public health: present and future* (ed. John Z. Bowers and Elizabeth Purcell), pp. 11–14. Josiah Macy Jr. Foundation, New York.

[104] Ibid., 12.

[105] Leathers, W.S. (1931). Undergraduate instruction in hygiene and preventive medicine to medical students. 8 July, 4, RFA, loc.cit. (note 15).

'socialized medicine', and, more on emotional than logical grounds, from social medicine, were probably hampered by the fact that many of the strongest advocates of preventive medicine and public health in the 1930s and 1940s were also committed to the concept of national health insurance as a means of solving the chronic problems of access to medical care in the United States.[106]

Although the separation between medical and public health education seemed inevitable in the peculiar context of United States medicine, it was often perceived as a barrier to those trying to organize health services in developing countries. Luis Fernando Duque of Colombia bitterly attacked the rigid separation in the early development of schools of public health and medical education in Latin America:

The health professionals shut themselves up in their schools of public health, and the physicians stayed within the walls of the medical schools and hospitals. The latter felt that public health specialists 'were no longer doctors', while the health people believed themselves to be crusaders in a cause they had to win, imposing it if necessary on the community as well as on other physicians who did not understand them . . . [107]

Guillermo Arbona, the Secretary of Health of Puerto Rico, agreed that developing countries could not afford separate preventive and curative health services; for rationality and economy, they needed integrated health systems.[108] In the same vein, John B. Grant of the Rockefeller Foundation repeatedly argued that health services could be more efficiently and effectively provided if based on the concepts of regionalization, integration of preventive and curative services, and community health centres.[109] Grant insisted that medical education in developing nations should be oriented toward prevention, with training in administration, epidemiology, and the social sciences. He believed that a similar programme should be used to transform medical education in the United States and that it would make schools of public health unnecessary: 'This trend, it seems to us, will occur as much in the richer and more highly developed countries as in the developing areas of the

[106] See, for example, Fee, Elizabeth (1989). Henry E. Sigerist: from the social production of disease to medical management and scientific socialism. *Milbank Quarterly*, **67**, suppl. 1, 127–50.

[107] Duque, Luis Fernando (1974). The future of schools of public health in Latin America. In *Schools of public health in Latin America*, p. 3. Josiah Macy Jr. Foundation, New York.

[108] Arbona, Guillermo (1963). Future role of schools of public health. In *The past, present, and future of schools of public health*, pp. 81–9. University of North Carolina, Chapel Hill.

[109] Seipp, Conrad (ed.) (1963). *Health care for the community: selected papers of Dr. John B. Grant*. The Johns Hopkins University Press, Baltimore, Maryland.

world. It will leave no justification for the existence of separate schools of public health, as such'.[110]

The concepts of regionalization and the integration of curative and preventive services were, however, more often honoured in rhetoric than in practice. The relationship between schools of medicine and schools of public health would continue to be marked by tensions and distance, with sporadic efforts to create co-operative programmes of teaching and research. In summarizing the pragmatic case for the independence of schools of public health, Milton Roemer concluded that the academic environment of patient-oriented clinical medicine was simply not conducive to the growth of community-oriented public health disciplines.[111] The economic foundations of medicine and public health are fundamentally different: one dependent on government-funded salaried positions, the other on the entrepreneurial basis of private practice. Efforts to merge public health and medical education in the United States are hardly likely to be successful as long as the economic foundations of preventive and curative services are so strikingly opposed.

In predicting a conflict between the private practice of medicine and the public organization of public health, Wickliffe Rose had perhaps been a better prophet than William Henry Welch. Welch's optimistic assertion that physicians would be eager for opportunities in public health had proved unfounded, except perhaps during the Depression era, when many physicians struggling unsuccessfully to find patients capable of paying for private medical care found public health an attractive alternative. Federal and state funding and support for public health became more widely available with the programmes of the New Deal. For a time, the economic imbalance between medicine and public health seemed to have shifted in favour of public health programmes. The failure to enact national health insurance in the late 1930s, however, had also made it impossible to bring preventive and curative services together into a single national system.

Had Wickliffe Rose's plan for a national system of public health education been implemented, it could have helped build a strong constituency for public health both locally and nationally. It could have solved the problem of preparing sufficient numbers of qualified personnel for public health programmes; it would probably have improved both the quality of those programmes and the health of the population. The results of research in the Hopkins school, and the other schools founded on similar lines, could more readily have been implemented in practice.

---

[110] Grant, John B. Mutatis mutandis. In *Health care for the community*, (note 109), p.182.
[111] Roemer, Milton I. (1984). More schools of public health: a worldwide need. *International Journal of Health Services*, **14**, 493–4.

But it is also difficult to see how, in the United States context, Rose's vision could have been successful without the political will to devote major federal and state resources to funding public health education and a broader sphere of public health practice. Welch's plan for public health research-based education was thus successfully implemented, but Rose's more ambitious educational plan has still to be realized.

6

The public's health: philosophy and practice in Britain in the twentieth century

JANE LEWIS

1. Introduction

Public health in twentieth-century Britain has assumed a number of different guises. In the early part of the century its role as 'preventive medicine' was stressed, while in the 1940s and again in the 1970s, attempts were made radically to change its whole orientation, first through the practice of 'social medicine' and later through 'community medicine'. In contrast to the United States, public health in Britain has always been seen as a medical specialty and this has been reflected in the various new labels that have been attached to it during this century.

Because public health has been seen as part of medicine, its practitioners have always been concerned to define their work in relation to other medical specialties and have been very much involved in the politics of both the medical profession itself, and of the delivery of medical services.

When the concept of 'community medicine' was debated in the early 1970s there was an interesting division of views as to how far it represented a new departure. Sir John Brotherston argued that it did not: community medicine was merely 'the latest name for that ancient, honourable and essential responsibility which is concerned with the medicine and health of the group. This is public health with a new name and new opportunities'.[1] Others were not so sure.

English academics in the field were particularly anxious to disassociate themselves from the pre-1974 public health departments, which

---

[1] Brotherston, Sir John (1973). The specialty of community medicine. *The Journal of the Royal Society of Health*, **93**, 203.

they felt had become mere centres for the administration of particular services. The hope in 1974 was to raise the status of the specialty by providing a more rigorous training for community physicians based on epidemiology and to create a genuine specialty for population medicine that was immediately recognizable as significantly different from general practice and hospital medicine.

The recent government enquiry, chaired by the Chief Medical Officer, Sir Donald Acheson, into 'the future development of the public health function' has nevertheless concluded that the term community medicine is confusing because it is not clear whether 'community' refers to the whole population or a district, nor whether it includes the hospital. It is also unclear whether it means 'medicine in the community' as opposed to 'hospital' medicine. The enquiry has recommended that the specialty be called 'public health medicine'.[2] It seems that after experiments in social medicine during the 1940s and in community medicine during the past decade, experiments which also sought to make major changes in public health education and in the education of students more generally, the wheel has come full circle.

Yet public health is in many respects no less confusing a term than community medicine. The age of Chadwick, Farr, and Simon is associated with the struggles for clean water and against infectious diseases, but as these battles were won, twentieth-century public health has faced a continuing identity crisis. By the early twentieth century, public health doctors tended to regard the nineteenth century's preoccupation with sanitary engineering as somewhat degrading. During this period public health switched its attention away from environmental concerns and toward 'personal prevention', offering advice on the prevention of disease and the promotion of health to individuals through clinics.

However, the continuing thread of prevention provided but a poor means of distinguishing public health from the interests of other medical specialties; general practitioners, for example, also claimed to practise personal preventive medicine. Early twentieth-century public health also became increasingly involved in the organization and administration of medical services through the local authorities. Indeed, in some parts of North America, especially perhaps in Canada, public health and state medicine were often taken to be synonymous during the inter-war years. By the Second World War, it was often difficult clearly to differentiate the work of public health doctors from that of general prac-

---

[2] Department of Health and Social Security (1988). *Public health in England: the report of the Committee of Enquiry into Future Development of the Public Health Function*, Cmnd. 289. Her Majesty's Stationery Office, London.

titioners in particular, other than by their commitment to a different form of service delivery.

The idea of social medicine was primarily an attempt by academic teachers of the subject, first to rethink the philosophy of public health, emphasizing the 'social relations of health', and secondly, to change the whole orientation of medical education towards the public health point of view by placing 'medicine in the matrix of society'. The success of social medicine therefore depended in large measure on a re-orientation of the whole of medical education. In the event, it did not even succeed in convincing public health practitioners, who were far more concerned about the fact that the National Health Service (which came into being in 1948) had not used local government for service delivery, with the result that public health doctors found themselves outside the medical mainstream with their administrative responsibilities reduced. Their response was to seek to develop other medical administrative capacities, rather than take up the academics' invitation to social medicine.

Community medicine sought to fuse the two main strands that had developed in twentieth-century public health. One was concerned with administration, or, as community medicine preferred, the planning and management of health care services, and the more nebulous alternative, with advice on how to prevent disease and promote public health. Like social medicine, community medicine talked about populations, rather than individuals. Like social medicine, its success depended on its becoming the directive force within medicine.

Both social medicine and community medicine represented well-worked-out attempts to revitalize and rethink public health. Social medicine substantially failed to influence public posture and a new specialty, community medicine, has struggled. The fates of both have been governed by a central paradox: if public health is about the health of the people, then much more is involved than medicine (the report of the working group on 'inequalities in health', chaired by Sir Douglas Black for the Department of Health and Social Security, wrote of the need, for example, to improve housing, education, and the maintenance of income).[3] Yet any such widening of public health's focus threatened to weaken an already weak specialty further. This chapter will show that differing views about the nature of public health have derived as much from public health's status within the medical profession as from the

---

[3] Townsend, Peter and Davidson, Nick (1982). *The Black Report: inequalities in health.* Penguin, Harmondsworth, Middlesex. This is the published version of a report of a working party formed by the Secretary of State for Health and Social Security, 1977; after a change of government, it was submitted to his successor in 1980. Members were Sir Douglas Black, Chairman, J. N. Morris, Cyril Smith, and P. N. Townsend.

philosophy of the specialty. As a result, the direction of the specialty has in the end been determined more by the changes in the structure of health services than by academic leaders and practitioners in the field.

2. Before the First World War: The shift to personal prevention

C-E. A. Winslow, the early twentieth-century American authority on public health (see Chapters 1 and 4), identified three phases in the development of the field in his country: the first, between 1840 and 1890 was characterized by environmental sanitation; the second, from 1890 to 1910 by developments in bacteriology, resulting in an emphasis on isolation and disinfection; and the third, beginning about 1910, by an emphasis on education and personal hygiene, often referred to as personal prevention.[4] This sequence of events is broadly congruent with developments in Britain. The pioneers of public health mounted heroic battles for sewerage and clean water and against infectious disease, as industrialization and rapid urbanization made more extensive and more formal protection of the community's health a major concern of government. 'Slum' and 'fever den' were terms used interchangeably in the nineteenth century. Both they and their inhabitants were feared as agents of infection before it was understood how this occurred.[5] Indeed state intervention went furthest in matters of health policy, largely because of the threat such diseases as cholera and smallpox posed to the whole community; vaccination against smallpox was the only measure that central government made the obligatory responsibility of local authorities.

The focus of nineteenth-century health policy was pre-eminently environmental: all dirt was considered to be dangerous. By the end of the century, social investigators were convinced that physical well-being was a necessary prerequisite for further social progress. The nineteenth-century vision of health policy was convincingly broad. In particular, the public health Acts were also housing Acts. As Sutcliffe has perceptively argued, the urban variable acted as a spur to state intervention because a large number of social questions concerned with poverty and housing as well as health were packed into the fear of urban degeneration and physical deterioration.[6] The urban environment was

---

[4] Starr, Paul (1982). *The social transformation of American medicine*, p. 191. Basic Books, New York.

[5] Wohl, Anthony (1983). *Public health in Victorian Britain*, p. 45. Harvard University Press, Cambridge, Massachusetts.

[6] Sutcliffe, Anthony (1983). In search of the urban variable. In *The pursuit of urban history* (ed. D. Fraser and A. Sutcliffe). Arnold, London.

feared to be producing a race of degenerates, physically stunted and morally inferior. The view of the Victorian commentators on social science that there was increasingly a relationship between social and moral categories, only served to intensify fear of contamination. Fear, together with religious zeal and civic pride (albeit often moderated by rate-payer parsimony) combined to produce the sanitary reform associated with nineteenth-century health reform.

By the early twentieth century, views began to change about health and about what reforms might be made. Above all they were characterized by an increasing concern with personal preventive medicine—which was to be called applied physiology by the public health journals. In 1908, the editor of *Public Health* reflected on the way in which it was generally acknowledged that modern public health work was the province of the pathologist and the physician rather than the sanitary engineer, and how increasingly public health was concerned with the application of general principles to individual personal differences. He continued, 'the most effective work is that which is individualized, and the consideration of the individual human unit will become a matter of increasing importance in our system of public health administration, with the increase and development in that system of the work of the physician'.[7] This shift was consolidated by scientific advances, particularly in bacteriology, but it must also be related to changes in the philosophy and practice of state intervention in the early twentieth century.

Increasingly, emphasis was placed on what the individual should do to ensure personal hygiene. The campaign to reduce infant mortality provides an especially clear example of this approach.[8] The campaign to 'glorify, dignify and purify' motherhood began in earnest after the Boer War. Epidemiological studies of the problem conducted in the late 1900s by people like Arthur Newsholme, at the local government board, revealed the death rate to be highest in poor inner city slums; however officials and public health doctors tended to view maternal and child welfare in terms of a series of discrete personal health problems, to be solved by the provision of health visitors, infant welfare centres, and better maternity services. Before the First World War, the bulk of their attention was focused on health education, and encouraged mothers to breast-feed and strive for higher standards of domestic hygiene. Clinic work was seen as a new kind of personal preventive clinical medicine which was provided free for those who could not pay.

Once it was realized that dirt *per se* did not cause infectious disease, the

---

[7] Editorial (1908). The functions of the doctor in public health. *Public Health*, **21**, 89.
[8] Lewis, Jane (1980). *The politics of motherhood; child and maternal welfare, 1919–39.* Croom Helm, London.

broad mandate of public health to deal with all aspects of environmental sanitation and housing as a means to promote cleanliness disappeared. As Starr has put it, the concept of dirt narrowed, thereby proving considerably cheaper to clean up.[9] On the one hand, 'germ theory' deflected attention from the primary cause of disease in the environment and from the individual's relationship to that environment, thus making a direct appeal from mortality figures to social reform much more difficult. On the other hand, social policy issues, such as housing and poverty, were, by the turn of the century, entering the realm of high politics in their own right; public health was no longer the prism through which urban reform of many and various kinds was enacted. The Edwardian years saw the introduction of a wide range of legislation in the field of social policy, the centrepiece being national insurance for periods of sickness and unemployment. Social policy became increasingly compartmentalized and unlike nineteenth-century Public Health Acts legislation, was thus more formally separated from welfare and at the same time the mandate of public health was narrowed.

Thus the vision of public health narrowed in the early twentieth century and the concept of personal prevention was harnessed to the movement for national efficiency. Sidney and Beatrice Webb were among those who stressed that any diminution in the prevalence of disease among the working class could be categorized as an economy measure.[10] They rightly pointed out that both public health reform and medical treatment under the nineteenth-century Poor Law shared the hope that better health would save the nation money. Edwin Chadwick, after all, had been inspired to action on health reform by the idea that disease brought large numbers to seek support from the Poor Law. In their work for the 1909 Royal Commission on the Poor Laws, the Webbs argued strongly for a system of health care that ensured the poor adopted hygienic habits. This early appeal to healthy lifestyles was broadly shared by social investigators, policy makers, and public health doctors in the early twentieth century. Only thoroughgoing eugenicists (referred to as the 'better-dead-school' by contemporaries) remained convinced that personal habits were determined by heredity rather than environment, and therefore held out against the idea that some further effort should be made to improve the health status of a population whose low level of physical fitness had been exposed in the course of recruitment for the Boer War, and investigated at length by the 1904 Interdepartmental Committee on Physical Deterioration.

---

[9] Paul Starr, op. cit., 189, (note 4).
[10] Webb, Sidney and Beatrice (1901). *The state and the doctor*. Longman's, London.

Strongly influenced by their contact with public health doctors, the Webbs campaigned vigorously in favour of extending the role of public health departments as opposed to making provision for care under the Poor Law. They considered any reform of the Poor Law medical services to be impossible because an increase in efficiency or in humanity or in preventive services would merely tempt more people to accept the status of pauper so as to obtain badly needed medical relief. Local authority public health departments served to create 'in the recipient an increased feeling of personal obligation and even a new sense of social responsibility . . . the very aim of the sanitarians is to train the people to better habits of life'.[11] The new state services proposed by the Webbs would have set charges in order not to make paupers of their recipients. Ill-health, like sweated labour and unemployment, was to the Webbs a barrier to national efficiency. The Webbs' vision was of medical officers of health and their public health departments teaching hygienic habits of health to the poor with the explicit intention of improving not merely the health but also 'the character of the race'. They regarded the educational work of health visitors and local authority infant welfare clinics as models for the future. In the event, this work comprised a small proportion of the medical officer of health's time. Statutory responsibilities for cleansing and sanitation, food and drink, and for infectious diseases proved to be far more time consuming, especially for medical officers of health in smaller districts.

The Liberal government of 1906–14 chose to extend health care provision on the basis of national insurance rather than limit it to local departments of public health. Like Chadwick, Lloyd George believed that sickness caused poverty and that insurance offered a two-pronged attack on the problem. First, it offered a means of income maintenance for wage earners during periods of sickness, and secondly, access to medical care that might restore wage-earning capacity. The Webbs felt that insurance would only 'intensify the popular superstition as to the value of medicine [i.e. drugs] and the popular reluctance to adopt hygienic methods of life'.[12] They believed that the inevitably deterrent nature of the Poor Laws prevented early diagnosis and the giving of medical advice, while insurance merely increased reliance on bottles of medicine and permitted malingering rather than encouraging hygienic habits. Only the public health service provided a genuinely preventive medical service because of its free availability and because it sought to change the people's habits. What seems not to have been realized was

[11] Ibid., 206.
[12] Ibid., 259.

that in practice the model of applied physiology, derived from clinical medicine and adopted by the public health doctor, was hard to distinguish from that of the ordinary general practitioner.

Despite public health's failure to provide the model for extension of health service reform in 1911, the public health service grew in size and importance during the inter-war years, but the fundamental difficulty in determining a firm sense of direction for the specialty remained. Public health doctors were perceived by other doctors, not unjustifiably, as providing an alternative model of health service delivery and one that independent practitioners were determined to reject.

3. The inter-war years: Personal preventive medicine and the place of public health in relation to general practice

By the First World War, bacteriology occupied a position of preponderant importance in the training for the Diploma in Public Health. Commentators on writings in public health education which appeared in *Public Health* and the *Medical Officer* during 1913 and 1914 were agreed that too much of the curriculum was occupied by courses in chemistry that equipped the medical officer of health to do the job of public analyst, which enabled him to measure the amount of margarine in butter and of chicory in coffee (see also Chapter 8). However, opinion was somewhat divided on the importance of bacteriology training. The Medical Officer of Health for Leith, William Robertson, felt it to be essential, but Professor H. R. Kenwood felt that there was not enough room in the curriculum for teaching preventive medicine and hygiene, especially in relation to infant welfare, which, after all, had been a consequence of the establishment of the 'germ theory'.[13] One solution to this difficulty suggested by the editor of *Public Health* in 1913 and strongly advocated by Sir George Newman, the first Chief Medical Officer to the Ministry of Health, in a series of books, pamphlets, and memoranda beginning in 1918, was to give preventive medicine a greater place in the education of every medical student: 'In fact it [preventive medicine] is not so much a separate subject of the curriculum that is required as a pervading influence, an attitude of mind, permeating and guiding all clinical study and practice'.[14]

[13] Robertson, William (1914). The training for the candidate for the public health qualification. *Public Health*, **27**, 398–400; Kenwood, H.R. ibid., 400–4.

[14] Newman, Sir George (1923). *Recent advances in medical education in England*, Memorandum to the Ministry of Health, p. 126. Her Majesty's Stationery Office, London.

This view was broadly supported by public health doctors who welcomed any wider recognition of the importance of the ideas they promoted. However, if it could be argued that a preventive consciousness was something that all doctors should have, it became additionally difficult to distinguish the core of public philosophy and practice. Throughout the inter-war years there was considerable antagonism between public health doctors and general practitioners accusing medical officers of encroachment. However, in terms of medical politics, public health doctors felt themselves to be in a position of strength during this period. Although the greater part of the responsibilities of most medical officers of health continued to consist of negotiating with the elected members of the local authority which employed them, of managing a department of health workers, and of fulfilling their statutory responsibilities, the Ministry of Health began substantially to extend their sphere of action. Governments of the inter-war years failed to extend health service provision under the National Insurance Act of 1911, and instead added piecemeal to services provided by the local authorities via public health departments. By 1939, local authorities were permitted to provide maternal and child welfare services, including obstetrical and gynaecological specialist treatment; a school medical service, including clinics treating minor ailments; dentistry; school meals and milk; tuberculosis schemes, involving sanatorium treatment, clinics, and aftercare services; health centres, the most elaborate being that built by the Finsbury Borough Council in 1938; and they had responsibility for developing local regional cancer schemes. The most important addition to the medical officer of health's responsibility came in 1929 when local authorities were permitted to take over administration of the Poor Law hospitals and many medical officers of health found themselves taking on the role of medical superintendent. From a position of growing strength in terms of the tasks they were being called upon to perform, medical officers of health spoke with increasing confidence of the importance of the public health service in leading the way in preventive medicine, primarily through the work of educating in personal hygiene, and of the importance of educating the general practitioner to play his part. However, at the end of the day, it might be argued that public health failed adequately to distinguish the content and direction of its work from that of other practitioners, especially general practitioners, which made its position extremely vulnerable when in the post-war reorganization of health services, government decided not to put the responsibility for administering the new National Health Service in the hands of the local authority. In addition, public health's preoccupation with first, the hygiene of the individual, and second, the administration of a growing number of services, resulted in a neglect of the medical officer of health's traditional task of 'community watchdog', in respect of sources of danger to the people's health, particularly poor nutrition levels, during a period of high mass unemployment.

There was considerable discussion as to the meaning of preventive medicine in the public health journals during the inter-war years. However, new thinking about health as opposed to sickness and about the determinants of both came not so much from the public health practitioners as from privately funded experiments in the provision of health services, and most important, from academics in medical and social science. In the 1940s, they began to consider the importance of a concept they called 'social medicine' rather than public health. It is significant that medical officers of health were at first puzzled by the discussion of this concept and by the late 1940s had rejected it.

The most influential voice within public health, 20 years previously, however, had been that of Sir George Newman who insisted that public health was no longer primarily concerned with sewerage, disinfection, the suppression of nuisances, the notification and registration of disease, and the implementation of by-law regulations, but rather was about 'the domestic, social and personal life of the people'.[15] It was therefore necessary for the public health doctor to have personal contact with the individual in order to provide health education. In his memorandum on the practice of preventive medicine, first issued in 1919, he argued for a new synthesis and integration in medicine, and in particular a closer integration between preventive and curative medicine. He was convinced that 'the whole science and art of preventive medicine is . . . essentially clinical in origin and purpose' and he emphasized the importance of a clinical training for medical officers of health.[16] Thus in stressing the idea that the prevention of disease had become less a matter of removing external and environmental 'nuisances' and more a personal concern, Newman brought the practice of public health very close to that of the general practitioner.

The 1919 Report on Medical and Allied Services, chaired by Lord Dawson, and set up in response to the Ministry of Health's request for a scheme for the provision of medical services, actually recommended passing the personal preventive health services developed by local authorities in the fields of infant welfare, venereal disease, and tuberculosis control to general practitioners. In the view of the Report:

[15] Idem. (1928). *The foundation of national health.* Ministry of Health, London.

[16] Idem. (1926). *An outline of the practice of preventive medicine,* Memorandum to the Ministry of Health, paras. 43–50. Her Majesty's Stationery Office, London. Idem. op.cit., 156 (note 14).

Preventive and curative medicine cannot be separated on any sound principle, and in any scheme medical services must be brought together in close coordination. They must likewise be both brought within the sphere of the GP, whose duties should embrace the work of communal as well as individual medicine. It appears that the present trend of the public health service towards the inclusion of certain special branches of curative work is tending to deprive both the medical student and the practitioner of the experience they need in these directions.[17]

Thus the Report made the general practitioner the key figure in its scheme for the delivery of medical services and argued for a system of medical organization based on the health centre that would end the general practitioner's intellectual isolation and provide him access to laboratory and radiology services, operating rooms, and a dispensary. By implication, the Report confined the medical officer of health to the environmental and sanitary duties that had characterized nineteenth-century public health work. Lord Dawson himself was both vehemently opposed to a state medical service and firmly committed to promoting the cause of the independent general practitioner over and above that of the salaried public health doctor.

The Times declared itself in favour of the Dawson proposals, condemning Newman's ideals as socialistic. However, it is doubtful as to whether Newman's commitment to public health stemmed from a commitment to what *The Times* chose to call 'state medicine'. Rather, the essence of his thoughts was his strong belief in the power of preventive medicine as health education.[18] In 1925, he had advocated the education of working-class mothers as being the only way of bringing down the infant mortality rate, and he remained convinced that the decline in infant deaths was due to this cause alone.[19] He was ready to acknowledge the general practitioner as being the pivot of the medical service and was anxious to see him practise preventive medicine too, doubting only that the medical curriculum of the 1920s provided him with enough knowledge to do so. Thus, Newman and the Ministry of Health ignored the Dawson Report, in part because it left so many controversial issues open, particularly in respect to finance, in part because the Ministry experienced severe financial constraints soon after the publication of the Report, in part because local authority public health departments provided a convenient administrative framework for extending the scope of state provision of particular health services and in

[17] Parliamentary Papers (1920). *Report of the Consultative Council on Medical and Allied Services*, Cmnd. 693, para.6, xvii.
[18] Editorial (1921). Health services. *Public Health*, **34**, 159.
[19] Lewis, op. cit., 29–30, 95, 104 (note 8).

part because of Newman's belief that the medical officer of health alone received any systematic training in the importance of personal preventive medicine. In this he was largely correct, although the extent of such training in a Diploma in Public Health curriculum that showed a heavy bias in favour of bacteriology and sanitation throughout the inter-war years was by no means great. Throughout the 1920s, public health departments were able to sustain their claim that 'public health work is mainly clinical medicine but clinical medicine of a special kind' by following the principles of Newman. The division of labour between medical officers of health and general practitioners rested on the separation of health education and advice from treatment. The evidence suggests that public health departments were, in fact, careful not to offer any treatment other than for the mildest ailments, but the boundary between the two types of provision was obviously hard to draw and indeed was sustained largely by a system of health services in which treatment was not free at the point of access. Philosophically, public health had boxed itself into a narrow corner where it was hard to distinguish it from curative medicine.

During the 1920s, general practitioners continually raised the spectre of encroachment by public health doctors on their private practices. Dr A. Cox, the Secretary of the British Medical Association, was asked to investigate the matter in 1927 and he reported in 1928. Although Cox favoured the cause of the general practitioner he acknowledged that general practitioners lacked training and interest in preventive medicine and that medical officers working in clinics were scrupulous in trying to get patients to consult a private doctor and only gave treatment for minor conditions.[20] The British Medical Association's Committee on Encroachments on the Sphere of Private Practice by the Activities of Local Authorities took a rather stronger line. It claimed that the private general practitioner had a wider range of clinical experience and a more direct knowledge of home conditions than the medical officer and stated firmly that medical practice with individuals, whether sick or requiring advice on how to maintain their health, 'naturally belongs to, because it is best provided by, private practitioners'. It concluded by recommending a complete separation between the work of general practitioners and medical officers of health in much the same manner as the Dawson Report: 'the main sphere of the private practitioner is the giving of medical advice and treatment to individuals; the main sphere of the

---

[20] *British Medical Journal* (1928). Report by the Medical Secretary on investigation into the operation of maternal and child welfare centres and school clinics in certain areas. **2**, Suppl. 194.

public health medical officer is the promotion of healthy conditions for the community'.[21]

The response of public health doctors was muted, in part because the increasing reliance of the Ministry on them for the provision of particular services placed them in a position of strength, and in part because, paradoxically, the Society of Medical Officers of Health relied on the British Medical Association regarding salary negotiations. In 1929, the British Medical Association successfully opposed the local authorities' argument that public health doctors should be paid on an administrative scale.[22] Medical officers of health never escaped the professional opprobrium that resulted from their status as salaried employees of local government. Nevertheless, the rapid increase in the size and responsibilities of the public health departments during the inter-war period, and particularly in the wake of the 1929 Local Government Act, made medical officers of health reasonably confident about the future. Dr Buchan, the Medical Officer of Health for Willesden, where the wide range of personal medical services provided by the local authority had roused particular ire among general practitioners, was led to remark that 'the very large provisions and concentrations in respect of public health and medical work made by the Local Government Act of 1929 are likely to lead to a State Medical Service'.[23] Thus even if Newman's idea of personal prevention had not encompassed the concept of a state medical service on public health lines, medical officers of health later came to look upon it as such.

Thus, during the 1930s, public health's sphere of influence grew substantially, but as ever with little philosophical underpinning. The Society of Medical Officers of Health took up Newman's campaign to extend the teaching of preventive medicine in the general curriculum, but did not devote much attention to the public health curriculum, other than to recommend the re-jigging of its component parts, which was substantially achieved by the General Medical Council's new regulations of 1937. In terms reminiscent of Newman before them and of the advocates of social medicine after them, the Society's Committee on the Training of Medical Students in Preventive Medicine argued in 1930 that:

[21] *British Medical Journal* (1929). Report on the encroachments on the sphere of private practice. **1**, 132.

[22] Archives of the British Medical Association (1929). Report of meeting of the representatives of the County Councils Association, Association of Municipal Corporations, Urban District Councils Association, Rural District Councils Association, Association for Environmental Control, Mental Hospitals Association, British Medical Association and the Society of Medical Officers of Health. 14 February, item 1859.

[23] Buchan, G. (1931). British public health and its present trend. *Public Health*, **45**, 9.

The medical student lives in the atmosphere of the dissecting room, the laboratory, the operating theatre and the hospital ward. His whole attention is directed to what is abnormal and he is taught to think almost entirely in terms of individual sick persons and never at all to regard himself as a member of a profession with great communal responsibilities.[24]

The Committee's Final Report, recommending that more attention be given to prevention in the medical curriculum, was submitted to the General Medical Council in 1931, but the Council decided that there was no cause to change its regulations on this point.

Medical officers of health were, on the whole, considerably less radical in their thinking and practice in the field of public health education than of general medical education, and indeed were outstripped both in terms of new ideas about health and in the performance of their traditional role of community watchdog by a number of pressure groups, social scientists, and a few more socially aware specialists within the medical profession. Above all, medical officers of health were preoccupied in the 1930s by their new administrative responsibilities for the former Poor Law medical institutions. Fears were expressed that the work of hospital administration was diverting the medical officer of health from his main task of prevention. The editor of the *Medical Officer* wondered whether medical officers of health would be able to return 'from the pursuit of pathology to their proper allegiance to physiology', commenting that 'much recent public health work seems to aim at converting it into a gigantic hospital.'[25] However, at least one medical officer of health produced a spirited defence of the medical officer of health's involvement as being very much a part of preventive work:

I understand there is a common belief that Medical Officers of Health during recent years have devoted so much time to the development of the growing municipal hospital schemes that they have become divorced from the practice of preventive medicine. It is correct to define preventive medicine as including all measures devised to prevent premature death and to maintain optimum health. I suggest that the development of the municipal hospital services represents a development of preventive medicine almost as revolutionary as the growth of the maternal and child welfare services and of school medical services in the latter part of the last century.[26]

The writer was undoubtedly correct in thinking that preventive medi-

---

[24] Archives of the Society of Medical Officers of Health (1930). *Minutes of the Society of Medical Officers of Health*. 11 April, A12. Wellcome Historical Unit, Oxford.

[25] Editorial (1930). Medicine and the state. *Medical Officer*, **44**, 21. Editorial (1931). Preventive medicine. *Medical Officer*, **45**, 1.

[26] Ferguson, J. (1935). Hospital policy in relation to preventive medicine. *Public Health*, **49**, 42.

cine had to be defined more widely than the traditional interests of public health doctors. That was the logic of the position of the Society of Medical Officers of Health when it argued that preventive medicine should occupy more space in the general medical curriculum. However, this medical officer of health was obviously content to define public health merely in terms of the tasks it had to assume.

Sir William Savage, the Medical Officer of Health for Somerset, was not content that this should be so. In his presidential address to the Society of Medical Officers of Health in 1935, he criticized public health by deploring the effects of the 1929 Public Health Act in the following terms:

We have become administrators of beds largely occupied by the end products of disease and supervisors of defectives [under mental illness legislation]; in a word, largely enmeshed in functions which are not our proper business.[27]

Savage also condemned the clinical work that absorbed so much of the medical officers' time as dull and routine and went on to call for more epidemiological research. He pointed out that while vast sums had been spent on isolation hospitals and while medical officers of health were intimately concerned with their administration, they worried less about putting into practice the kind of modern medical knowledge that rendered such hospitals unnecessary.[28]

The history of diphtheria immunization gives point to Savage's criticism. The responsibility for immunization rested very much with the individual local authorities and each medical officer of health, whose task it was to persuade his Public Health Committee to pursue an active immunization campaign in each locality. This often required special persistence in the financially straitened circumstances of the 1930s. Effective immunization agents were available by the early 1920s and reports of successful trials in Canada and the United States were published at the end of the decade. Yet between 1927 and 1930 the medical journals showed that many were preoccupied with more traditional approaches to the disease and were deeply distrustful of immunization. A significant number seem to have concentrated their efforts on swabbing throats and noses in an effort to identify carriers, and on confining victims in hospitals. Public health doctors employed as tuberculosis officers tended to identify with the institutional treatment of the disease. In the case of diphtheria the result was that while the death rate in Canada fell steadily

---

[27] Savage, Sir William (1935). Our future. Presidential address to the Society of Medical Officers of Health. *Public Health*, **49**, 42–7.
[28] Ibid.

in the 1920s and 1930s, in Britain the rate showed no decline until 1941, when a national immunization scheme was eventually implemented.[29] In 1939, R.M.F. Picken, Professor of Preventive Medicine at the Welsh National School of Medicine, felt that the medical officer of health had taken on too much administrative work to be an effective proponent of preventive medicine:

Public health might have developed on very different lines. It might well have remained purely preventive, grown out of sanitation to be concerned mainly with the problems of the nutrition of the people, their physical fitness, and public education generally, and kept away from any sort of medical advice and treatment of the individual . . . we have moved a long way in quite a different direction. I think, for instance, that one of the reasons why the United States of America has been far more successful in diphtheria immunization than we have is that their public health departments have not been burdened with the great variety of medical work with which we have been saddled . . . [30]

In this view medical officers of health had certainly been guilty of encroachment as well as failing to develop their traditional responsibility for the health of the people.

Recent research provides considerable evidence that medical officers of health neglected many aspects of their duties as community watchdogs during the 1930s, both in respect to the more traditional areas such as immunization, and to new concerns over the effects of long-term unemployment on nutritional standards and levels of morbidity and mortality.[31] For the most part medical officers of health filed optimistic annual reports on the health of their communities. For its part, the Ministry consistently refuted evidence provided by pressure groups and social scientists as to the existence of a relationship between high unemployment and deteriorating health standards, reserving particular condemnation for the handfuls of medical officers of health who expressed similar opinions. Dr K. Fraser, the Medical Officer of Health for Cumberland concluded that there 'was really very little malnutrition due to actual lack of food—there are a number of poorly-nourished looking children; but in nearly all of them it is a case of poor general physique rather than malnutrition'.[32] Some 50 local authorities, mainly in the depressed areas, sent in returns to the Ministry of Health suggesting that

[29] For a fuller description of these points see Lewis, Jane (1986). The prevention of diphtheria in Canada and Britain, 1914–1945. *Journal of Social History*, **20**, 163–76.

[30] Picken, R. M. F. (1939). The changing relations between the medical officer of health and the medical profession. *Public Health*, **52**, 262.

[31] Webster, Charles (1982). Healthy or hungry thirties? *History Workshop Journal*, **13**, 114.

[32] K. Fraser, cited by Charles Webster, op. cit. (note 31).

they were experiencing less than half the average incidence of subnormal nutrition. Some medical officers of health were philosophically opposed to giving nutritional supplements despite the apparently good results in this regard achieved by the National Birthday Trust among pregnant women in South Wales.[33] It is hard to avoid Charles Webster's conclusion that in adopting an optimistic point of view, medical officers of health were telling the Ministry of Health what it wanted to hear.[34]

During the 1930s, the lead in raising questions concerning the health status of the population was taken by political lobby groups, such as the Children's Minimum Council, the Committee Against Malnutrition, and the National Unemployed Workers Movement, all of which called for a higher level of unemployment benefit to enable families to secure the minimum nutritional requirements set out by the British Medical Association. Groups such as the Women's Health Enquiry surveyed the health status of some 1250 working-class wives and found that only 31.3 per cent could be considered to be in good health.[35] A professional social scientist, Richard Titmuss, undertook a survey of infant mortality and concluded that the decline in overall infant mortality rate was not matched by a narrowing of the gap between social classes.[36] Finally, a small number of consultants, particularly obstetricians and gynaecologists, attempted to draw attention to the high levels of maternal mortality and morbidity. Sir James Young estimated that 'about 69 per cent of hospital gynaecology is a legacy from vitiated childbearing'. He despaired of 'the apathy of organised medicine towards the positive value of health ideals', and 'the profession's devotion to disease [which] has blinded us to the duties of health'.[37]

G.C.M. McGonigle was one of a very small number of medical officers of health who attempted to link public health more to these ideas of positive health, rejecting the idea of 'personal preventive clinical medicine'. In 1920, McGonigle referred to the importance of 'understanding the normal biology of the human being' and of getting away from 'the conception of our science as being in preventive medicine, and [visualizing] it as the science of maintaining normality'.[38] In its essentials this

[33] Lewis, op. cit. (note 8).

[34] Webster, op. cit. (note 31).

[35] Spring Rice, M. (1981). *Working class wives*. Virago, London. (1st edn, 1939.)

[36] Titmuss, Richard (1943). *Birth, poverty and wealth*. Hamish Hamilton, London.

[37] Young, Sir James (1929). The woman damaged from childbearing. *British Medical Journal*, **I**, 891–5; idem. (1933). The medical schools and the nation's health. *The Lancet*, **ii**, 119–20.

[38] McGonigle, G. C. M. (1930). The biological concept of preventive medicine. Presidential address to the Northern Branch of the Society of Medical Officers of Health. *Public Health*, **43**, 239–45.

was a very similar view to that of the pioneer Peckham Health Centre, which, during the 1930s, tried to develop a philosophy of health as distinct from the practice of medicine and the delivery of medical services.[39] McGonigle was virtually alone among public health doctors in insisting that the general decline in infant mortality began long before the advent of child welfare work, thereby questioning the value of the whole idea of 'applied physiology'. Like Savage, he called for epidemiological research and in his own district of Stockton-on-Tees undertook an influential study of a group of families who were moved from slum houses to a new housing estate and showed that their health status deteriorated relative to those who stayed behind, largely because a greater proportion of their income was absorbed by the higher rents that were charged on the new estate.[40] Essentially, McGonigle was defining public health's task as a concern with the determinants of health and their promotion, and in this view he was far in advance of most of his colleagues. The Ministry of Health, however, dismissed his views as those of a budding labour politician.[41]

The majority of medical officers of health were content to expand the range of services provided by their public health departments, expecting that the balance of medical care provision would soon swing in favour of a state service, whereupon the medical officer of health as the only salaried doctor would come into his own. However, the British Medical Association remained resolutely opposed to such a vision as its 1938 document, 'A general medical service for the nation', made clear.[42] It favoured the extension of national health insurance and a central role for the general practitioner. The Ministry showed no inclination toward either an extension of insurance or a fully fledged state-salaried service. For all Newman's willingness to add in an *ad hoc* manner to the powers of local authorities, he was not prepared to argue that the balance of medical care provision should be swung in favour of the public health service. It was this that rendered public health doctors' apparent willingness to allow the content and direction of public health to be defined by its tasks a fragile basis for future prosperity.

[39] Lewis, Jane and Brookes, Barbara (1983). A reassessment of the work of the Peckham Health Centre, 1926–51. Symposium on Health and Society. *Millbank Mermorial Fund Quarterly*, **61**, 307–50.

[40] McGonigle, G. C. M. and Kirby, J. (1936). *Poverty and public health*, pp. 108–27. Gollancz, London.

[41] Public Records Office, Ministry of Health 56/56, Sir Arthur Robinson to the Minister, 11 January (1934).

[42] British Medical Association (1938). *A general medical service for the nation*. British Medical Association, London.

4. The Second World War: Public health and social medicine

The term 'social medicine' was not widely used until the mid-1940s, after John Ryle had resigned the Regius Professorship of Physic at Cambridge and had, in 1942, accepted an invitation to become first Professor of Social Medicine at Oxford. The roots of social medicine were to be found in the work of social investigators and pressure groups concerned about health status during the 1930s. Ryle himself paid tribute to the work of the Peckham Health Centre and the Women's Group on Public Welfare, which had investigated the health and welfare of children evacuated during the early stages of the war. Social medicine was very much a part of the committed discussion of health planning and reconstruction that was carried on during the war. Ryle made no bones about telling his medical students in Cambridge in 1940:

by one means or another you must develop the social conscience which has in the view of many of us, been too little evident in the years preceding the War . . . medical students and doctors as a body . . . have held themselves too much aloof from the larger social problems . . . I do not ask you necessarily to ally yourself to any particular creed but I do ask you to be seriously interested in man's environment and the possibilities for its improvement.[43]

Richard Titmuss, who was appointed Professor of Social Administration at the London School of Economics in 1946, played a major part in developing the concept of social medicine and in 1942 he drafted a paper explaining that this was not as:

yet another stage in the growing recognition of the social relations of health. Our vision is broadening; men are being pictured against a man-made environment; the multiple factor in disease and disorder is replacing the single causation concept; the study of life is replacing a morbid concentration on death.[44]

However, after the establishment of the Oxford Chair in 1942, the development of social medicine was conditioned by its location within the universities and, in the search for academic credibility, it moved further away from a concern with health policy and social science. Thus, social medicine failed in two crucial respects to fulfil its early promise. In part because of this, and in part because of their own narrowness of vision, public health practitioners did not take up the idea of social medicine. This in turn resulted in a damaging rift between teachers and practitioners in the field.

[43] Ryle, J. A. (1942). Today and tomorrow. *British Medical Journal*, **2**, 801.
[44] Titmuss Papers (1942). Untitled paper on social medicine. TS, 21 December. Some of the late Professor Titmuss' papers are open at the British Library of Economics and Political Science in the London School of Economics.

From the first, the concerns of social medicine were defined primarily by academics. Ryle defined it as applied aetiology:

social medicine is clinical medicine activated in its aetiological enquiries by social conscience as well as scientific interest and having its main purpose the education of progressive and lay thought, and the direction of legislation on behalf of national health and efficiency.[45]

By the late 1940s, it seems that Ryle's commitment to clinical medicine was exercising more influence over his thinking than his commitment to the importance of a social conscience. Like Newman in the 1920s and 1930s, Ryle was concerned to reform the way clinicians studied aetiology to include social and environmental factors, although he insisted that social medicine was more comprehensive than previous ideas of preventive medicine. In practice, the concept of social medicine remained vague. F.A.E. Crewe, who was Professor of Social Medicine in the University of Edinburgh, stressed the importance of medical statistics and of developing a social biology, but looking back in 1949 he was not convinced that social medicine had developed theoretically beyond the earlier German concept of social hygiene.[46]

Increasingly, the concept of social medicine was narrowed in order to stake a claim for respectability in the academic world. Ryle's own later work emphasized not only the links with clinical medicine and epidemiology at the expense of social science and health policy, but also the importance of the study of social pathology—the quantity and cause of disease—at the expense of the more radical and difficult aim of promoting health. As an American observer remarked in 1951, the Oxford Institute of Social Medicine concerned itself more and more with factors affecting mortality and morbidity, and shied away from both 'the allegedly sentimental aspects of social medicine . . . often stigmatized as the "unmarried mother" category of social problems', as well as from organizational and operational problems of the health service.[47] For example, Ryle criticized J.N. Morris and Richard Titmuss' study of the epidemiology of rheumatic heart disease for paying too much attention to the 'poverty factor'.[48] In both Oxford and Birmingham, social medicine increasingly came to mean medical statistics and Sydney Leff was essentially correct in his perception that one of its main weaknesses lay

[45] Ryle, J. A. (1942). Letter. *British Medical Journal*, **2**, 801.

[46] Crewe, F. A. E. (1949). Social medicine as an academic discipline. In *Modern trends in public health* (ed. A. Massey), p. 73. Butterworth, London.

[47] Weinerman, E. Richard (1951). *Social medicine in Western Europe*, pp. 12–13. University of California, School of Public Health, Berkeley.

[48] Ryle, J. A. (1943). Letter to R. M. Titmuss, 13 October. Titmuss Papers (note 44).

in the arbitrary selection of problems that were often related to the practice of medicine or to the life of the community.[49] Most academics involved in the field of social medicine were convinced that the public health departments were old fashioned in their approach. W. Hobson, Professor of Social and Industrial Medicine in the University of Sheffield, commented on their 'woeful lack of data on which to base a scientific approach to the planning of health services'.[50] Medical officers of health responded angrily. They had greeted the concept of social medicine in 1942 with considerable enthusiasm, the general reaction being that its proponents were taking up issues that public health departments had always been concerned about. Enthusiasm turned to puzzlement and impatience with the vague definition of social medicine's aims and objectives, its high academic tone, and its reluctance to consider practical questions about the health services. Only a few medical officers of health embraced the ideas of social medicine. J.Kershaw, the Medical Officer of Health for Accrington in Lancashire, was one seeing social medicine as 'the development of medicine in relation to social life'. However, he also noted that 'the biggest danger facing the new specialty was that it might become too academic'.[51] By 1947, the public health journals were rejecting social medicine as being too clinical and showing too much interest in social pathology as opposed to health; they also saw it as being too keen to dismiss the contribution of the public health departments. The *Medical Officer* was particularly incensed by the Oxford Institute's attack on mass radiography and infant welfare clinics on the grounds of poor cost effectiveness.[52] Thus, instead of trying to convert medical officers of health to the practice of social medicine, exponents of social medicine became increasingly alienated from the practice of public health. (Acheson discusses other aspects of the social medicine movement in Chapter 8).

At the same time, social medicine failed to have the kind of impact in the medical schools that Ryle had hoped for. The Report of the Inter-Departmental Committee on the Medical Schools of 1944 recommended the development of departments of social medicine, seeing them as a means of reorienting the whole medical curriculum: 'to the neglect of the promotion of health, medical practice and consequently medical education has been concerned primarily with disease, chiefly as it affects individuals. A radical reorientation of medical education and

---

[49] Leff, Sidney (1953). *Social medicine*, pp. 12–13. Routledge & Kegan Paul, London.

[50] Hobson, W. (1949). What is social medicine? *British Medical Journal*, **2**, 125.

[51] Kershaw, J.D. (1943). The task of social medicine. *Medical Officer*, **70**, 197–9.

[52] Editorial (1951). The Oxford Institute of Social Medicine. *Medical Officer*, **85**, 12.

practice is essential'.[53] But commenting that there was no accepted definition of social medicine, the Report gave no clear idea as to how the subject was to be developed and confined itself to stressing the importance of health promotion and of training clinicians in social diagnosis. Most medical schools responded by slightly modifying their departments of public health, but without fundamentally changing their approach to medical education. Indeed, Ryle's Chair was not filled when he died in 1950.

For all its problems, social medicine represented one of the few moments when the nature of medical education, research, and care was constructively challenged and for that reason public health doctors were wrong to dismiss it. If they had taken up the original idea of synthesis between social science and medicine, based on epidemiology, public health might have faced the post-war world on a firmer philosophical footing. As it was, the schism between social medicine academics and public health practitioners widened to a dangerous extent; this was one of the major problems which attracted the attention of the Royal Commission on Medical Education, which was chaired by Lord Todd and reported in 1968. That Commission was to recommend that a new specialty to be called 'community medicine' be established in order to bridge this gap between university teachers and service practitioners.

5. 1948–1974: Searching for direction

Medical Administration

When the government's White Paper on the National Health Service was published in 1944, one reviewer in the *Lancet* condemned the proposals on the grounds that they were concerned with medical services rather than with health services. Commenting specifically on the White Paper's proposals regarding the establishment of health centres (which were destined to come to nought), the reviewer wrote:

a real health service must surely concern itself first with the way people live, with town and country planning, houses and open spaces, with diet, with playgrounds, gymnasia, baths and halls for active recreation, with workshops, kitchens, gardens and camps, with the education of every child in the care and use of his body, with employment and the restoration to the people of the right and opportunity to do satisfying and creative work. The true 'health centre' can

[53] Ministry of Health (England) and Department of Health for Scotland (1944). *Report of the Inter-Departmental Committee on Medical Schools*, para. 20. Her Majesty's Stationery Office, London.

only be a place where the art of healthy living is taught and practised: it is a most ominous and lamentable misuse of words to apply the name to what is and should be called a 'medical centre'.[54]

This commentator was not alone in observing that the National Health Service appeared to be more a national sickness than a national health service. Indeed, the National Health Service can be viewed as freezing in place a health care system dominated by the hospital. General practitioners succeeded in defending their status as independent contractors and the teaching hospitals retained full control of their affairs under their separate boards of governors, in spite of nationalization. Only the public health service appeared to lose, something that was inevitable once the government had decided not to opt either for a salaried service or for unification under the local authorities. Facing the loss of their powers in respect of the municipal hospitals and the inevitable decline in their clinical work once the population was given universal access to general practitioner services, most medical officers of health felt profoundly gloomy and bemoaned the reduction in their empires both in public health journals and in their annual reports for 1948.

The *Medical Officer* tried to strike a positive note when it remarked that the medical officer of health would at last be free of his duties in hospital administration and would be able to devote himself to epidemiology. The journal added that the responsibilities for hospital administration had in all probability diverted officers from the business of prevention, which accounted for 'the "discovery" of social medicine which had for a century been the daily work of the Medical Officer of Health'.[55] Fred Grundy, who was Professor of Preventive Medicine in the National University of Wales (and previously had been Medical Officer of Health for Luton), urged that medical officers of health should begin to develop information services, carry out epidemiological research, and serve as the effective link between the three parts of the National Health Service, namely hospitals, general practice, and public health.[56] However, the immediate inclination of public health doctors was not to follow Grundy's injunction to reorient their work towards the gathering of local health statistics and information and the promotion of effective integration, but rather to look for new services to administer, especially under Section 28 of the National Health Service Act of 1966, which referred to the possibility of providing welfare services for preventing illness, helping those suffering from illness, or for

[54] An urban practitioner (1944). The White Paper reviewed. VI. *Lancet*, **i**, 443.
[55] Editorial (1948). The medical officer of health and the hospital board. *Medical Officer*, **79**, 258–9.
[56] Grundy, F. (1953). New paths for public health. *Public Health*, **63**, 190–2.

providing aftercare services. Responsibility for running ambulance services, home helps, and old people's homes became particularly time-consuming tasks.

As a result, local authorities' associations expressed the view that medical officers of health were only administrators with medical knowledge, implying that they had no connection with the mainstream of medicine and were fulfilling a largely executive function. Public health doctors spent much of the 1950s and 1960s fighting the insistence of local authorities that they should be paid on a scale comparable to other administrative officers rather than to other doctors; the argument was that coping with the hierarchical nature of the public health service was closer to the somewhat rigid working of the unreformed local government system than to the medical profession. In particular, promotion invariably was gained only through dead men's shoes. But while they resisted attempts at lay control from within the local authority structure, the character and future of public health departments were nevertheless closely bound up with local government. Public health work was necessarily constrained by the complicated structure of the authorities and was in large part dependent on the achievement of local government reform, which came too late to help.

During the 1950s and 1960s, medical officers of health found themselves increasingly squeezed between pressures from within, namely the local government hierarchy and the desire on the part of sanitary inspectors, health visitors, and social workers for greater professional freedom, and pressures from without. The latter were from general practitioners with whom they had to share responsibility for services outside the hospital, and from academics and social scientists who expressed increasing impatience in respect of the perceived failure of the public health departments to deliver effective community care. There is evidence of considerable frustration and confusion on the part of medical officers of health as they struggled to come to terms with the new structure and to forge new relationships. In commenting on the difficulty the medical officers of health and sanitary inspectors had in working together during the 1950s, Dr E. Hughes, the Medical Officer of Health for Reading, looked back to an earlier, simpler age, when the objectives of public health had been clearer. He felt that while some of the problems arising from these working arrangements were:

undoubtedly due to empire building on the part of a few public health inspectors . . . I suggest that there may well be other reasons. The sanitarians [57] . . .

---

[57] The word 'sanitarian' in Britain can cause difficulties. It was originally applied to Southwood Smith, Chadwick, and their colleagues who, through the 1830s and the

knew a great deal about such matters as housing, drainage, pure milk supplies and infectious diseases and were able to gain the respect of sanitary inspectors. Now there seems to be a tendency for them to be replaced by the social medicine addicts who are quite happy to leave things to the public health inspector and then complain if there are symptoms of separationism.[58]

The comment is more interesting for the evidence it provides of the continuing antagonism of many practitioners towards academic social medicine than it is for its analysis of the cause of the problem.

Most medical officers of health undoubtedly took the idea of promoting co-operation between the parts of the health service in the delivery of community care very seriously, but in their dealings with general practitioners the issue of encroachment was far from dead. Although general practitioners no longer had cause to fear encroachment from the local authority on their private practices, they continued to be suspicious of local authority control regarding the promotion of health centres, for example.

Similarly, the moves of some medical officers of health to attach health visitors to general practices often met with opposition.[59] In Buckinghamshire, Margot Jefferys found some general practitioners looking back nostalgically to the days when the district nurse was the only social service.[60] It must be pointed out that there was an absence of both coherent principle and planning in respect of community care. As Alan Walker has observed, community meant different things at different times, and in relation to different groups in need.[61] Regarding the elderly, for whom it was originally intended to mean domiciliary care, it was reinterpreted to include local authority residential care. Thus, both the Hospital Plan of 1962 and the local authorities' Health and Welfare Plans of 1963 envisaged the expansion of residential provision. In the meantime, the shortage of beds in both sectors resulted in increasing confusion as to the boundaries between the two types of health care. With the failure either firmly to distinguish community care from

1840s, as Pelling put it, 'sought on a national scale [to establish] the simple correlation between insanitary conditions and disease and its practical connotations' (Pelling, Margaret (1978). *Cholera, fever and English medicine*, pp. 6 and 7. Oxford University Press). In the United States, and very occasionally in the United Kingdom, it has also meant a non-medically trained expert in sanitation. Other names for people in this post have been sanitary inspector, public health inspector, and currently, environmental health officer. (*ed.*)

[58] Hughes, E. (1961). Administration and organization of the environmental health services. *Public Health*, **75**, 147.

[59] Robinson, J. (1982). *An evaluation of health visiting*, p. 19. London, Centre for the Education and Training of Health Visitors.

[60] Jefferys, Margot (1965). *An antomy of social welfare services*. Michael Joseph, London.

[61] Walker, Alan (1982). The meaning and social division of community care. In *Community care*, p. 17. Blackwell, Oxford.

institutional provision or to increase the flow of resources to domiciliary
care, the Ministry resorted to exhorting the three parts of the National
Health Service to co-operate and co-ordinate their work. Medical officers of health were seen as the principal co-ordinators, and increasingly
found themselves condemned as unimaginative and narrow in their
approach. In the view of Titmuss and Morris, for example, the description of administrators with medical knowledge was broadly accepted
and medical officers of health were seen primarily as managers of services doing little to investigate properly the health status of their populations and so to provide a basis for planning services. The public image of
the medical officer of health was unhappily personified at that time in
the dreary and obstructionist character of Dr Snoddy in the popular
British television series, Dr Finlay's Casebook, which was concerned
with the daily work of a general practitioner.

Academics in departments of social medicine and of public health,
began, along with social scientists, as early as the 1950s, to urge substantial reform in the training of public health recruits and in public health
practice, in order to reinvigorate the specialty. In particular, a case was
made for medical administration as specialized work, not in the sense of
institutional administration, as was the case in the 1930s, but rather in
the hope that medical officers of health would become broadly based
health strategists. However, to practitioners, administration tended to
continue to mean the day-to-day administration and co-ordination of
services. Dr E.D.Irvine, the Medical Officer of Health for Manchester,
was an early advocate of medical administration. He disagreed with the
view expressed by Dr R.H.Parry that the new order gave the medical
officers of health the chance the cut the Gordian knot of administration
and devote themselves to epidemiology and prevention, believing rather
that public health doctors had to control the organization.[62] In line with
his fairly traditional ideas about administrative control, a pamphlet put
out by the Society of Medical Officers of Health in 1954 on the functions
of the medical officer of health fell just short of claiming the right to
administer all local health and welfare services.[63]

As early as 1946, Professor J.M. Mackintosh, who held the Chair of
Public Health in the London School of Hygiene and Tropical Medicine,
complained that the more flexible regulations for the Diploma in Public
Health (DPH), introduced in 1937, were already out-of-date in respect
of the small space they allowed for the teaching of administration. In the
post-war period, the theoretical framework for the DPH was couched

[62] Irvine, E. D. (1954). Medical administration. *Public Health*, **67**, 172–5.
[63] Archives of the Society of Medical Officers of Health (1954). The functions of the
medical officer of health. Wellcome Historical Unit, Oxford.

only in the broadest terms, making it possible for universities to modify the orientation of courses and so keep in line with changing needs. Nevertheless, impatience with the failure of any clear pattern of training to emerge was widely expressed. In the Universities of Bristol and Manchester respectively Professors Wofinden and Fraser Brockington felt strongly that the DPH had got out of step with the new structure of the health services.[64] In the late 1950s, academics began to push for courses in medical administration by which they meant not day-to-day administration but the larger problems of health care delivery. In 1958, Grundy described the trend in public health teaching as moving from the traditional emphasis on sanitary science, public health administration, epidemiology of infectious disease, and vital statistics, to the indeterminate type of curriculum which added personal health services and health education, and finally to a comprehensive course. This both enlarged the scope of the curriculum and changed its emphasis to include medical sociology; the organization of health and welfare services, medical care and social services; statistics; epidemiology; personal hygiene and environmental hygiene.[65] More traditional professors of public health were quick to question Grundy's sense of the direction the field was taking. J. Johnstone Jervis declared himself 'disappointed, disillusioned and disheartened' by it and continued for some years to argue that the primary concern of public health was, and should be, environmental. He blamed social medicine for diverting public health from its true path.[66] Jervis's arguments were presented in such a way that they sounded at best defensive and at worst reactionary. He was Professsor of Public Health at Leeds, but his was certainly a minority opinion among academic leaders in the field. Nevertheless, many recent commentators on community medicine would argue that he was right to warn medical officers of health against neglecting their traditional tasks of environmental control.

Most leaders saw the development of medical administration as having the potential to give the medical officer of health both specialist status and a more central place in the medical care system. Professor Wofinden was reflecting this view when in 1959 he referred to public health doctors as 'being out of step with this age of medical specializa-

---

[64] Brockington, C. Fraser (1962). Training for public health and medical administration. *Medical Officer*, **106**, 97–8; Wofinden, R. C. (1958). Medical administration: the appropriate forms of training. *Public Health*, **73**, 343–53.

[65] Grundy, F. (1958). The teaching of social medicine and public health. *Public Health*, **73**, 29–33.

[66] Jervis, J. Johnstone (1958). The teaching of medicine and public health. *Public Health*, **73**, 123–33.

tion' and urged them to plan for a future, not in a 'subservient executive role within social administrations', but rather as 'broad advisers' to the health service.[67] It is important to note that in this view of the future of public health there was very little or no room for the clinical medical officer. It was assumed that these doctors would cease to practise as general practitioners took over the work of clinical prevention. Professor J.N.Morris, who was a leading proponent of social medicine, and would be influential in formulating the role of the new community physician, argued in a University of London Chadwick Trust Lecture in 1957 that prevention and cure should be integrated in the work of the general practitioner.[68] Many medical officers of health agreed that the days of the clinical medical officer were numbered. Certainly the *Medical Officer* saw something rather attractive in the prospect of the general practitioner taking over the clinical work and wondered whether this would not then allow the medical officer of health to emerge 'as a co-ordinator and overseer of the health services of his community', rather than being 'confined to the administration of the smallest part of them'.[69] Clinical medical officers continue to practise to this day, the significant difference being that, since 1974, a gulf has widened between them and the service community physicians. With this, an acute problem of an inadequate career structure has developed.

By the mid-1960s the vision of the medical officer of health as a medical administrator was being more clearly articulated. M.D.Warren, a senior lecturer in preventive and social medicine at the London School of Hygiene and Tropical Medicine, wrote about the need to separate the clinical and administrative components of public health: 'for the future we want to graft preventive medicine onto curative medicine [in the shape of the general practitioner], link community medicine with institutional medicine [by relocating the remaining clinic doctors in hospitals] and develop the specialty of medical administration'.[70] In 1962 the Porritt Report on the organization of medical services recommended that health services be unified under the area health boards and that the medical officer of health become a consultant in environmental health to new departments of social health based in the hospitals.[71] Although the Report was not implemented, its publication quickened discussions and

[67] Wofinden, op. cit. (note 64).

[68] Editorial (1957). Medical care. *Medical Officer*, **97**, 104.

[69] Editorial (1962). Towards a measure of care. *Medical Officer*, **108**, 93.

[70] Warren, M. D. (1966). Possible developments in training for community health and medical administration. *Medical Care*, **4**, 177–80.

[71] Committee to Review Social Assay for Medical Services (Chairman: Sir Arthur Porritt) (1962). *A review of the medical services in Great Britain*, pp. 66–7. Her Majesty's Stationery Office, London.

disagreements about the future direction of public health, for it was recognized by both academics and Ministry officals that medical officers of health would have a broader training if they were to stake a claim to advise on more than environmental health issues.

In an influential article on the future of the family doctor, also published in 1962 (at the height of the crisis over general practice), Titmuss fuelled the debate about the future of the medical officer of health by asking whether, if the general practitioner became more of a community doctor, there would still be a case for the medical officer of health.[72] Sir John Reid, at that time Medical Officer of Health for Northamptonshire, immediately replied that the answer was to capitalize on the medical officer of health's expertise in epidemiology and to transform him into a specialist whose knowledge and techniques would be available to his colleagues in all branches of medicine.[73] Like Wofinden, Reid wanted to make the medical officer of health a broad adviser to the health service. Reid was exceptional among medical officers of health in taking up the call for a new training and a new role; he went on to become a leading advocate of community medicine and the community physician.

The first diploma in medical services administration was offered in 1959 by the Department of Social Medicine at the University of Edinburgh. In a letter to The *Lancet*, the Professor of Social Medicine there, Stuart Morrison, linked medical administration to social medicine, arguing that it involved the practice of medicine in relation to populations and groups rather than individuals.[74] However, in its submission to the Royal College of Physicians Committee on Departments of Social and Preventive Medicine, the Society of Medical Officers of Health had some doubts as to whether medical administration could be 'taught in a university course or whether it can only be learned on the spot through doing under wise guidance',[75] thus revealing that the majority of medical officers of health were still thinking of administration in a much narrower sense. The course at Edinburgh aimed to train doctors in community diagnosis, and included epidemiology, statistics, medical sociology, preventive medicine, and economics, politics, and the law in relation to health problems in the community. As such it closely resembled

---

[72] Titmuss, Richard (1965). The role of the family doctor today in context of Britain's social services. *Lancet*, **i**, 2.

[73] Reid, Sir John (1965). A new public health—the problems and the challenge. *Public Health*, **79**, 183–96.

[74] Morrison, S. L. (1965). Letter. *Lancet*, **i**, 392.

[75] Archives of the Society of Medical Officers of Health (1965). Memorandum for the Medical Administration Committee of the Royal College of Physicians, 11 June. Wellcome Unit for the History of Medicine, Oxford.

Grundy's comprehensive model for public health education. A similar approach focusing on the government of health services, human behaviour and motivation, and the epidemiology of health and disease was strongly supported by Brockington in his case for remodelling the DPH rather than developing a separate Diploma of Medical Administration. By 1967, the Royal College of Physicians had given their blessing to the hope that in future senior medical administrators would be more clearly equated with consultants and a working party set up by the Nuffield Provincial Hospitals Trust on training in medical administration took as given the idea that ultimately clinical work would go to the general practitioners and the hospitals and, for the first time, linked the work of the medical officer of health in medical administration to that of the administrators employed by the hospital boards. The essentials of this idea, which necessarily involved a separation between senior public health doctors and clinical medical officers, was carried through into the reorganized National Health Service in 1974.[76]

In these debates over the possibilities of medical administration, the relationship between medical administration and social medicine, and between the executive (or management) and advisory role inherent in the term medical administrator was never made clear. These issues were to continue to bedevil the conceptualization of community medicine and the role of community physician. Nevertheless, efforts to reform the public health curriculum in the late 1960s emphasized epidemiology as the core element in public health education, with the intention that medical officers of health would become broad advisers to the health service. In Edinburgh in 1965, S. L. Morrison announced his intention of merging the DPH with the Diploma in Medical Administration to become a Diploma of Social Medicine or Community Health in order to train medical officers of health to become epidemiologists rather than administrators of departments, and advisers rather than managers.[77] In Manchester, the DPH was transformed to cover epidemiology and statistics, behavioural sciences, principles of administration and management, and advances in medicine. It could be argued that such reform was a case of too little too late. Certainly the material collected in the late 1960s by the Committee on Personal Social Services (Seebohm Com-

[76] Royal College of Physicians (1966). *Committee on Medical Administration, Report 4.* Royal College of Physicians, London; Nuffield Provincial Hospitals Trust, Vocational Training Medicine (1967). *Reports of three working parties on vocational training for the general practitioner, psychological services and the administration of hospital and public health services,* p. 42. Nuffield Provincial Hospitals Trust, Oxford.

[77] Morrison, S. L. (1965). Postgraduate training for a career in public health. *Public Health,* **79**, 280–90.

mittee) seemed to provide more evidence to explain the failure of public health departments either to analyse or deal effectively with the new health problems associated with the changing patterns of mortality and morbidity. The need of the chronically sick for community care was of particular pertinence.

Community Medicine

In the context of the strong arguments for reform and revitalization being provided by the academics, the recommendations of Seebohm's Committee and of the discussion paper the government circulated before the reorganization of the National Health Service (the Green Paper), both published in 1968,[78] provided the final push. J. N. Morris was the only medical member of the Seebohm enquiry and both he and Titmuss were convinced of the weakness of local authorities in general and public health departments in particular, in achieving progress in the field of community care and in developing new approaches to social work. In recommending the establishment of new social service departments, the Seebohm Report threatened to remove the fastest growing services that came under the medical officer of health's control as well as removing a large portion of his staff, namely the social workers. It was no coincidence that the Green Paper sought to reassure public health doctors that they would find a new, expanded, albeit unspecified, role as community physicians within the reorganized National Health Service.

It was J. N. Morris who first defined the role of the community physician. He believed strongly that the principles of modern epidemiology should provide a firm grounding for public health practice. His extremely influential monograph on epidemiology identified the major uses of the subject as historical study, community diagnosis, analysis of the workings of health services, analysis of individual risks and chances, the identification of syndromes, and the completion of the clinical picture.[79] From this he developed the concept of a community physician responsible for community diagnosis and thus providing the intelligence necessary for efficient and effective administration of the health services.[80]

Morris did not agree with the attempt of some American epidemiolo-

[78] Ministry of Health (1968). *National Health Service: the administrative structure of the medical and related services in England and Wales.* Her Majesty's Stationery Office, London; Parliamentary Papers (1967–68). *Report of the Committee on Local Authority and Allied Personal and Social Services,* **157**, Cmnd. 3793, xxxii.

[79] Morris, J. N. (1969). *The uses of epidemiology,* 3rd edn. Livingstone, Edinburgh. (1st edn, 1957.)

[80] Idem. (1969). Tomorrow's community physician. *Lancet,* **ii**, 811–16.

gists to rescue epidemiology from public health and bring it back to the laps of practising physicians,[81] but he nevertheless approached prevention through the needs of the individual, believing that a multi-causal epidemiological approach would ensure the consideration of socio-economic and environmental variables and eliminate the danger of 'blaming the victim' for his illness. Using the example of coronary heart disease, he argued that the barriers between prevention and cure were crumbling and that 'public health needs clinical medicine—clinical medicine needs a community'.[82] In a manner reminiscent of Ryle, Morris emphasized the importance of co-operation with clinicians.

His ideas were fed directly into two crucial policy documents of the late 1960s. The first was the report of the Seebohm Committee (of which he was a member), and the second that of the Todd Commission on Medical Education. He was not a member of the latter, but his views were expressed by Richard Titmuss. The Todd Commission clearly articulated the two main components of Morris's formulation of community medicine in its definition: 'the specialty practised by epidemiologists and administrators of medical services'.[83] It also recommended closer links with clinical medicine and between academics and practitioners in the field of community medicine. Like the Seebohm Committee, Todd's Royal Commission envisaged environmental health services (and hence the sanitary inspectors) and social work services leaving a public health department but remaining under the auspices of local government, while the community physician would move away from clinical work as he found his new role within the National Health Service.[84]

Medical officers of health were attracted to the idea of community medicine and the position of the community physician chiefly because they understood that it meant a substantial rise in status for the specialty. They showed considerable awareness of the problems of coming under the control of central government and of forging working relationships with other doctors in the health service, particularly those in the hospital sector; both these issues were to become important after 1974. However, medical officers of health had little influence over the basic decisions as to the final shape of the reorganized National Health Service.

This was particularly crucial because it would seem that policy

[81] Paul, J. R. (1958). *Clinical epidemiology*, p. 40. University of Chicago Press.

[82] Morris, op. cit., 814 (note 79).

[83] Parliamentary Papers (1967–68). *Report of the Royal Commission on Medical Education [The Todd Commission]*. Cmnd. 3569, para. 133, xxv.

[84] County Medical Officer of Health Archives (1968). File A21, especially notes of a discussion on 20 September. Wellcome Institute for the History of Medicine, London.

makers' understanding of the role of the community physician differed in emphasis from that of academics. The Department of Health and Social Services Report on Medical Administrators, chaired by Lord Hunter, was the first document to spell out the position of the community physician in the new National Health Service.[85] The community physician was seen as the key to effective integration of the health services, linking lay administrators to clinicians and co-ordinating the work of the National Health Service with that of the local authorities. The community physician was recognized as a specialist adviser, with particular skills in epidemiology. However, the Committee felt that he had to be more than an adviser if his expertise was to be put to proper use; thus a substantial number would be given management responsibilities in the new consensus management teams. The Report talked of epidemiology only as a means of assessing health needs, which were narrowly defined in terms of service provision.

The Report on Management Arrangements for the Reorganized National Health Service, published in 1972, defined three roles for the community physician as specialist, adviser, and manager.[86] All three were closely geared to ensuring the effective operation of the reorganized National Health Service. As a specialist, the community physician would stimulate integration and link the various parts of the service (no mention was made here of epidemiological skills); as adviser, he would liaise with the local authorities; and as a manager, he would be responsible for planning, information, evaluation of service effectiveness, and co-ordination of preventive care services. The roles of specialist/adviser and manager formed the core of subsequent definitions of the community physician's role.[87] However, the debate over both training and practice in the decade after 1974 centred on whether these roles were intended to be of equal importance. It seems clear that the newly formed Faculty of Community Medicine favoured that of specialist/adviser and stressed the complementary nature of community and clinical medicine, while policy makers stressed the importance of recommending changes in management and in the deployment of resources.

The medical officers of health moved into the role of community physician having been told that they were to be the linchpin of the new

[85] Department of Health and Social Security (1972). *Report of the Working Party on Medical Administrators (Chairman: Lord Hunter)*, para. 18. Her Majesty's Stationery Office, London.

[86] Department of Health and Social Security (1972). *Management arrangements for the reorganised health service*, para. 4.1(b). Her Majesty's Stationery Office, London.

[87] Eskin, Frada (1979). The role of management training in community medicine. *Community Medicine*, **1**, 236–42.

National Health Service, co-ordinating and administering services, but in the early months most were distraught, insecure, and confused. They had little idea as to the meaning of the part they were to play in the new management structure or indeed of the place of management in the scheme of things.

6. Conclusion

There are many themes running through the story of twentieth-century public health training and practice. Above all there is the tendency for public health to have defined itself in terms of the functions it undertook at any particular point in time. During a period of expansion like the 1930s, this resulted in a feeling of confidence, but morale fell when a major change in the structure of health services in 1948 reduced the range of the medical officer of health's activities. Public health departments responded by looking for new tasks to fill the gap. In 1974, the concept of community medicine had been brought forward initially by academics, if not by service practitioners, but was again defined principally by its place in the new structure.

It has proved very difficult to give public health a firm direction in terms of its aims and objectives in training recruits. The slowness in adapting curricula in the 1960s proved crucial in this respect. However, even if new methods of practice had been inculcated into trainees as someone like Morris would have wished, there remained the difficulty of maintaining any dynamic connection between academics and practitioners. To some extent these difficulties were due to a failure on the part of public health practitioners to recognize the need for a coherent philosophy, and in part to the difficulty that academics and practitioners experienced (and continue to experience) in defining terms like management and social medicine. However, it must also be acknowledged that if public health attempts to adopt a broad mandate—to secure, for example, healthy public policy—it inevitably encounters wider political conflicts with the medical profession, government, and industry.

For all that, a desire to improve the health of the people by preventing disease and promoting health has characterized public health thinking and practice throughout the twentieth century. But there has been little progress in developing a body of knowledge, as opposed to a continually changing list of tasks and goals, linked in the mind of the practitioner to the bureaucratic concept of managing the health of populations. Both social medicine and community medicine proposed a reorientation of medical thinking and practice whereby public health became the sun and other specialties the planets, but this did not happen. Social medicine failed in its bid to dominate the medical curriculum, and community medicine in its bid to become the linchpin of the National Health Service. As reorganizations of the National Health Service subsequent to that of 1974 (i.e. 1982 and 1984) put increasing emphasis on line management, especially within the hospital sector, so the role of the community physician as the integrator of health services was lost from view before the capacity to offer wide-ranging medical advice had been properly developed. In advocating a return to public health with more emphasis on the prevention of communicable disease, the 1988 government enquiry into the Public Health Function, chaired by Sir Donald Acheson, represents an attempt to retrench and to secure a separate, but firm, niche for public health within the National Health Service. Gone for the present is any attempt to make public health central among medical specialties. Yet many of the old tensions remain. The interdisciplinary and wide-ranging nature of public health's concerns is acknowledged in the Report's call for multidisciplinary awareness in public health education. On the Committee's recommendation the future name for the specialty is, nevertheless, 'public health medicine'. The definition of public health is couched in terms of prevention and promotion; yet a curriculum is described which gives the pride of place to the analysis of health service needs. Concern about public health status as a medical specialty and ambivalence about its role within a national health service which focuses on the development of curative medical services thus remain strong.

7

Professional education for public health in the United States

ELIZABETH FEE AND BARBARA ROSENKRANTZ

1. The years between the wars

The federal structure of the United States has meant that the public health function is divided among a multitude of state, city, and local health departments, with a relatively weak centralized authority. The most important federal organization in public health is the United States Public Health Service, an agency that has often aided the development of state health departments by lending expert personnel and providing advice and consultation on specific problems.[1] The proper balance of responsibility for public health among federal, state, and local health departments has been a rather contentious question; taking the long view, it has shifted in the course of the twentieth century in the direction of greater federal responsibility for research, regulation, and financing of public health activities.

In the 1920s and early 1930s, the Surgeon General, Hugh Cumming, expanded the research activities of the Public Health Service but opposed any increase in federal support for state and local health programmes.[2] The Public Health Service grew slowly over these years until the crisis of the Depression in the 1930s. The New Deal programmes

---

[1] The standard history of the Public Health Service is Williams, Ralph C. (1951). *The United States Public Health Service, 1798–1950*. United States Public Health Service, Washington, DC.; see also Schmeckebier, Laurence F. (1923). *The Public Health Service, its history, activities and organization*. Johns Hopkins Press, Baltimore, Maryland; Furman, Bess (1973). *A profile of the United States Public Health Service, 1798–1948*. U.S. Department of Health, Education, and Welfare, Washington, DC. For a condensed, updated, and livelier account, see Mullan, Fitzhugh (1989). *Plagues and politics: the story of the United States Public Health Service*. Basic Books, New York. See also Koop, C. Everett and Ginzburg, Harold M. (1989). The revitalization of the Public Health Service Commissioned Corps. *Public Health Reports*, **104**, 105–10.

[2] For the early development of research in the Public Health Service, see Harden, Victoria A. (1986). *Inventing the NIH: federal biomedical research policy, 1887–1937*. Johns Hopkins University Press, Baltimore.

and the Social Security Act of 1935 marked a considerable expansion of federal involvement in both social welfare and in public health. The Social Security Act provided old-age benefits, unemployment insurance, workers' compensation, and grants for maternal and child health services. It also provided matching grants to the states for the development of state and local health services and offered funds and fellowships for training the new personnel needed. The National Health Survey of 1935–36 documented the high incidence of chronic disease and disability in the population and provided a basis for the National Health Plan of 1938, which made an unsuccessful case for an expanded public health system and a national medical care programme supported either by taxes or insurance. Beginning with the Committee on the Costs of Medical Care in 1927–32, there had been continuing attempts to solve the problem of the organization and financing of health services so as to guarantee greater access to care for all Americans.[3] The repeated efforts throughout the 1930s and early 1940s to develop a system of national health insurance never garnered sufficient political strength to overcome the determined opposition of the medical profession and the American Medical Association.[4]

As Surgeon General, Thomas Parran was head of the Public Health Service during its most activist period from 1936 to 1948. Already famous for his leadership of the venereal disease programmes of the Public Health Service, Parran presided over the dramatic growth in the research capabilities of the National Institutes of Health, the expansion of the Commissioned Officer Corps in the Public Health Service during the Second World War, the beginnings of the Communicable Disease Center, the early years of the World Health Organization, and the considerable development of state and local health department programmes in the United States.[5] In 1945, Harry S. Mustard, Director of the School of Public Health at Columbia University, declared:

---

[3] The Committee on the Costs of Medical Care (CCMC) was an effort by 50 representatives of the public health and medical professions, funded by major foundations, to make national recommendations for the strengthening of public health and the coordination of all health services. For a general account of these efforts, see Falk, I.S. (1973). Medical care in the USA—problems, proposals and programs from the Committee on the Costs of Medical Care to the Committee for National Health Insurance. *Milbank Memorial Fund Quarterly*, **51**, 1–39. See also the reprint of the CCMC report (1970). *Medical care for the American people: the final report of the Committee on the Costs of Medical Care.* United States Government Printing Office, Washington, DC.

[4] See, for example, Hirshfield, Daniel S. (1970). *The lost reform: the campaign for compulsory health insurance in the United States from 1932 to 1943.* Harvard University Press, Cambridge, Massachusetts.

[5] The Communicable Disease Center (CDC) changed its name to the Center for Disease Control in 1970 and to the Centers for Disease Control in 1980. Elizabeth Etheridge

The United States Public Health Service occupies an enviable and commendable position in its relationships with the health authorities of the several states . . . through high standards of performance and through demonstration and efficiency, the Public Health Service has raised the level of work performed in every county, city, and state health department with which it has had even indirect contact.[6]

Although the Public Health Service played the starring role, many public health activities were scattered throughout the federal bureaucracy. About 40 agencies were active in public health; by 1945, these included the Department of Agriculture (home economics, entomology, plant quarantine), Department of Commerce (Bureau of the Census and Vital Statistics), Department of the Interior (Office of Indian Affairs in sanitation and medical care, Bureau of Mines in industrial hygiene), Federal Security Agency (Pure Food and Drug Administration, Office of Education), and the Department of Labor (Division of Maternal and Child Health, Children's Bureau, Bureau of Labor Statistics).

The state health departments had developed greatly in the 1920s and 1930s. During the First World War, they had been miserably understaffed when so many of their sanitarians, doctors, and nurses went off to join the Armed Forces. The great influenza epidemic of 1918 had infected five million people in the United States and killed 500 000, providing a bitter lesson of the continuing need for public health and infectious disease control. After the war, state and municipal health departments actively recruited replacement personnel and expanded their programmes with new organizational units and increased staffing, especially of public health nurses. Bacteriological laboratories continued to be important, while divisions of tuberculosis, child and maternal health, venereal diseases, public health administration, and health education played a major role in most state and city health departments, along with divisions of sanitation and vital statistics. After the first flush of enthusiasm for the achievements of bacteriology, many health departments were now paying more attention to community-based health activities and popular health education. When federal funds, matched with those provided locally, became available for maternal and child health services, many divisions expanded their services for mothers and infants. In 1923, Charles-Edward A. Winslow went so far

---

is currently completing a history of the CDC, *The believers: a history of the CDC* (tentative title), to be published by California University Press.

[6] Mustard, Harry S. (1945). *Government in public health*, p. 59. The Commonwealth Fund, New York.

as to announce the ending of the bacteriological age and to describe popular health education as the keynote of the 'new public health':

The dominant motive in the present-day public health campaign is the education of the individual in the practices of personal hygiene. The discovery of popular education as an instrument in preventive medicine, made by the pioneers in the tuberculosis movement, has proved almost as far-reaching as the discovery of the germ theory of disease.[7]

Public health practice varied greatly throughout the states and cities across the country. Differences in state health organization, surveyed by Charles Chapin in 1915, remained in the 1920s, with some states mounting extremely energetic and efficient programmes and others doing relatively little for their populations.[8] In many states, public health activities were fragmented and disorganized; a 1941 survey of state health departments would find a multitude of agencies, state boards, and commissions involved in public health activities, with as many as 18 different agencies in a single state.[9] The money spent for public health work also varied widely, ranging from $0.13 per capita in Ohio to $1.68 in Delaware. In most cases, states that spent the largest sums put most of the money into hospital services rather than into prevention.

An American Public Health Association survey of municipal public health department practice, published in 1923, gives a similar view of the wide variation in public health organization across 83 United States

---

[7] Winslow, Charles-Edward A. (1923). *The evolution and significance of the modern public health campaign*, pp. 53, 55. Yale University Press, New Haven, Connecticut. See also, Winslow, C–E.A. (1926). Public health at the crossroads. *American Journal of Public Health*, **16**, 1075–85.

[8] Chapin, Charles V. (1915). *A report on state public health work, based on a survey of state boards of health*. Council on Health and Public Instruction. American Medical Association, Chicago. It is interesting to note that Chapin finds it necessary to argue that state health officers should have some practical knowledge of sanitation (p. 68):
'No man should be elected to the important position of state health officer who has not had good training in sanitation, not necessarily university training, but certainly training in some subordinate position in the department, or in municipal work . . . It is not a qualification for holding such an office that a man is a party worker or can manipulate his medical society, or poll a majority of the state board of health.'
For an analysis of public health in one of the most progressive states, see Rosenkrantz, Barbara (1972). *Public health and the state: changing views in Massachusetts, 1842–1936*. Harvard University Press, Cambridge, Massachusetts.

[9] Mountin, Joseph W. and Flook, Evelyn (1941). Distribution of health services in the structure of state government: the composite pattern of state health services. *Public Health Reports*, **56**, 1676; Mountin, Joseph W. and Flook, Evelyn (1943). Distribution of health services in the structure of state government: state health department organization. *Public Health Reports*, **58**, 568.

cities at that time.[10] The major categories of expenditure were administration, communicable disease control, tuberculosis, venereal diseases,
infant welfare, school health supervision, public health nursing, sanitary
inspection, food inspection, and vital statistics, with a group of miscellaneous activities ranging from provision of public baths to morgues.
Expenditures ranged from $0.12 to $1.05 per capita, with most of the
health departments reporting a doubling of expenditure between 1910
and 1920.[11]

In most rural parts of the country, efficient provision of public health
services depended on county health organizations, smaller and simpler
units than the larger state and municipal health departments. The
Rockefeller Sanitary Commission, which initiated the control of hookworm in the southern states had been a major force in the promotion of
local health units, and many tended to see the rapid organization of
county health units as a panacea for all the problems of rural health.[12]
Staffing such units, however, was a major problem as there were never
enough adequately trained people available. Despite considerable effort
and money spent on the development of local health services from about
1910, only 541 counties out of the 3070 counties in the United States had
any form of public health service by 1934. Then came the Social Security Act of 1935, which provided funds to the states, on a matching basis,
to encourage them to set up comprehensive local public health services.
Under this impetus, both federal and state funding for public health
doubled in the decade of the Depression. By June 1942, 1828 counties—
almost two-thirds of the total—could boast of health units directed by a
full-time public health officer.[13]

In 1942, the American Public Health Association worked out a plan

---

[10] *Report of the Committee on Municipal Health Department Practice of the American Public Health Association, in cooperation with the United States Public Health Service* (1923). Public Health Bulletin, no. 136. United States Government Printing Office, Washington, DC.

[11] Ibid., 36. It is interesting to note that only 21 of the 83 health officers in the survey held a bachelors degree; 73 out of the 83 were graduates in medicine, two were graduates in engineering, and two graduates in law as well as medicine. Ten of the 83 had special-ized training in public health, three holding the doctorate of public health, the others dip-lomas and certificates. Of these, one had been trained in the University of Oxford and held the British Diploma in Public Health. Ibid., 21.

[12] Ferrell, John A. and Mead, Pauline A. (1936). *History of County Health Organizations in the United States, 1908–1933, prepared by Division of Surgeon General.* United States Government Printing Office, Washington, DC.

[13] Kratz, F. K. (1943). Status of full-time local health organizations at the end of the fiscal year 1941–1942. *Public Health Reports,* **58,** 345–51. Much of this gain would be lost during the war; by the end of the war only 1322 counties had an organized health service. See Corwin, E.H.L. (ed.) (1949). *Ecology of health,* p. 125. The Commonwealth Fund, New York; Mustard, Harry S. (1945). *Government in public health,* p.190, The Common-wealth Fund, New York.

for providing a comprehensive system of local health services covering the whole nation.[14] Haven Emerson, in a report, *Local health units for the nation*, estimated the cost of a modest but adequate basic health service for each of 1197 proposed new health units. He stated that communities over 50 000 should be able to provide reasonably adequate local services at the cost of one dollar per capita; a superior service could be furnished for two dollars per capita.[15]

The push for development of local health departments stimulated the already strong demand for trained public health personnel. The existing schools of public health at Johns Hopkins, Harvard, Yale, Columbia, Michigan, and North Carolina provided a relatively sophisticated education in the scientific basis of public health at the masters and doctoral level.[16] They produced a small number of public health specialists with a thorough knowledge of such subjects as administration, epidemiology, statistics, bacteriology, and communicable disease control. The main source of financial support for private schools of public health was the Rockefeller Foundation, and for state schools, their respective state governments. Even taken together, however, these élite schools of public health were completely unable to fill the demand for large numbers of trained public health personnel to fit the needs of state, municipal, and local health department programmes.

In 1935, for the first time, the federal government provided funds for public health training. It offered funds to states to employ new public health professionals but required that the states establish minimum qualifications for new professional personnel, all of whom were to have some specialized public health training. The consequence was an energetic and growing demand for public health courses, preferably ones which produced a large and steady stream of graduates with the minimum acceptable credentials. The new federal funding thus helped to expand the training possibilities for public health personnel, even if this training was often less than fully adequate.

Several state universities opened new schools of public health and existing schools increased their enrolments to capacity. By 1939, 45 different institutions were offering 18 different degrees in public health. Many of the new programmes provided very short intensive courses lasting only a few weeks or months, targeted at employed people who

[14] Emerson, Haven (1945). *Local health units for the nation*. The Commonwealth Fund, New York.

[15] Ibid., 2.

[16] Leathers, W.S. *et al.* (1937). Committee on Professional Education of the American Public Health Association. Public health degrees and certificates granted in 1936. *American Journal of Public Health*, **27**, 1267–72.

needed credentials, but who did not have the leisure for full-time study. Within three years, from 1935 to 1938, more than 4000 individuals, including about 1000 doctors, had received some public health training with the new federal funds. Public health leaders agreed that one year was the minimum time necessary to provide the basic educational background for public health practice; they argued that the short training courses were a necessary stop-gap measure until more comprehensive educational programmes could be developed.

On 26 April, 1941, representatives from the leading schools of public health, namely those at Columbia, Harvard, Johns Hopkins, Michigan, North Carolina, Toronto, and Yale, met to organize the Association of Schools of Public Health, 'to promote and improve the graduate education and training of . . . professional personnel for service in public health'.[17] The members clearly disapproved of the new, fast training courses and limited the membership of the association to those involved in graduate education.[18] They wanted an accreditation mechanism to establish standards for public health training—a wish that had to be postponed until after the war emergency. The Association of Schools of Public Health established an office in Washington, DC, which served as a base for lobbying members of Congress on legislation of interest to the schools.

In the late 1930s and 1940s, other federal funding programmes in public health were intended to control specific diseases or to provide services for special population groups, such as pregnant women and children. This tendency to fund separate programmes for different diseases or for different population groups has been termed the 'categorical' approach to public health. It had the disadvantage of leading to fragmented programmes with little integrated planning. It had the advantage of being politically popular; Members of Congress were often willing to allocate funds that supported vertical programmes for specific diseases or for particular groups—health and welfare services for

[17] Lowell J. Reed of Johns Hopkins was elected President, Milton J. Rosenau of North Carolina Vice-President, and Henry F. Vaughan of Michigan, Secretary-Treasurer. Minutes of the organization meeting of the Association of Schools of Public Health, Baltimore, Maryland, April 26, 1951, 1. Enclosure to minutes of the meeting of the Association of Schools of Public Health, 11–12 April, 1951. Baltimore, Maryland. Alan Mason Chesney Archives, Johns Hopkins University, RG 1, Box 48. The University of Minnesota was soon added to the list of accredited graduate programmes.

[18] In the 1920s, there were four schools of public health in the United States, all at private universities: Johns Hopkins, Yale, Columbia, and Harvard. In the 1930s, four state universities entered the field: Michigan, Minnesota, North Carolina, and California at Berkeley.

children were especially appealing—even when they displayed little interest in general public health or administrative expenditures.[19] Although state health officers often felt constrained by vertical programmes, they rarely refused federal grants-in-aid and thus they adapted their services to the available pattern of funds. Federal grants came in turn for maternal and child health services and crippled children (1935), venereal disease control (1938), tuberculosis (1944), mental health (1947), industrial hygiene (1947), and dental health (1947). Many of these programmes, such as maternal and child health and venereal disease control, included funds for specialized training programmes and student support grants. This pattern of vertical or categorical funding, started in the 1930s, would continue to shape the organization of public health departments through the post-war period. As institutionalized in the National Institutes of Health, it would also shape the future patterns of biomedical research.

2. Public health and the Second World War

Mobilization for war acted as a major force behind the expansion and development of public health in the United States. Public health was declared a national priority for the armed forces and the civilian population engaged in military production. As James Stevens Simmons, Brigadier General and Director of the Preventive Medicine Division of the United States Army, declared:

A civil population that is not healthy cannot be prosperous and will lag behind in the economic competition between nations. This is even more true of a military population, for any army that has its strength sapped by disease is in no condition to withstand the attack of a virile force that has conserved its strength and is enjoying the vigour and exhilaration of health.[20]

Politicians were now willing to vote appropriations for public health as essential to national defence.[21] As the federal government began planning and organizing new health programmes, state and local

---

[19] Corwin, E.H.L. (ed.), op.cit., *xii* (note 13).

[20] Simmons, James Stevens (1943). The preventive medicine program of the United States Army. *American Journal of Public Health*, **33**, 931–40. After the war, Simmons became Dean of the Harvard School of Public Health.

[21] Mustard, Harry S. (1941). Editorial. Yesterday's school children are examined for the army. *American Journal of Public Health*, **31**, 1207.

governments were also urged to orient their activities to the war effort.[22] Joseph W. Mountin, Assistant Surgeon General, underlined the sense of urgency: 'If a machine is idle because the worker who should tend it is sick, that machine is doing a job for Hitler'.[23] Health departments again suffered from a critical shortage of personnel as doctors, nurses, engineers, and other trained and experienced professionals left to join the armed services.[24]

In 1940, the United States Public Health Service expanded its programme of grants to states and local communities, sending personnel to particularly needy areas. The Community Facilities Act provided $300 million in funds for construction of public works, which included sanitary and health facilities, in communities with rapidly expanding populations because of new military camps and war industries. The Office of Defense Health and Welfare Services, created as part of the Office for Emergency Management, co-ordinated efforts to protect the health of the nation at war, while the Office of Scientific Research and Development organized the national research effort.[25]

The shock of the discovery that many of the young men being called into the Army were physically unfit for military service provided a powerful impetus for increased national attention to public health, mirroring the British experience in the Boer War and the American experience in the First World War. The Selective Service examinations represented the most massive health survey ever undertaken, with over 16 million young men examined; fully 40 per cent of them were declared physically or mentally unfit for service.[26] The leading causes of rejection were defective teeth, visual problems, orthopaedic impairments (e.g. from polio), diseases of the cardiovascular system, nervous and mental diseases, hernia, tuberculosis, and venereal diseases. As G. St. J. Perrott of the United States Public Health Service noted, mortality from tuberculosis and some other infectious diseases had declined since the First World War, but morbidity rates had changed little, if at all: both wars

---

[22] See, for example, Burgdorf, Alfred L. (1943). War and the health department. *American Journal of Public Health*, **33**, 26–30; for the disarmingly pessimistic view of a local health officer, see Swartout, Hubert O. (1944). Wartime problems of a county health officer. *American Journal of Public Health*, **34**, 379–82.

[23] Mountin, Joseph W. (1942). Evaluation of health services in a national emergency. *American Journal of Public Health*, **32**, 1128.

[24] Idem. (1943). Responsibility of local health authorities in the war effort. *American Journal of Public Health*, **33**, 35–40.

[25] Sullivan, Frances (1942). Public health planning for war needs: order or chaos? *American Journal of Public Health*, **32**, 831–6.

[26] Perrott, G. St. J. (1944). Findings of selective service examinations. *Milbank Memorial Fund Quarterly*, **22**, 358–66; idem. (1946). Selective service rejection statistics and some of their implications. *American Journal of Public Health*, **36**, 336–42.

had made visible the appallingly poor health of the American population.[27] The Selective Service examinations also made obvious the fact that the health of black recruits in the segregated army was far worse than that of white servicemen.

Major population shifts had occurred with the mobilization for war and the movement of workers to areas with defence industry plants. Peaceful villages near army camps had turned into boom towns and some cities had doubled their population within a couple of years.[28] In many cases, the existing infrastructure of water supplies and sewage systems were completely inadequate to cope with these population movements.[29] Army training camps in the South had often been placed in areas with pleasant climates, where the *Anopheles* mosquito already bred in profusion and malaria was endemic. In order to control malaria, the Public Health Service established the Center for Controlling Malaria in the War Areas. After the war, when substantial funds were made available for malaria eradication efforts, this organization was transformed into the Centers for Disease Control which would come to play a central role in the effort to control both infectious and non-infectious diseases throughout the nation.

During the war, the schools of public health provided short training courses for the medical officers of the armed services in such subjects as parasitology, tropical medicine, sanitation, and venereal disease control. Many of the faculty as well as the graduating students joined the war effort, especially in preventive medicine and infectious disease control programmes. The schools of public health emerged from the war years in a weakened position, with many of their faculty gone and their programmes disrupted.

3. Schools of public health: 1945

In the autumn term of 1945, 396 graduate students were enrolled in the seven major schools of public health in the United States.[30] One half of

[27] Idem. (1946). Selective service statistics and some of their implications. *American Journal of Public Health*, **36**, 341–2; Underwood, Felix J. (1942). The role of public health in the national emergency. *American Journal of Public Health*, **32**, 530.

[28] Maxcy, Kenneth F. (1942). Epidemiologic implications of wartime population shifts. *American Journal of Public Health*, **32**, 1089–96.

[29] For wartime concern with water supplies, see, for example, Goudey, R.F. (1941). Wartime protection of water supplies. *American Journal of Public Health*, **31**, 1174–80; Weir, W.H. (1945). Lessons learned from the internal security program of the War Department. *American Journal of Public Health*, **35**, 353–7.

[30] The largest classes were at those at Michigan, North Carolina, Columbia, Johns Hopkins, and Harvard. California, Minnesota, Michigan and North Carolina also had

the physicians and two-thirds of the sanitary engineers came from outside the United States; most of these would become public health officers in their own countries or in international health agencies.[31] The students from the United States represented a variety of professional groups, including physicians, engineers, dentists, veterinary surgeons, statisticians, physiologists, bacteriologists, administrators, health educators, and nurses.[32]

In 1946 the American Public Health Association established an accreditation mechanism, the Committee on Professional Education, chaired by William P. Shepard, to monitor the standards of education at schools of public health. The committee visited all schools of public health between 1945 and 1947 and formally accredited 10 schools for the Masters of Public Health (MPH) and seven for the Dr.P.H. degree. The ten schools accredited for the MPH were California, Columbia, Harvard, Johns Hopkins, Michigan, Minnesota, North Carolina, Toronto, Vanderbilt, and Yale.[33] A number of other schools offered some public health training but were not formally accredited; these included Chicago, Indiana, Massachusetts Institute of Technology, New York University, Oregon, Pennsylvania, Rutgers, St. Louis, Simmons, Syracuse, Washington, Wayne, and Western Reserve.[34]

The curriculum of schools of public health was heavily focused on the biological sciences, epidemiology, biostatistics, and public health administration. The largest number of hours of instruction for graduate students was given in public health administration; next in order came biostatistics, environmental sanitation, microbiology, hospital administration, public health education, epidemiology, and tropical public

large numbers of undergraduate students. Student data; eight accredited Schools of Public Health, Fall term 1945; data supplied by Deans of Schools for use of Surgeon General's Committee on Postwar Training of Public Health Personnel, April 1946. Alan Mason Chesney Archives, Johns Hopkins University, Record Group (RG) 3, Series a, Box 87.

[31] The largest numbers of foreign students attended Michigan, Johns Hopkins, North Carolina, and Harvard.

[32] Physicians and health educators made up almost two-thirds of all graduate students in public health. Physicians were the most numerous group at Michigan, Columbia, Johns Hopkins, and Harvard, and health educators at North Carolina, Yale, California, and Minnesota. The largest numbers of health educators and sanitary engineers were being trained at North Carolina and Michigan, the largest numbers of laboratory workers at Johns Hopkins and California, and the largest number of statisticians at Columbia.

[33] In 1948/49, Vanderbilt was dropped from the list and Tulane added. The seven schools accredited for the Dr.P.H. were California, Columbia, Harvard, Johns Hopkins, Michigan, North Carolina, and Yale. In 1950, Pittsburgh was added to the list of accredited schools for both the MPH and the Dr.P.H..

[34] Degrees offered by certain schools of public health, 1946. Alan Mason Chesney Archives, Johns Hopkins University, RG 3, Series a, Box 76.

health.[35] Charles-Edward A. Winslow of Yale University, as head of the Committee on Professional Education, commented that schools of public health paid too little attention to the environmental, social, and economic aspects of public health and that too few schools taught the history of public health, mental hygiene, or public health nursing—all fields he believed essential for the education of public health specialists.[36]

By the time of the American Public Health Association's survey of schools of public health in 1950, the existing schools had become crowded to capacity.[37] Together, the schools were training over 1200 students per year and reported that they could double the number with additional financial support. Financial constraints were the limiting factor in growth; many of the schools needed new teaching and clinical facilities and all wanted to employ more faculty members. The major problem was to find money for operating expenses and salaries. In all schools, tuition fees represented a small proportion of income—less than 15 per cent. The public schools depended on state appropriations, while private schools relied on endowments, gifts, and research grants. Overall, the income from research grants was directly related to the size of the faculty. On average, faculty members spent 40 per cent of their time on teaching, 40 per cent on research, 10 per cent on administration and

[35] A survey of all accredited schools of public health in 1950 listed the following subjects as commonly offered:

- public health administration or practice
- biostatistics or vital statistics
- public health education
- environmental sanitation
- epidemiology
- hospital administration
- industrial hygiene
- maternal and child health
- medical economics and medical care administration
- microbiology and bacteriology
- public health nursing
- nutrition and biochemistry
- physiological hygiene and physiology
- tropical public health and parasitology

A category of 'other' included cancer control, public health dentistry, experimental medicine, mental hygiene, personal health, tuberculosis, and venereal disease control. Rosenfeld, Leonard S., Gooch, Marjorie, and Levine, Oscar H. (1953). *Report on schools of public health in the United States based on a survey of schools of public health in 1950*. Public Health Service, United States Department of Health, Education, and Welfare, Publication no. 276, p. 16. United States Government Printing Office, Washington DC.

[36] Winslow, Charles-Edward A. (1949). The preparation of professional workers in the field of public health. In Corwin, op.cit., 161–70 (note 13). See also Shepard, William P. (1948). The professionalization of public health. *American Journal of Public Health*, **38**, 151.

[37] Rosenfeld *et al.*, op.cit. (note 35).

10 per cent on community service. Of all the faculty active in research, 40 per cent were based at Johns Hopkins and Harvard.

In 1950, somewhat over half of the students in schools of public health enrolled with professional qualifications. About one-third of the students were physicians and a smaller proportion were nurses. Like the students, the faculty represented a variety of professions. About 40 per cent of the faculty were physicians, with most of the others holding doctorates in various scientific fields. About 25 per cent of the faculty held doctorates of public health and a larger number held masters of public health degrees.

4. The epidemiological transition

In the post-war years, the public health community came clearly to understand that the disease patterns of the country had changed: in 1900, the leading causes of death had been tuberculosis, pneumonia, diarrhoeal diseases, and enteritis; by 1946, they were heart disease, cancer, and accidents. The importance of the chronic diseases was becoming recognized during the 1930s, but this knowledge had been temporarily eclipsed by the urgent demands of infectious disease control during the war. With the return to peace, public health officers now realized that they must come to terms with the problems and prevalence of chronic diseases.[38] Communicable disease control no longer provided a sufficient *raison d'être* for health departments; the major infectious disease problems of the early twentieth century, such as tuberculosis, poliomyelitis, syphilis, typhoid, and diphtheria seemed to have been effectively controlled.

The transition from dealing with infectious diseases to non-infectious diseases was not an easy one. Too little was known; health officials had no clear idea of how to prevent cancer or heart disease. Where there was agreement about the relatively simple methods of bacteriology and vector control in preventing infectious disease, there was only complexity, confusion, and disagreement about the relative importance of nutritional, behavioural, occupational, and environmental health factors in controlling chronic diseases.

When federal grants were made available for cancer control in 1946 and for heart disease in 1948, the one widely accepted approach to prevention was through screening and early diagnoses. This seemed to place chronic disease prevention in the domain of individual medical

[38] Fox, Daniel M. (1989). Policy and epidemiology: financing health services for the chronically ill and disabled, 1930–1990. *Milbank Quarterly*, **67**, suppl. 2, 1–31.

care and some public health officials were worried about becoming directly involved in the provision of medical services. In 1945, Harry Mustard warned that if medical care became the responsibility of public health departments, 'Many comfortably established routines would be rudely shaken and it is possible that a hypertrophied medical-care tail would soon wag the none too robust public health dog'.[39]

In their turn, private practitioners who wanted to provide preventive medical services to their patients argued that public health departments should have nothing to do with chronic diseases. They saw private medical practice as the appropriate locus for prevention: 'For example, disturbances of the climacteric, cancer, metabolic disorders, such as diabetes, cardiovascular disease, and the like are utterly beyond the influence of public health measures . . . prevention, early detection, and control of these disorders are and will continue to be individualistic and not *en masse*'.[40] To most physicians, preventive medicine meant periodic examinations—and they preferred to keep the state out of the doctor's office.

Some believed that the chronic diseases provided an opportunity to integrate preventive and curative medicine. In the immediate post-war period, considerable optimism and energy were devoted to the possible reorganization of public health and medical care.[41] In the late 1940s and early 1950s, a small group of physicians and academics felt enthusiastic about the concept of social medicine as seeming to offer a fresh perspective on the problems of chronic illness. Iago Galdston, Secretary of the New York Academy of Medicine, organized the Institute on Social Medicine in 1947, later publishing the papers as *Social medicine: its derivations and objectives*.[42] The social medicine discussions seem to have had little long-term effect on either public health or medical practice but they constitute an interesting intellectual movement which illustrates, if it did not solve, the tensions between public health, preventive medicine, and clinical practice in this period.

There were several versions of the social medicine idea, some of

[39] Mustard, Harry S. (1945). *Government in public health*, p. 191. The Commonwealth Fund, New York.

[40] Stieglitz, Edward J. (1945). *A future for preventive medicine*, pp. 32–3. The Commonwealth Fund, New York.

[41] Stern, Bernard J. (1946). *Medical services by government: local, state, and federal*, pp. 31–2. The Commonwealth Fund, New York. Viseltear, Arthur J. (1972). *Emergence of the Medical Care Section of the American Public Health Association, 1926–1948: a chapter in the history of medical care in the United States*. American Public Health Association, Washington, DC.; Fox, Daniel M. (1986). *Health policies, health politics: the British and American experience, 1911–1965*. Princeton University Press, New Jersey.

[42] Galdston, Iago (ed.) (1949). *Social medicine: its derivations and objectives*. The Commonwealth Fund, New York.

which are reflected in Chapters 6 and 8. John Ryle linked social medicine to clinical preventive medicine rather than to public health. Public health, he said, was concerned with environmental improvement, while social medicine extended its view to 'the whole of the economic, nutritional, occupational, educational, and psychological opportunity or experience of the individual or of the community'.[43] Edward J. Stieglitz responded that social medicine was simply 'public health maturing . . . The maiden, public health, has married sociology and changed her name'.[44]

The new effort to deal with the chronic diseases seemed to demand a reformulation of epidemiological methods and a closer association of the biological and social sciences. At the time, academic epidemiology was the epidemiology of infectious diseases; academic preventive medicine was the science of the prevention of infectious diseases; both had been brought to a high level of technical sophistication based on the biological and laboratory sciences. The idea that public health and epidemiology should be concerned with the relation of health to social structure had received little more than occasional rhetorical attention. The concept was easier to state than to put into practice. Ernest L. Stebbins, Dean of the Johns Hopkins School of Public Health, consistently argued that epidemiology was the essential discipline for dealing with both chronic and infectious diseases and that chronic disease epidemiology would have to involve the social sciences.[45] Margaret Merrell and Lowell J. Reed, statisticians from the Hopkins school, made a similar point in a brief paper that was to become a classic statement on 'the epidemiology of health'.[46] Their suggestion that health could be quantitatively measurable, and that health could be advanced in the total absence of disease, provided a conceptual break with the disease-oriented model of infectious disease epidemiology.

Epidemiology, broadening its scope to place more emphasis on the social environment, now became newly fashionable as 'medical ecology'.[47] John E. Gordon, professor of preventive medicine and epidemiology at the Harvard School of Public Health and a prominent exponent of the 'newer epidemiology', argued that the triumvirate of

[43] Ryle, John. Social pathology, in Galdston, op.cit., 64 (note 42).

[44] Stieglitz, Edward J. The integration of clinical and social medicine, in Galdston, op.cit., 80–1 (note 42).

[45] Stebbins, Ernest L. Epidemiology and social medicine, in Galdston, op.cit., 101–4 (note 42).

[46] Merrell, Margaret and Reed, Lowell J. The epidemiology of health, in Galdston, op.cit. 105–10 (note 42).

[47] The term 'ecology of health' was also popular. See, for example, Corwin, op.cit. (note 13).

'environment, host, and disease' could be applied to non-communicable organic diseases such as pellagra, cancer, psychosomatic conditions, traumatic injuries, and accidents.[48] The new epidemiologists firmly rejected the notion of a single cause of disease (the agent) in favour of multiple causation.[49]

For some, the ideas associated with social medicine brought optimism about new approaches to the chronic diseases, the possible integration of preventive and curative medicine, and the extension of comprehensive health programmes to the whole population.[50] Others were more cautious. Eli Ginzberg, for example, warned that neither personnel nor resources were available for implementing the new programmes being discussed.[51] In New York State, an excess of $1.5 billion was being spent annually on medical budgets, whereas the combined public health budgets amounted to only $36 million, or 2.4 per cent of the total.[52] Ginzberg warned optimistic thinkers of an 'anti-government attitude' in the United States and the prevalent assumption that health depended on medical care, with the ever-increasing provision of doctors and hospital beds. He and others, whose views ranged across the political spectrum, urged public health professionals to do a more effective job of persuading the public that advances in diet, housing, and public health nursing were far more important to health than the construction of hospitals. While hospitals were being built across the country, local health officer positions stood vacant because communities refused to provide reasonable salaries.[53]

The more pessimistic prognoses for public health, however defined, proved correct in the political climate of the 1950s. High hopes and aspirations were not translated into effective health programmes; acute care facilities and biomedical research expanded dramatically in the post-war period, while public health departments struggled to maintain their programmes on inadequate budgets and with little political support. Post-war reconstruction meant massive expenditures for biomedical

---

[48] Gordon, John E. (1950). The newer epidemiology. In *Tomorrow's horizon in public health*, pp. 18–45. Transactions of the 1950 Conference of the Public Health Association of New York City, Public Health Association, New York. Idem. (1953). The world, the flesh and the devil as environment, host and agent of disease. In *The epidemiology of health*. (ed. Iago Galdston), New York Academy of Medicine. pp. 60–73.

[49] Stebbins, Ernest L. Epidemiology and social medicine, op.cit., 101–4 (note 45).

[50] Smillie, Wilson G. (1950). The responsibility of the state. In *Tomorrow's horizon in public health: transactions of the 1950 conference*, pp. 95–102. Public Health Association of New York City, New York.

[51] Ginzberg, Eli. Public health and the public, in *Tomorrow's horizon in public health*, op.cit., 104 (note 50).

[52] Ibid., 106.

[53] Ibid., 101–9.

research and hospitals, the partial payment for medical care by expanding private insurance coverage, the relative neglect of public health services, and a complete failure to implement the more radical efforts to reorganize medical care through focused attention to the social determinants of health and disease.

5. Hospital construction: The Hill–Burton Act

The two major accomplishments of the post-war period were in hospital construction and the creation of the biomedical research establishment. The American Hospital Association and the American Medical Association, with support from the American Public Health Association, strongly supported the Hospital Survey and Construction Act of 1946, more popularly known as the Hill–Burton Act, after Senators Lister Hill of Alabama and Harold H. Burton of Ohio. Hospital construction, especially in rural areas, promised to bring the benefits of medical science to all the people—without in any way disturbing the freedoms of the medical profession or the patterns of paying for their services. One-third of the costs of building hospitals would be paid by the federal government, with $75 million set aside for each of the first five years.[54] No health programme had ever been so generous or so popular. The act did include funds for building public health centres, but the public health component of the bill was far overshadowed by the emphasis on acute care facilities. Hill-Burton was a symbol of the national demand for access to medical care but it in no way challenged the private organization of medical practice nor the relative disregard of public health services. The United States could have been completely covered by local health departments for a fraction of the cost of Hill-Burton, but there was no strong political constituency for public health that could effectively compete for resources with curative medicine.

6. Biomedical research and high technology medicine

There are many reasons why the United States moved toward ever more sophisticated biomedical research and high technology medicine in the post-war era. Stephen Strickland, among others, has examined the politics of research funding and shown how the priorities of research were set by the basic sciences and clinical medicine.[55] Perhaps the more

[54] Feshbach, Dan (1979). What's inside the black box: a case study of allocative politics in the Hill–Burton program. *International Journal of Health Services*, **9**, 313–39.

[55] Strickland, Stephen P. (1972). *Politics, science, and dread disease*. Harvard University Press, Cambridge, Massachusetts.

idealistic visions of social medicine, of the integration of the social and biomedical sciences in relation to health, and of the integration of preventive and curative services in a reorganized health system, were unrealistic given the balance of political forces both inside and outside medicine.[56] However, some of the blame for the neglect of public health must be shared by the public health profession for failing to articulate its goals and programmes, build the political support it needed, communicate more effectively to the general public, and promote a strong and persuasive case for adequate funding of public health services.

In retrospect, it seems clear that public health failed to claim—or be given—sufficient credit for controlling infectious diseases. Two major scientific achievements of the war, the first effective uses of penicillin and DDT, were especially relevant to public health. In popular perception, however, scientific medicine took credit both for the specific wartime achievements and for the longer history of controlling epidemic diseases; in public relations terms, medicine and biomedical research seized the public glory, the political interest, and financial support available for further anticipated health improvements in the post-war world.

Besides claiming a share of the credit for declining infectious diseases, public health departments needed to move quickly to develop programmes for the chronic diseases. Most health departments, however, were slow to start anything new; it was a lot easier simply to continue running the same categorical programmes and clinics within already established bureaucratic structures. It was one thing to call for leadership and another to provide the money. The political atmosphere of the 1950s did not support aggressive new programmes, and health department budgets were stagnant; state legislatures were not responsive to the advocates of expensive new health programmes.

Health departments did implement, or try to implement, one important, new, and very cost-effective public health measure: the fluoridation of water supplies to protect children's teeth. However, despite strong support from scientific authorities and professional organizations, fluoridation was effectively halted in many cities and towns through determined local opposition. As such a simple and obviously effective measure could be so energetically opposed, health departments must have become aware of the difficulties of instituting more adventurous or expensive interventions. One great triumph of the 1950s was the successful development of the polio vaccine and its implementation on a

---

[56] Report of the New York Academy of Medicine, Committee on Medicine in the Changing Order (1947). *Medicine in a changing order*, p. 109. The Commonwealth Fund, New York.

mass scale. The success of the polio campaign was, however, in large part due to private funding and a massive public relations campaign by the Foundation for Infantile Paralysis which raised public awareness and developed public support, interest, and enthusiasm. The appeal for crippled children proved extremely popular and the polio vaccination campaign, despite some major setbacks, was a remarkable success.

Despite such public success, in the 1950s the real expenditures of public health departments failed to keep pace with the increase in population.[57] Federal grants-in-aid to the states for public health programmes steadily declined, the total dollar amounts falling from 45 million in 1950 to 33 million in 1959. Given inflation, the decline in purchasing power of these dollars had been even more dramatic.[58] At a time when public health officials were facing a whole series of new health problems, poorly understood, they were also underbudgeted and understaffed. Jesse Aronson, director of local health services in New Jersey, offered an honest if rather devastating account of the state of small public health departments:

The full-time health officer is frequently, because of inadequate budget and staff, limited in his activities to a series of routine clinical responsibilities in a child health station, a tuberculosis clinic, a venereal disease clinic, an immunization session, and communicable disease diagnosis and treatment. He has little or no time for community health education, the study of health problems and trends, the initiation of newer programs in diabetes control, cancer control, rheumatic fever prophylaxis, nutrition education, and radiation control. In a great many areas the health officer position has been vacant year after year with little real hope of filling it. In these situations, even the pretence of public health leadership is left behind and local medical practitioners provide these services on an hourly basis.[59]

By the mid 1950s, public health had become caught in a downward spiral. Lack of funding meant a lack of new initiatives and programmes, which led to the health departments being looked upon as dull and unenterprising; this unexciting reputation meant they could neither attract new funding nor the people who might have brought new energy and new ideas. Health departments seemed dull bureaucracies, devoted to necessary functions, running tuberculosis clinics and other largely routine operations. When state legislatures wanted to build nursing homes, abate water pollution, or promote mental health, they often

[57] Sanders, B.S. (1959). Local health departments: growth or illusion? *Public Health Reports*, **74**, 13–20.

[58] Terris, Milton (1959). The changing face of public health. *American Journal of Public Health*, **49**, 1119.

[59] Aronson, Jesse B. (1959). The politics of public health—reactions and summary. *American Journal of Public Health*, **49**, 311.

simply bypassed state health departments as not active or not interested in these issues. Public health officials were expressing 'frustrations, disappointments, dissatisfactions, and discontentments' said John W. Knutson, in his presidential address to the American Public Health Association.[60] To change this dreary situation, public health officials, he said, must develop more imagination, political skills, and knowledge of human motivation and behaviour. 'Our graduate students', he said, 'need a better understanding of the social and political forces swirling about them as they work professionally. In place of rapidly outdated factual information, I would have them gain from graduate education in public health a fundamental knowledge of four broad fields: cultural anthropology, human ecology, epidemiology, and biostatistics'.[61] Yet even with the best possible preparation, the bureaucratic controls and poor funding of state health departments tended to ensure conformity and to discourage young professionals from initiating or taking responsibility for new programmes.

The annual meeting of the American Public Health Association for 1955 adopted the theme 'Where are we going in public health?' In a rousing speech, Leonard Woodcock, international vice-president of the United Auto Workers, both praised public health and damned public health departments.[62] State divisions of occupational health were hopelessly underfinanced, he said, workplace inspections were rarely carried out, and occupational disease reporting was totally inadequate. The labour movement had the impression that health departments had no leaders with the passion and commitment for which Alice Hamilton had been so admired. The labour unions, said Woodcock, wanted public health departments to assess the quality of medical services, evaluate pre-payment plans, and provide comprehensive preventive services; above all, not to stand aside and let commercial insurance companies dictate the future of medical care.[63]

Most commentators agreed that public health departments should become active in new areas of public health: the chronic diseases, including rehabilitation, mental health, industrial health, accident prevention, environmental issues, and medical care organization. The New York

[60] Knutson, John W. (1957). Ferment in public health. *American Journal of Public Health*, **47**, 1489.

[61] Ibid., 1490–1.

[62] Woodcock, Leonard (1956). Where are we going in public health? *American Journal of Public Health*, **46**, 278–82.

[63] Ibid., 280. Subsequent discussions showed that many of those present at the APHA meetings admitted the truth of Woodcock's critique. Leavell, Hugh R. (1956). Where are we going in public health? Association Symposium. Part II. Resolving the basic issues, **46**, p. 408.

State Commissioner of Health, Herman E. Hilleboe, was one of the few to report new programmes of research on the chronic diseases. The New York State Health Department was examining all male state employees between the ages of 40 to 55 to learn how best to detect cardiac disease at an early stage and thus develop effective and economical methods of health screening for cardiac problems.[64] This department had built research facilities, a hospital, laboratories, and animal farms at the Roswell Park Memorial Institute in Buffalo to support research on the causes and treatment of cancer. Other new state chronic disease programmes included multiple screening efforts in Virginia and pilot studies of atherosclerosis and nutrition in Minnesota. Hilleboe urged state health departments to undertake research on more effective methods of public health practice and chronic disease control.[65]

A few years later, Milton Terris offered a forceful summary statement of the dilemma of public health. The communicable diseases were disappearing; their place had been taken by the non-infectious diseases which the public health profession was ill-prepared to prevent or control.[66] The public understood that research was crucial, and federal expenditures for medical research had multiplied from $28 million in 1947 to $186 million 10 years later. Most of this money, however, was being spent for clinical and laboratory research; few appreciated the importance of epidemiological studies in addressing these problems. Schools of public health had been slow to deal with these issues, as had health departments, with a few notable exceptions, as in the case of New York and California. Yet even the comparatively small sums spent on epidemiological research had produced dramatic successes: the discovery of the role of fluoride in preventing dental caries, the relation of cigarette smoking to lung cancer, and the suspected relation of serum cholesterol and physical exercise to coronary artery disease.[67]

7. Schools of public health: 1955

Of the 10 accredited schools of public health in the United States in 1955, four were associated with state universities and six with privately

[64] Hilleboe, Herman E. (1955). Public health in a changing world. *American Journal of Public Health,* **45**, 1517–24.

[65] Idem. (1957). Editorial: research in the public health practice. *American Journal of Public Health,* **47**, 216–17.

[66] Terris, Milton (1959). The changing face of public health. *American Journal of Public Health,* **49**, 1113–19.

[67] Ibid., 1114.

endowed universities—and none of them had adequate budgets.[68] Faculty salaries were so low that advertised positions went unfilled and about 10 per cent of all faculty positions remained vacant.[69] As federal support was limited almost entirely to research grants, the research budgets in most of the schools were increasing, while the teaching budgets were static or declining.

In the 1950s, schools of public health expanded their research base in the basic biological sciences. The schools' main source of growth was the new federal research grant programmes of the National Institutes of Health. As federal funding supported basic research in the biomedical sciences more than in the applied sciences, the laboratory sciences in the schools of public health became stronger. Money flowed for basic biological research rather than for teaching, administration, or practice. As a result, many schools of public health seemed ready to turn into research institutes, oriented to the priorities of the National Institutes of Health and their associated scientific communities, rather than to the practical problems and needs of health departments. Those selected and rewarded for their abilities in research were often relatively uninterested in the immediate problems and activities of public health officers.

Some schools defended their interest in research as educating for state, national, and international leadership—as Cecil Sheps later put it, 'the difference between a center of academic excellence, in terms of research and advanced scientific training, and the crasser problem of producing manpower for vocational purposes'.[70] At Johns Hopkins, however, Stebbins, who had served as Commissioner of Health of New York City, urged the faculty in schools of public health not to shut themselves up in their laboratories but to be actively involved in service to their local communities. He argued the importance of field research, research into administrative practice, and research in the social sciences. 'Knowledge of the natural history, the basic etiology, and means of prevention of heart disease', he contended, 'may come from sociologic studies rather than from the biological laboratory'.[71] Manifestos and proclamations had, however, less impact than the research dollars which flowed

[68] The 10 accredited schools were at Berkeley, Columbia, Johns Hopkins, Harvard, Michigan, Minnesota, North Carolina, Pittsburgh, Tulane, and Yale.

[69] Smillie, Wilson G. and Luginbuhl, Martha (1959). Training of public health personnel in the United States and Canada: a summary of ten years' advance in schools of public health. *American Journal of Public Health*, **49**, 456.

[70] Sheps, Cecil G. (1974). Trends in schools of public health in the United States since World War II. In *Schools of public health: present and future*. (ed. John Z. Bowers and Elizabeth F. Purcell), p. 8. Josiah Macy Jr. Foundation, New York.

[71] Stebbins, Ernest L. (1957). Contribution of the graduate school of public health—past, present, and future. *American Journal of Public Health*, **47**, 1511.

more readily into the laboratories than into community-based sociological research.

The numbers of students being trained at schools of public health fell by half in the period from 1946 to 1956. Whereas most students entering medical careers anticipated good incomes, economic security, and social prestige, public health practitioners had no such expectations.[72] Some schools were so concerned about the decline in numbers and quality of the students seeking the MPH degree, they considered limiting admissions to doctoral students, essentially deciding to train only those interested in research careers.[73] Doctoral candidates studying for the D.Sc. or Ph.D. in specialized scientific fields were unlikely to be interested in traditional public health officer positions. The complaints continued that schools of public health were more dedicated to research than to training students for public health practice—but those who complained never had the funding to shift the priorities.

The relationship of public health to medicine continued to be a problem for schools of public health. Although an MD degree was still considered essential for public health leadership positions, public health was simply failing to attract medical graduates in the competition with the lucrative and interesting careers possible in medical research and private medical practice. Over the 10 years from 1948 to 1958, there had been no increase in the number of physicians obtaining MPH degrees and no increase in the number of Dr.P.H. degrees awarded to physicians. George Rosen noted that despite the growing research accomplishments of schools of public health, they were unable to fill the need for trained public health officers.[74] For a partial explanation of this failure, he quoted a comment made by Parran in 1943:

It is discouraging that ordinary medical graduates have not taken public health courses and that no considerable number of students in public health schools pay their own way. This reflects the fact that public health as a career, except in limited categories, does not offer rewards so substantial or such security as to induce students to make their own investment in this postgraduate training.[75]

A number of schools, particularly the state-supported schools, were

[72] Stiles, William W. and Watson, Lois C. (1955). Motivations of persons electing public health as a career. *American Journal of Public Health*, **45**, 1563–8.

[73] Smillie, Wilson G. and Luginbuhl, Martha. op.cit., 457 (note 69).

[74] Rosen, George (1963). The school of public health: its derivation and objectives. In *The past, present and future of schools of public health*, pp. 26–38. Dedication programme addresses, School of Public Health, University of North Carolina, Chapel Hill.

[75] Parran, Thomas (1944). Public health schools and the nation's health. Dedicatory address, School of Public Health, University of Michigan, 1943–44, Ann Arbor, Michigan, 7–14. As cited by Rosen, op.cit., 33 (note 74).

now admitting non-physicians to the MPH degree; overall, somewhat more than half of all MPH candidates were non-physicians. And about half of the physicians studying for the MPH came from countries other than the United States. In the United States, public health, while not attracting large numbers of physicians, was appealing to many other students interested in social reform issues and in the particular scientific fields and issues relevant to public health. Nationally, the major increase in the student body came from public health nurses, health educators, sanitarians, and other non-medically trained specialists. The problem was that these groups had relatively little political or economic clout compared to the medical profession; in public health departments, state legislatures, and in communicating with the general public, the voices of physicians were given much more credence than those of non-medical public health specialists.

8. Federal funding for public health

In 1956, the United States Congress finally realized that public health departments were suffering from a severe shortage of trained personnel. The Senate Committee on Labor and Public Welfare noted a 'startling and shocking drop' in the annual number of public health trainees between 1947 and 1955.[76] The Health Amendment Act of 1956 authorized the Public Health Service to fund traineeships in public health for physicians, nurses, sanitary engineers, nutritionists, medical social workers, dentists, health educators, veterinary surgeons, and sanitarians.

The Association of Schools of Public Health now took on the task of garnering desperately needed financial aid for schools of public health. Ernest Stebbins of Johns Hopkins and Hugh Leavell of Harvard walked the halls of the United States Congress urging its members to support public health education. They gained an especially interested and sympathetic audience in Senator Lister Hill and Representative George M. Rhodes. In 1958, Congress enacted a two-year emergency programme authorizing $1 million a year in federal grants to be divided among the accredited schools of public health.

---

[76] Senate Committee on Labor and Public Welfare, 29 May 1956. As cited in *Report of the National Conference on Public Health Training to the Surgeon General of the Public Health Service, July 28–30, 1958*, p. 1. United States Department of Health, Education and Welfare, Washington, DC.

The First National Conference on Public Health Training, 1958

The first National Conference on Public Health Training was intended to evaluate the effectiveness of the traineeship programme.[77] The 63 invited participants included representatives of state and local health departments, graduate schools of public health, schools of nursing, medical schools, research institutions, hospitals, foundations, industrial medical departments, and voluntary health agencies. As expected, the report of the conference to the United States Congress declared a grave shortage of qualified public health personnel: the official public health agencies had well over 2500 professional job vacancies in 1958. In some areas, there were as many as four vacant positions for every trained applicant, and many vacancies were taken up by untrained people.[78] Over 20 000 of the professional workers employed by governmental and voluntary health agencies had no specialized training in public health.[79]

The new funds for public health training had undoubtedly helped address a critical situation. More than 1000 new traineeships had been provided in 1957 and 1958. The new funds had stimulated state training programmes, increased general interest in the field of public health, and improved morale and work performance in health agencies. For the first time since 1951, the numbers of trainees supported by state and local health authorities had increased.

The Conference now requested that $15 million be appropriated in construction costs for new teaching facilities and that teaching grants be made to institutions educating public health engineers, public health nurses, nutritionists, sanitarians, and laboratory scientists. It asked that funding be set aside to support teaching positions at schools of public health and that additional funds be given to state health departments to allow personnel to take short courses in public health programming, administration, and management. It urged the Public Health Service to assist states with in-service training by making available its specialist personnel, laboratories, and programmes for training purposes. It advocated freer exchange of personnel between the Public Health Service, educational institutions, and state and local health departments. The report concluded with a stirring appeal to value public health training as essential to national defence:

[77] *Report of the National Conference on Public Health Training to the Surgeon General of the Public Health Service, July 28–30, 1958*, p. 1. United States Department of Health, Education and Welfare, Washington, DC.

[78] Ennes, Howard (1957). Manpower—the Achilles' heel in public health. *American Journal of Public Health*, **47**, 1390.

[79] Senate Committee on Labor and Public Welfare, 29 May 1956, loc. cit., 2 (note 76).

The great crises of the future may not come from a foreign enemy . . . 'D' day for disease and death is everyday. The battle line is already in our own community. To hold that battle line we must daily depend on specially trained physicians, nurses, biochemists, public health engineers, and other specialists properly organized for the normal protection of the homes, the schools, and the work places of some unidentified city somewhere in America. That city has, today, neither the personnel nor the resources of knowledge necessary to protect it.[80]

Representative Rhodes now introduced the Public Health Training Act of 1959 to implement the recommendations of the National Conference on Public Health Training.[81] Stebbins noted in his testimony to Congress that the alumni roster of just one of the 11 schools, Johns Hopkins, included a Surgeon General, a Deputy Surgeon General, at least two Assistant Surgeon Generals of the United States Public Health Service, Directors and Assistant Directors of the National Institutes of Health, state health officers of the largest states, innumerable city and county health officers, research scientists in federal, state, and university research centres, and those responsible for preventive medical services in the army, the navy, and the air force. Stebbins argued that not only were these people responsible for the health of the nation—public health was also essential to international relations and America's reputation abroad:

As a part of the program of aid to friendly nations of the free world, many physicians and other health scientists have been brought to the United States under the sponsorship of the Federal Government for education in the field of public health and preventive medicine. There is increasing evidence that this program has contributed materially to the improvement of health in other countries and has been an important factor in furthering friendly relations among the countries of the world.[82]

On 9 September 1960, President Eisenhower signed the Hill–Rhodes bill and a supplemental appropriations bill with $2.5 million to implement the Hill–Rhodes Act in 1961. The Act authorized $1 million annually in 'formula' training grants for accredited schools of public health, $2 million annually for five years for project training grants to schools of public health, public health nursing, and public health

---

[80] *Report of the National Conference on Public Health Training to the Surgeon General of the Public Health Service, July 28–30, 1958*, p. 15. United States Department of Health, Education and Welfare, Washington, DC.

[81] George M. Rhodes to James L. Crabtree, undated, Alan Mason Chesney Archives, Johns Hopkins University, RG 1, Box 48.

[82] Statement by Stebbins on the need for financial assistance for the School of Hygiene and Public Health, 1959, 1–2. Alan Mason Chesney Archives, Johns Hopkins University, RG 1, Box 48.

engineering, and up to $70 000 annually for administrative costs to the public health service.[83]

Between 1957 and 1963, the United States Congress appropriated a total of $15 million to support public health trainees. In 1961, it raised the ceiling on formula grants from $1 million to $2.5 million per year.[84] It provided project grants to develop new curricular areas; over the first three years, for example, it gave $5.4 million for programmes in air and water pollution, radiological health, accident prevention, chronic diseases, health economics, and medical care administration.[85]

The downward trend in public health enrolments was reversed. However, there were still serious shortages of personnel, with an estimated 5000 vacant positions in 1962. Only 51 per cent of those already employed by public health departments were judged to have had an adequate level of training.[86]

Second National Conference on Public Health Training, 1963

The second National Conference recommended that the ceiling on formula grants be raised from $2.5 million to $5 million, that grants-in-aid for training be made to state health departments, that special fellowships be made available to schools of public health for faculty development, and that construction grants be provided to schools of public health and nursing schools. It also recommended that project grants be extended to departments of preventive medicine in medical schools. The problems of public health were magnified in the departments of preventive medicine in medical schools. A survey of such departments found that the 62 departments responding had 53 full-time budgeted vacancies for assistant, associate, or full professors.[87] Another study revealed that among physicians 35 years of age and under, only 33 were receiving residency training in public health; the comparable figures were 1827 in psychiatry, 3718 in general surgery, and 4375 in internal medicine.[88]

Over the years, Leavell and Stebbins had been very effective in gaining Congressional support for schools of public health in both the

---

[83] Spaulding, Roger B. (1960). Memorandum to the Deans of Schools of Public Health, 9 September. Alan Mason Chesney Archives, Johns Hopkins University, RG 1, Box 48.

[84] These funds were allocated according to a complex calculation: one-third of the money was allotted equally among the 12 eligible schools of public health and two-thirds were allotted according the numbers of federally sponsored students, to offset part of the difference between income from tuition and the costs of instruction.

[85] Report to the Surgeon General (1963). *Second National Conference on Public Health Training, August 19–22, 1963.* United States Public Health Service, Washington, DC.

[86] Ibid., 9–10.

[87] Ibid., 24.

[88] Ibid., 20.

Senate and the House. They were also successful in gaining support from organizations and influential individuals.[89] Lister Hill championed schools of public health in the Senate and John E. Fogarty, of Rhode Island, became their main supporter in the House.

9. The curricula of schools of public health

In the early 1960s, schools of public health were actively expanding and developing new curricular areas, partly in response to the new federal project grants. The Association of Schools of Public Health discussed the 'ferment' in schools of public health around the new, or newly recognized, problems of chronic illness, mental disorders, air pollution, medical care organization, ageing, accidents, and radiation hazards.[90] James L. Troupin, Director of Professional Education for the American Public Health Association, also noted a dramatic growth in the numbers of courses in hospital administration, behavioural sciences, and mental health.[91]

The schools of public health were continuously engaged in self-examination and curricular revision, and this resulted in variations in organization between the different schools.[92] Virtually all schools of public health had departments of public health administration, environmental health, biostatistics, and epidemiology. About half had departments of occupational health, health education, nutrition, tropical medicine, microbiology, and public health nursing, and about one third had departments of hospital administration, mental health, maternal and child health, and physiology. A few schools also had departments of behavioural sciences, biochemistry, personal health, and social welfare.[93]

[89] Snyder, John C. (1964). Memorandum on future legislative activities to the Deans of the Schools of Public Health in the U.S. and Puerto Rico, 31 March, p. 2. Alan Mason Chesney Archives, Johns Hopkins University, RG 1, Box 48.

[90] Statement for committee by Drs. Breman, Gilbert, Rosen and Tems (1959). 6 February. Association of Schools of Public Health, Alan Mason Chesney Archives, Johns Hopkins University, RG 1, Box 49.

[91] Troupin, James L., Director of Professional Education, American Public Health Association. Analysis of teaching staff in schools of public health, 1958–59. Alan Mason Chesney Archives, Johns Hopkins University, RG 1, Box 41; Troupin, James L. (1960). Schools of public health in the United States and Canada, 1959–1960. *American Journal of Public Health*, **50**, 1770–91.

[92] At Johns Hopkins in 1964, the major departments were biochemistry, biostatistics, chronic diseases, environmental medicine, epidemiology, maternal and child health, mental hygiene, pathobiology, public health administration, radiological science, and sanitary engineering.

[93] Troupin, James L. Schools of public health in the United States and Canada, 1960–61. Alan Mason Chesney Archives, Johns Hopkins University, RG 1, Box 41.

The budgets of most schools continued to grow throughout the 1960s, with the increases coming in sponsored research grants rather than in general operating funds. The proportion of institutional income from research grants rose from 38 per cent in 1959/60 to 40 per cent in 1960/61, 43 per cent in 1961/62, and 46 per cent in 1962/63.[94] In 1960, research grant funds to the schools were slightly larger than teaching funds: by 1965, research grants on average were more than 50 per cent larger.[95] Many argued that the concentration on research was an unhealthy development for the educational mission of schools of public health:

Current preoccupation with research, together with the relatively easy availability of grants for this purpose, has tended to distort the picture of teaching staffs in educational institutions. Many grant projects operating in schools of public health include persons of faculty rank who are supported entirely out of grant funds.[96]

Students, faculty, and administrators all had their complaints about this system of funding the schools largely through research grants; students complained that they were not getting sufficient faculty time and attention; faculty complained of the pressures and stresses of being expected to bring in research funds, conduct research, and also teach; and administrators complained that since most of the funding went to support specific research projects, there was little flexibility in their budgets—the funds could not be used for general purposes.

Growing research budgets, however, meant growing numbers of faculty and students, with especially marked increases in the period between 1958 and 1965.[97] Most of the new faculty appointments were made in public health administration, medical care, behavioural sciences, rehabilitation, demography and human ecology, radiological health, public health social work, and international health. In the 1960s, many schools added programmes in demography, international health, mental health, medical care, and hospital administration. As one

[94] During this period the proportion of funds derived from teaching grants remained relatively stable at about 28 per cent and the proportion representing university appropriations at about 14 per cent.

[95] Troupin, James L. Schools of public health in the United States and Canada, for the year ending June 1965, p. 5. Alan Mason Chesney Archives, Johns Hopkins University, RG 1, Box 41.

[96] Idem. Schools of public health in the United States and Canada, 1960–61, p. 10.

[97] The proportion of women on school faculties also increased rapidly, although most were clustered at the lower levels of the academic hierarchy. By 1965, 10 per cent of the full professors were women, 33 per cent of associate professors, 25 per cent of assistant professors, and 50 per cent of lecturers and instructors. Idem, *Schools of public health in the United States and Canada, for the year ending June 1965*, p. 17.

commentator noted, 'Biomedical research, the provision, financing and management of personal health care, consumer protest, and politics seem to have taken the play away from classic public health services, its officers, and their organizations'.[98]

Between 1960 and 1964, the total numbers of applicants to schools of public health more than doubled and the total numbers graduating increased by 50 per cent, from 708 in 1960, to 998 in 1964, to 1142 in 1965.[99] The majority of students, about 70 per cent, studied for the MPH degree, the basic qualification for public health practice.[100] In 1965, the professional backgrounds of students were listed in order of frequency as physicians, health educators, nurses, administrators, and sanitarians, followed by some 22 other groups of specialists.[101]

The largest professional group among the students, and the one watched with considerable interest, was the physician group: the proportion of physicians among the total graduates had dropped to 27.5 per cent in 1959/60 then increased again, with the new funding for traineeships from the Public Health Service, to 35 per cent in 1961 and 38 per cent in 1962; it then again fell to 34 per cent in 1963, 31 per cent in 1964, and 29 per cent in 1965. Gaylord W. Anderson, Director of the School of Public Health at the University of Minnesota, criticized schools of public health for focusing their attention on physicians:

If public health is indeed a synthesis of the contributions of diverse professional disciplines, each of which focuses its special competencies upon the many facets of a community problem, then it must follow that a true school of public health

[98] Nelson, Russell A. (1974). Organizational relationships of schools of public health. In *Schools of public health: present and future.* (ed. John Z. Bowers and Elizabeth F. Purcell), p. 11. Josiah Macy Jr. Foundation, New York. See also Hume, John C. The future of schools of public health: The Johns Hopkins School of Hygiene and Public Health, ibid., 64.

[99] Troupin, James L. *Schools of public health in the United States and Canada, for the year ending June 1964*, pp. 10–11. Alan Mason Chesney Archives, Johns Hopkins University, RG 1, Box 41; Idem, Schools of public health in the United States and Canada, for the year ending June 1965, p. 11. Alan Mason Chesney Archives, Johns Hopkins University, RG 1, Box 41. By 1965, the schools graduating the largest numbers of students were, in order, Michigan, Berkeley, North Carolina, Minnesota, Johns Hopkins, and Harvard.

[100] The proportion of women students stayed fairly constant in the early 1960s at between 25 and 30 per cent, and the proportion of foreign students also remained fairly steady at about 20 per cent of the total enrolments.

[101] Troupin, James L. Schools of public health in the United States and Canada, for the year ending June 1965, p. 29. op.cit. (note 99). The other 22 groups of specialists referred to in the text were, in order of frequency: bacteriologists, statisticians, engineers, nutritionists, veterinary surgeons, dentists, chemists, social workers, biologists, physicists, physical therapists, social scientists, industrial hygienists, pharmacists, dental hygienists, accountants, economists, lawyers, architects, historians, optometrists, and physiologists.

cannot restrict its instructional programme to one or two professional groups, rejecting the rest as though they did not exist or, if existing, deemed unworthy of the attention of the school and its faculty.[102]

The degree to which nurses were welcomed into schools of public health varied across the institutions. Johns Hopkins and Harvard gave clear preference to physicians; at Michigan, Minnesota, and North Carolina, nurses were said to be more fully accepted as equal citizens.[103] At Johns Hopkins and Harvard, about 60 per cent of the students were physicians and 12 per cent nurses; among the Johns Hopkins faculty, although 50 per cent of all professors and associate professors were physicians, only one of the 65 was a nurse.[104] Public health nurses were usually a minority, sometimes a small minority, in schools of public health, whereas in health departments, they constituted about half of all public health workers.

In 1962, about 300 nurses were enrolled in masters level programmes of public health nursing; one third of these were in schools of public health and two-thirds in schools of nursing. The deans of schools of public health felt that nursing schools should carry out education to the baccalaureate level, training practitioners, and that schools of public health should take over at the graduate level, educating higher level teachers and administrators.[105] Their view of medical schools and engineering schools was similar; ideally, students would get their basic professional training in these other institutions, and come to schools of public health for postgraduate degrees.

Health education was a growing specialty and a major aspect of the curriculum in many schools of public health, especially at Michigan, North Carolina, the University of California at Berkeley, and the University of Puerto Rico. By 1964, 1800 persons specializing in health

---

[102] Anderson, Gaylord W. (1963). Schools of public health—past—present—future: the present. In *The past, present, and future of schools of public health*, p. 68. University of North Carolina, Chapel Hill.

[103] Report on the teaching of public health nursing in schools of public health to Association of Schools of Public Health, Chapel Hill, North Carolina, 9 April, 1963. Alan Mason Chesney Archives, Johns Hopkins University, RG 1, Box 48.

[104] At the upper ranks, there were nine statisticians, seven biologists, six chemists, four engineers, two physiologists, two economists, and two social scientists. American Public Health Association, Committee on Professional Education, Report of accreditation visit, Johns Hopkins University, School of Hygiene and Public Health, March 24–26, 1964. Alan Mason Chesney Archives, Johns Hopkins University, RG 1, Box 46, 1.

[105] Minutes (1963). Association of Schools of Public Health, Chapel Hill, North Carolina, 9 April, 6–9. Alan Mason Chesney Archives, Johns Hopkins University, RG 1, Box 48.

education had earned masters degrees in schools of public health, and these health educators were much in demand.[106] The Association of Schools of Public Health recommended that all schools of public health appoint full-time faculty with doctoral degrees in health education but stopped short of suggesting that all schools develop specialized health education programmes.[107]

By 1962, the number of schools of public health in the United States had risen to 12. The two most recent were in Puerto Rico, and California (Los Angeles). There were also two Canadian schools of public health—Toronto and Montreal. With expanding research activities and increasing numbers of students, most of the schools were complaining of lack of space and physical plant. Funds for new construction under the Hill–Rhodes Act led to an acceleration of building in seven of the schools.[108] Between 1960 and 1964, the average space occupied by the schools increased by 50 per cent.[109] Within the same period, the number of faculty members also increased by 50 per cent, while the average income of the schools doubled from $1 300 000 to $2 600 000.[110]

In 1963, the dedication of a new building at the School of Public Health at the University of North Carolina at Chapel Hill provided an occasion for public health leaders to reflect on the state of education for public health. Despite the inspiring and generally laudatory remarks that might be expected on such an occasion, the speakers also used the gathering as a forum for wide-ranging criticism. Stebbins, the Dean at Hopkins, argued that most of the problems stemmed from a lack of adequate funding; the schools of public health were like two-thirds of the population of the world, 'ill-housed and ill-fed', without the physical facilities

[106] Boatman, Ralph H. (1965). Professional preparation in health education in schools of public health. A report prepared for the 1965 Annual Meeting of the Association of Schools of Public Health, 22–23. Alan Mason Chesney Archives, Johns Hopkins University, RG 1, Box 48.

[107] Minutes (1965). Association of Schools of Public Health, Report on Health Education. 13 April. Alan Mason Chesney Archives, Johns Hopkins University, RG 1, Box 48. The following year, John Hume, who was Professor of Public Health Administration at Johns Hopkins, reported that his school had been unsuccessful in its 'strenuous efforts' to recruit a full-time faculty member in health education, and that it was 'unlikely' that Hopkins would ever launch a programme of training health educators at the masters level. John C. Hume to Ralph H. Boatman, 12 March 1966. Alan Mason Chesney Archives, Johns Hopkins University, RG 1, Box 48.

[108] Troupin, James L. Schools of public health in the United States and Canada, for the year ending June 1962, p. 5. Alan Mason Chesney Archives, RG 1, Box 41.

[109] Idem. Schools of public health in the United States and Canada, for the year ending June 1964, p. 4. Alan Mason Chesney Archives, Johns Hopkins University, RG 1, Box 41.

[110] Ibid., 5–6.

or finances to train adequate numbers of public health officers.[111] Myron Wegman, Dean of the School of Public Health at the University of Michigan, argued that the schools of public health must do much more to integrate the social and biological aspects of health, while Ruth B. Freeman, a nurse and health administrator from Johns Hopkins, argued for the importance of public health practice: 'All too often the school works on the community instead of in it. The community is seen as a research laboratory, rather than . . . as a reality test for the philosophy and methods being taught'.[112]

Most speakers stressed the need for breadth of intellectual vision; schools should be educating for leadership, not training technicians. Leaders, they agreed, were needed to identify and tackle new problems; their view of public health must be broad and intelligently integrated. In perhaps the most striking statement of this common perception, Ira Hiscock, professor emeritus of public health at Yale who had *de facto* been Dean there, quoted Charles-Edward A. Winslow, his mentor, as follows:

You can train a dog to come to heel, you can train a vine to grow on a wall, you can train an engineer to use a slide rule, you can train a doctor to recognize the rash of measles . . . Education is not learning tricks—techniques . . . An educated person is a person who has learned certain principles and viewpoints, certain criteria that make it possible to go on learning; to go on changing, to go on developing . . . a person isn't much educated unless he is constantly developing vision.[113]

David E. Price, Deputy Surgeon General, provided an encouraging note in stating that community health research was moving up on the federal policy agenda. As its first major item of health legislation, the new administration of John F. Kennedy had passed the Community Health Services and Facilities Act of 1961, authorizing federal project grants for community studies and demonstrations to improve the delivery of out-of-hospital services, especially for the chronically ill.[114] The Health Professions Educational Assistance Act provided grants for the construction of new schools of medicine, dentistry, public health,

---

[111] Stebbins, Ernest L. (1963). The present role of a school of public health. In *The past, present, and future of schools of public health*, p. 57. University of North Carolina, Chapel Hill.

[112] Wegman, Myron E. School of public health—Present, in op.cit. 75 (note 111); Freeman, Ruth B. Schools of public health: the future from the standpoint of a producer of public health personnel, ibid., 93.

[113] Winslow, C–E.A. (1944). Unpublished seminar talk, 9 June. Cited by Hiscock, Ira V. The beginning of our school of public health. In ibid., 40–41.

[114] Price, David E. Federal responsibilities in education for public health, ibid., 153–60.

and nursing and made loans to students with a forgiveness feature which provided incentives to practise in public agencies.

With increased funding for public health at home, there was also growing interest in public health abroad. The newly created Agency for International Development encouraged schools of public health to develop centres for international health training and believed that United States students who entered careers in international health would become 'ambassadors of American science'.[115] Jacques May of the Agency for International Development told the Association of Schools of Public Health that his agency was becoming increasingly concerned about international nutrition and population control.[116] John Hume and Timothy Baker argued the need for three or four centres in the United States with multidisciplinary faculties for research and teaching in international health.[117]

By 1965, the whole nation seemed to have become concerned about the 'population explosion'. Stebbins testified to the Senate Government Operations Subcommittee on Foreign Aid Expenditures in favour of funding for population programmes: 'The health, well-being, and even the peace of the world, is threatened by what has been called the Population Explosion'.[118] Senator George McGovern introduced a bill to give universities long-term funding to provide technical assistance to developing countries.[119] He argued in the Senate that such technical assistance should be regarded as a profitable national investment:

Technical assistance is not an entirely charitable undertaking. It is good

[115] Minutes (1964). Executive session, Association of Schools of Public Health, 7–8 April, University of Toronto School of Hygiene, pp. 6–7. Alan Mason Chesney Archives, Johns Hopkins University, RG 1, Box 48.

[116] Minutes (1965). Association of Schools of Public Health, 12 April, Yale University, p. 4. Alan Mason Chesney Archives, Johns Hopkins University, RG 1, Box 48.

[117] Hume, John C. (1974). Future roles of schools of public health in relation to tropical medicine. In Bowers and Purcell, op.cit. 107–111 (note 98). See also Baker, Timothy D. (1972). Teaching and research in tropical medicine in the United States. *Bulletin of the New York Academy of Medicine*, **48**, 1255–61.

[118] Stebbins, Ernest L. (1965). A statement on Senate Bill S1676, 18 August, p. 3. Alan Mason Chesney Archives, Johns Hopkins University, RG 1, Box 49. John D. Rockefeller III also testified:

Today, in my judgment, no problem is more urgently important to the well-being of mankind than the limitation of population growth. As a threat to our future, it is often compared to nuclear warfare. Population growth is like a lingering, wasting illness; nuclear destruction is like a sudden act of violence. But both endanger the future of life on our planet, or more important perhaps, life as we want it to be.

Statement by John D. Rockefeller III, New York City Chairman of the Board of the Population Council, Inc., before the Senate Government Operations Subcommittee on Foreign Aid Expenditures, 28 July 1965.

[119] Gardner, John W. AID and the universities, pp. 14–15, 47–50. Alan Mason Chesney Archives, Johns Hopkins University. RG 1, Box 49.

business. It is one of the best economic, political and moral investments we can make and we have, in our colleges and universities, institutions with proved ability to get us a high return on our investment.[120]

10. The 1960s and the war on poverty

At home, the 1960s saw the growing power of the civil rights movement, riots in the urban black ghettos, and federal support for the 'war on poverty'. The anti-poverty effort and other Great Society programmes became deeply involved with medical care. Growing concern over access to medical care and hospitalization, especially by the elderly population, culminated in Medicare and Medicaid legislation in 1965 to cover medical care costs for those on social security and for the poor. Both programmes were built on a 'politics of accommodation' with private providers of medical care, thus increasing the incomes of physicians and hospitals, and leading to spiralling costs for medical services.[121] Other anti-poverty programmes, such as the neighbourhood health centres that were intended to encourage community participation in providing comprehensive care to underserved populations, fared less well because they were seen as competing with the interests of private care providers.[122]

The passage of Medicare legislation in 1965 generated considerable excitement in schools of public health.[123] State health agencies were concerned about monitoring and evaluating medical care services and hospital costs; they wanted schools of public health to provide the scientific basis for rational decision-making in health services delivery.[124] State health departments were calling for new administrative personnel at all levels and demanding special training for medical care administrators, financial managers, and survey teams. Milton Roemer of the University of California at Los Angeles estimated in 1966 that there were 6220 new

[120] McGovern, George (1965). A new basis for technical assistance through colleges and universities. *Congressional Record—Senate*, 19 February, p. 1965.

[121] Starr, Paul (1982). *The social transformation of American medicine*, pp. 374–8. Basic Books, New York. The Great Society programmes of the Johnson administration were concerned with social welfare, especially the needs of the poor.

[122] Davis, Karen and Schoen, Cathy (1978). *Health and the war on poverty*. Brookings Institution, Washington, DC.

[123] Report of the Special Study Committee (1966). The role of schools of public health in relation to trends in medical care programs in the United States and Canada. Association of Schools of Public Health, New Orleans, 6 April. Alan Mason Chesney Archives, Johns Hopkins University, RG 1, Box 48.

[124] Thompson, John D. Future roles of schools of public health in relation to state health services, in Bowers and Purcell, op.cit., 95–107 (note 98).

positions in medical care administration requiring graduate educational preparation, including 1370 positions in governmental agencies, 715 in public health agencies, 1515 in health insurance programmes, and 270 in academic institutions.[125] Very few of these new positions were likely to be filled by physicians but all wanted people trained at the masters or doctoral level at schools of public health.

The United States Public Health Service curtailed its usual grant application procedures to provide quick funding for schools of public health willing to provide short training courses in administration.[126] As in the 1930s, short courses would be developed to meet the urgency of the national demand. Seven of the 12 schools of public health already offered extension or continuing education programmes in health services administration—including evening courses, summer school courses, and short-term institutes. In addition to the Medicare and Medicaid programmes, the planning and development of regional centres for heart disease, cancer, and stroke involved five schools of public health affiliated with teaching hospitals.[127]

Schools of public health were now expected to provide trained personnel for the planning, organization, and management of the health care system and to conduct research on the financing and utilization of health services. In 1967, the Association of Schools of Public Health recommended that all schools strengthen their programmes in medical care administration and that every MPH graduate receive adequate instruction in medical care organization within the core curriculum.[128]

As usual, however, there were financial constraints. A slight decrease in Hill–Rhodes funding, together with increasing numbers of both schools and students, meant that each individual school was now receiving considerably less federal support. Herman Hilleboe warned of the urgent need to 'keep the story of the schools of public health before the Public Health Service, Congress, other educational institutions, and the health professions generally'.[129] The Third National Conference on Public Health Training in 1967 reiterated already familiar themes and

[125] Report of the Special Study Committee, p. 9 (note 123).

[126] Ibid., 8.

[127] The purpose of this legislation was to make possible more effective application of knowledge concerning these disorders, to increase the supply of trained manpower, to advance knowledge of the major chronic diseases, and to encourage demonstrations of new methods of patient care. University medical centres were to serve as the focal points of co-ordinated regional programmes of service, training, and research.

[128] Minutes of annual meeting, Association of Schools of Public Health, School of Hygiene, University of Montreal, Canada, May 8–10, 1967, pp. 4–5. Alan Mason Chesney Archives, Johns Hopkins University, RG 1, Box 48.

[129] Ibid., 22.

reported that, despite the gains that had been made, the gap between the demand and supply of appropriately trained public health professionals was still 'increasing at an alarming rate'.[130]

Many of the new health and social programmes of the 1960s had bypassed the structure of the state health departments and set up new agencies to mediate between the federal government and local communities. Medicare and Medicaid reflected the usual priorities of the medical care system in favouring highly technical interventions and hospital care while failing to provide adequately for preventive services. Neighbourhood health centres and community-based mental health services were established without reference to public health departments. When environmental issues attracted public concern and political attention in the 1960s and 1970s, separate agencies were also created to respond to these concerns. At the federal level, the Environmental Protection Agency was created to deal with such issues as solid wastes, pesticides, and radiation. At the state level, environmental agencies were often separate from public health departments and failed to reflect specific health concerns or public health expertise. Similarly, mental health agencies were often separate from public health departments. The broader functions of public health were again split between numerous different agencies; losing a clear institutional base, public health also lost visibility and clarity of definition. For a field that depends so heavily on public understanding and support, such a loss was dangerous.

The schools of public health responded to the new federal initiatives. They developed new programmes in medical care administration, mental health, international health, population control, and environmental health. Increasingly, the schools of public health were training students for a whole range of health programmes; state and local health departments had to compete for graduates with newer international, federal, and state programmes. The link between public health departments and schools of public health weakened as the schools found new and more powerful patrons in the federal government. Students also responded to the new national interest in an expanded definition of public health. In the 1960s, enrolments climbed. Between 1958 and 1973, enrolments in schools of public health quadrupled. The vast majority of students were in masters programmes, but the numbers of doctoral candidates also quadrupled between 1960 and 1971.

[130] *Third national conference on public health training, August 16–18, 1967, Report to the Surgeon General* (1967). United States Department of Health, Education, and Welfare. United States Government Printing Office, Washington, DC.

Beginning in the 1960s, students were attracted to international health, population control, and medical care administration by new federal grants in these areas.[131] Large numbers of students were going into health administration, hospital administration, mental hygiene, health education, maternal and child care, and family planning. About one third of the graduates in the 1960s were employed by public health agencies, one quarter by medical care facilities, one quarter by colleges and universities, and the remainder by international health agencies and voluntary organizations.[132] Seven new schools of public health were accredited between 1965 and 1972 at the Universities of Hawaii, Loma Linda, Oklahoma, Texas, Washington, Massachusetts, and Illinois, and five more schools between 1973 and 1989 at the Universities of South Carolina, Alabama, Boston, San Diego State, and South Florida. Other schools and programmes are currently being established and some are in process of applying for accreditation.[133]

The development of federal health programmes in the 1960s meant new growth for schools of public health but had also made them vulnerable to changes in federal priorities; if federal funds were cut, the schools would have difficulty maintaining their programmes.[134] Programmes could appear and disappear in response to changing federal fashions in research funding.[135] By the early 1970s, more than half the schools' financial support came from the federal government, and in some schools, the figure was as high as 85 per cent.[136]

Between 1966 and 1976, a large number of studies examined the changing role of schools of public health.[137] John Evans argued that schools of public health should educate health executives, planners, and

---

[131] Hume, John C. The future of schools of public health: the Johns Hopkins School of Hygiene and Public Health. In Bowers and Purcell, op.cit., 64 (note 98).

[132] Sheps, Cecil G. Trends in schools of public health in the United States since World War II, ibid., 1–10 (note 98).

[133] Information as of March 1990 from the Council for Education in Public Health, Washington, DC.

[134] Hogness, John R. The future of schools of public health in relation to government. In Bowers and Purcell, op.cit., 124–9 (note 98).

[135] Ramsey, Frank C. Observations of a recent graduate of a school of public health, ibid. 130–3 (note 98).

[136] Summary, ibid. 172–6 (note 98).

[137] Wren, G.R. (1967). Graduate education for hospital administration: a comparison of public health and business school programs. *Hospital Administration*, **12**, 33–64; T. Hall *et al.* (1973). *Professional Health Manpower for Community Health Programs*. School of Public Health, University of North Carolina, Chapel Hill; *Report of Commission on Education for Health Administration* (1975). Ann Arbor, Michigan; *Higher education for public health* (1976). Report of the Milbank Memorial Fund Commission, New York; *Education for health administration: A future agenda* (1977). Vol.3: Ann Arbor, Michigan.

policy makers and provide mid-career training for experienced individuals of different professional backgrounds.[138] He said they should shift the balance of teaching from the administration of institutions to the health of populations, and from the structural, bureaucratic, and financial aspects of health services to organizational behaviour, motivation of providers and consumers, and techniques to improve the quality and effectiveness of health care. The more successful of the schools expanded to include these and many other newer areas of concern, with dynamic new programmes in health policy, environmental and occupational health, international health, chronic diseases, and the problems of ageing.

11. Public health today

The organization of public health continues to show huge variation among the states: in some states, public health may be combined with mental health, with environmental services, with Medicare and Medicaid agencies, or with social welfare agencies. In the 1970s public health departments became providers of last resort of medical care for uninsured patients and for Medicaid patients rejected by private practitioners. By 1988, almost three-quarters of all state and local health department expenditures went for personal health services.[139] As Harry Mustard had predicted some 40 years earlier, direct provision of medical care absorbed much of the limited resources—in personnel, money, energy, time, and attention—of public health departments, leading to a slow starvation of public health and preventive activities.[140] The problem of care for the uninsured and the indigent loomed so large that it eclipsed the need for a basic public health infrastructure in the minds of many legislators and the general public.

In the Reagan revolution of the 1980s, federal funding for public health programmes was cut. Through the mechanism of block grants, power was returned to state health agencies, but in the context of funding cuts, this was the unpopular power to cut existing pro-

---

[138] Evans, John R. (1982). Measurement and management in medicine and health services: training needs and opportunities. In *Health and populations*, p. 19. (ed. M. Lipkin and H. Lybrand). Praeger, New York.

[139] Institute of Medicine, Committee for the Study of the Future of Public Health (1988). *The future of public health*, p. 110. National Academy Press, Washington, DC.

[140] Ibid., 52.

grammes.[141] Given general budget cuts, state health departments were often left the task of managing Medicaid programmes or of delivering personal health services to those lacking private health insurance. State health departments also had to attempt to deal with the adverse health consequences of reductions in other social programmes, and the problems of a growing poverty population, as evidenced in drug abuse, alcoholism, teenage pregnancy, family violence, and homelessness, as well as the health and social needs of growing populations of illegal immigrants.

As Daniel Fox has argued, the AIDS epidemic made obvious a national crisis of authority in the health system and revealed the structural contradictions and weaknesses of national and federal health policy.[142] For state and local health agencies, the AIDS epidemic exacerbated their existing problems and also gave a new visibility and urgency to public health efforts. The public health community agreed that a major national effort was needed in education and prevention. Much of the AIDS funding, when it did come, went into research and medical care; as usual, education and prevention received much less attention. At the same time, the mobilization of public concern provides an opportunity for renewed attention to public health and increased political support. The recent report by the Institute of Medicine, on *The future of public health* notes that:

In a free society public activities ultimately rest on public understanding and support, not on the technical judgment of experts. Expertise is made effective only when it is combined with sufficient public support, a connection acted upon effectively by the early leaders of public health.[143]

Despite the continuing political and economic problems of public health departments, schools of public health are still growing. In 1988, they graduated 3500 students, up from just under 3200 graduates in 1982.[144] These graduates are employed in international, federal, state, and local agencies, in universities, hospitals and medical care institutions, and in foundations, corporations, unions, and consumer organizations

---

[141] Omenn, G.S. (1982). What's behind those block grants in health? *New England Journal of Medicine*, **306**, 1057–60.

[142] Fox, Daniel M. (1988). AIDS and the Amercian health polity: the history and prospects of a crisis of authority. In *AIDS: the burdens of history*, 316–43. (ed. Elizabeth Fee and Daniel M. Fox). University of California Press, Berkeley.

[143] Institute of Medicine, Committee for the Study of the Future of Public Health. *The future of public health*, op.cit., 130 (note 139).

[144] Data on the graduates of schools of public health is available from the Association of Schools of Public Health, 1015 Fifteenth Street N.W., Washington, DC, 20005.

throughout the country. As in earlier years, the demand for public health graduates exceeds the supply.

12. Conclusion

The problems facing schools of public health in the United States have been described. Enormous growth in research grants has, at least in part, overshadowed the traditional commitment to teaching and community service. Research credentials, awards, and publications tend to be valued over public health practice. A declining proportion of faculty has any practical experience in public health and therefore, it may be plausibly argued, is better qualified to prepare students for research than for more practical careers. Solutions to these problems are not easy—it would help if there were funding for teaching programmes, practical internships, and community-based research and practice, which might involve part-time faculty who were prominent practitioners. Without disputing the importance of continuing research, we may note that while the growth in scientific productivity has been remarkable, our ability to implement that knowledge in terms of practical public health has been less impressive.

A continuing theme in the history of education for public health has been the relationship between medical and non-medical public health personnel. It is interesting to note that, of the total graduates of schools of public health in 1988, just over 22 per cent are physicians, 8 per cent nurses, 12 per cent hold other masters degrees, and 4 per cent other doctoral degrees.[145] The proportion of physicians varies considerably between schools, ranging from 5 per cent at the University of Massachusetts to 46 per cent at Harvard. About half of the students with prior medical training come from countries other than the United States, so that overall, about 12 per cent of the graduates of schools of public health are home-grown physicians.

Physicians are thus a minority group in public health and are likely to remain so, unless there is some dramatic shift in the relative reward structure between public health and private medical practice. This is an issue which raises the most fundamental questions of the nature of modern medical care, with its preference for high-technology medicine over funding for preventive services and basic public health. Without a deliberate change in these values, expressed as a willingness to direct financial resources to prevention, public health is unlikely to appeal to

---

[145] The proportion of physicians has been slowly increasing in recent years, up from 18 per cent in 1982.

large numbers of physicians. Those attracted to the field will continue to share with their non-medical colleagues a social commitment that often conflicts with the dominant priorities of the medical system and that transcends the care of the individual patient to focus on the health of populations.

8

The British Diploma in Public Health: heyday and decline

ROY ACHESON

1. The role played by the General Medical Council

By 1900, the struggles and confusion which had been characteristic of
the early years of the Diploma in Public Health had been resolved. In the
halcyon days which followed throughout the reign of Edward VII the
number of candidates successfully attempting the DPH more than doubled. In this chapter we shall see how by the onset of the First World
War new difficulties had developed. These were in the management of
the examination itself, in the adaptation of the syllabus to the changing
needs of the practical world for which it was designed and in its appropriateness for doctors working elsewhere in the British Empire.

Taking the Public Health Act of 1848 as a starting point nearly 30
years of unstructured practical experience were to elapse before any
training was required, and 20 more of plotting and planning before a
proper programme which fitted the professional needs of the medical
officer of health was developed. However, by the turn of the century,
the rules for the Diploma did fit the needs of an English medical officer
of health as a snail fits its shell or a lizard its skin. Just as any reptile
grows, the programme grew, and continued to try to grow but the skin
became stretched to bursting point, and a new skin could not be formed
to fit it. Over the next 75 years the DPH course and examination
became more and more amorphous and the medical officer of health's
working environment more heterogeneous. But neither the government nor the profession changed its view of how education in public
health should be controlled or directed. The General Medical Council
had in 1858 been brought into existence to ensure that young people
who set out to practise medicine were prepared to do so competently,
and that once they had started to practise, they behaved in a morally and
socially acceptable manner. Ten years later, before the Council had
come to terms with these issues of the 'what' and the 'how' of basic

medical education, they were faced with the different, and perhaps more difficult task. They agreed, at the request of the British Medical Association, to create and monitor a specialty which put little if any emphasis on clinical skills and so lay outside orthodox medicine. One reason for this was the marginal nature of public health itself which, as we have seen elsewhere in this book, is not regarded as a specialty of medicine in the United States. A second was that the professional role of the Medical Officer of Health changed more, and more frequently, than that of the clinical practitioner, and it was very much more difficult to draw up, and enforce, an appropriate course schedule. It is therefore hardly surprising that the regulations of the General Medical Council seemed incapable of yielding more than a little. The desire of the various examining boards to maintain autonomy and freedom from official control—especially when this caused extra trouble or expense—was important too. For instance, it was not until the Council's 'Resolutions and Rules' of 1911 introduced the requirement that each candidate had to produce evidence of having attended course(s) in 'sanitary law, vital statistics, epidemiology, school hygiene etc . . . given by a Teacher or Teachers in the Department of Public Health of a recognized Medical School'. Previously, so far as the Council was able to enforce control, it did not matter where or how candidates learned, provided they achieved the required standard in the examination. Another change in that year was to subsume the colourful term 'outdoor work' under 'practical work'—which included laboratory experience—but the substance of the original remained the same.[1] These criticisms notwithstanding, as Elizabeth Fee describes in Chapter 5, W. H. Welch was so impressed with the British system for training that with important modifications, he introduced it to the United States at the Johns Hopkins University.

The General Medical Council had first instituted Resolutions and Rules in 1889;[2] these were modified in 1900, and subsequent to 1911,

---

[1] General Medical Council (1911). *Minutes. Report by the Public Health Committee.* Appendix X: Resolutions and Rules for Diplomas in Public Health, pp. 377–80.

[2] In 1889, the Rules stipulated that:

- a period of at least 12 months should pass between registration, and the presentation of a candidate for the Diploma;
- each candidate, after registration, should have six months' laboratory instruction;
- each candidate should produce evidence of six months' practical instruction under a medical officer of health; and
- the examination, which should be conducted by specially qualified examiners, should comprise laboratory work as well as written and oral examinations.

See General Medical Council (1889). *Minutes.* Appendix V, p. 3; see also Chapters 2 and 3 above.

further reviews involving innovations followed in 1924, 1933, 1937, 1945, 1955, and 1967. Most of them simply attempted to adjust the programme to changes and developments of the role of the medical officer of health. Some of these were scientific, some legal and administrative, and some cultural and political. Recurring issues were whether or not to raise the age and professional maturity at which candidates were eligible to sit the examination, which as Porter indicates, had been an issue from the outset. Another chronic problem was whether or not to increase the duration of instruction in practical work. Successful changes tended to be in detail rather than in spirit. The review of 1955 was a major step backwards and we shall return to this. Finally, the revision of 1962 introduced fundamental changes which set the scene for a new era when the lizard irrevocably burst its skin.

The revision of 1924

The 1920s were a time of reassessment. In 1924, the Public Health Committee of the Council reacted strongly in favour of the report of Bruce Low, the second inspector. A few months after it had been submitted, the General Medical Council's Public Health Committee introduced changes in the Resolutions and Rules for the Diploma in Public Health. There were three principal considerations behind these changes, as follows:

(1) the course in public health was too short;
(2) the scope of study was too limited and should be extended; and
(3) the standard of the examination should be raised.

Allocation of time for teaching was prescribed in detail. It was proposed, not for the first time, that the curriculum should extend over 12 months not just three university terms; thus, if his period of clinical work was taken into account, the new diplomate would have to have two full years of postgraduate experience (Rule 1). Five months were to be spent studying bacteriology, parasitology, and chemistry and physics; 220 hours of them in the laboratory (Rule 3). Over and above this, 100 hours were required in other classroom work, such as public health and sanitation, epidemiology, vital statistics, meteorology, and climatology (Rule 4). To set out in detail the hours of teaching to be devoted to each subject was new, but was consistent with the Council's approach to basic medical education, and also to the requirement of 1911 that candidates must attend appropriate courses. Rule 5 required three months' experience in a hospital for infectious disease and Rule 6 at least six months outdoor work referred to as 'acquiring practical knowledge of the duties, routine and special, of Public Health Administration'. These duties were spelt out. Rules 7, 8, and 9 were concerned with the conduct of the examination.[3] Epidemiology, which had been considered to be of some importance in the earliest days of the diploma, but became overshadowed by bacteriology, at last emerged as a subject in its own right with a required 20 hours in the curriculum, to which were to be added 10 hours of vital statistics. This was just three years before Major Greenwood was to be appointed to the first chair in epidemiology and vital statistics in Britain at the London School of Hygiene and Tropical Medicine.

The revision of 1933

Next to that of 1967, the revision of 1933 was the most far-reaching. It was stimulated by the Royal Colleges of Physicians and Surgeons in London because of important new duties of medical officers of health which had been set out in the Local Government Act of 1929. These put vaccination, infant life protection, care of the mentally ill, and the power to develop their own hospital services in the hands of the local authorities.[4] As the chief medical officer to local government, the medical officer of health therefore now had added curative to the preventive services which were already under his control. In 1936, the Midwives Act appended to this formidable list control of the domiciliary service provided by trained midwives, who worked with general practitioners; thus there was a considerable extension of the size and nature of their practice. The General Medical Council had recognized the enlarged responsibilities by stating that as candidates passed from their state of pupillage as medical students, to that of established practitioners, they should be able to give mature consideration to the obligations and duties involved in the work of the Public Health Service. They should 'acquire direct experience of medical work in a responsible capacity, in general medical practice, in hospital or laboratory appointments, or in any branch of clinical work or study related to State Medicine'. The statement continues: 'In the public interest, the time has arrived to adapt the Diploma or Degree to candidates who are seriously intending to take up Public Health as a career'.[5] This recognizes the fact that previously a significant proportion of diplomates never registered their qualification, and therefore were ineligible to become medical officers of health in any but the small authorities (see figure 2.2 page 75).

No longer, so far as the Council is concerned, is the examination for

[3] General Medical Council (1921). *Minutes*. Report of the Public Health Committee, pp. 500–7.
[4] Ibid. (1931). Appendix VII, 363–6.
[5] Ibid. (1931). Appendix XIX, 432.

the Diploma simply a method of determining whether a candidate has enough skill and experience to accept the statutorily defined responsibilities of a single post. Instead, it is seen as being a step in the professional training of any doctor who wants to work in the general field of public health. Thus an important milestone in the history of postgraduate specialist training in Britain is passed, but it also makes an unhealable, if incomplete, rupture in the membrane containing the DPH.

These changes may seem trivial to us today, but they were not trivial in the eyes of the university schools where the teaching had to be done. Indeed, the time lapse between the passing of the 1929 Public Health Act, and the receipt by the Council of the letter from the Royal Colleges may very well have been occasioned by foot-dragging on the part of the universities. So, anxious to ensure that they were implemented undiluted, the Council took the unprecedented step in its history before and since, of promulgating them without previous discussion or consultation. The Council was roundly upbraided for this, but the new regulations stuck.

The prescription of study time was developed further. For Part I, laboratory and classroom study were increased from 100 to 280 hours (some of which still had to be devoted to meteorology and climatology in relation to Public Health, which was finally to be dropped six years later).[6] The Council, moreover, emphasized that its recommendations about duration of course work were minimal. They encouraged universities to extend them as they saw fit, and pointed out that, *in toto*, recommended instruction amounted to 630 hours which should be considered against a lower limit in the ordinary full academic year of 900 hours.[7]

Two innovations, which had a direct bearing on the new responsibilities of the medical officer of health, were required for Part I of the examination. The first was course work in radiology and electrology in relation to public health:

to enable him to be in a position to advise his Local Authority on the therapeutic purpose and utility of artificial light, radiology and electrology, on the appropriate equipment and installation, on the staffing, on the precautions necessary to fulfil the conditions of the National Physical Laboratory, on the selection and subsequent supervision of the patients, on the general management of a radiological and electrical department [in hospital].[8]

One reason for widespread objections to this was that new lecturers would be required, to which the Council replied 'medical schools

6 Ibid. (1937). Appendix VIII, 304–8.
7 Ibid. (1931). Appendix VII, 366.
8 Ibid., 364.

should have little difficulty in providing the type of practical instruction required'; another was that the newly required 280 hours for the course for Part I would be insufficient.[9] The second innovation was the introduction of physiology and biochemistry in their application to nutrition and hygiene. This, of course, was to prepare the medical officer of health for his new concern for, in the words of the legislature, 'infant life protection'. But as the Council pointed out, physiology and biochemistry had 'practical application in the promotion of the general health' and 'an intimate relation . . . [with] . . . the various applications of Radiology'.

The emphasis in clinical and curative medicine was extended. To instruction in maternal and child health and school health, which was required by the 1924 revision, was added in 1933 a requirement to be familiar with mental hygiene, mental health services, and hospital services. Once all attempts to restrict the DPH to its original purpose were abandoned, there was pressure for changes which were a little more far-reaching, but the nature of the Council's responsibilities was such that they were always cautious. The indignation of the Irish schools, who continued to look towards the General Medical Council for the setting and enforcement of standards, was justifiable because the Irish Free State had been independent from Britain for over a decade and the Local Government Act of 1929 had no relevance there.

The revision of 1946: the Certificate in Public Health

During the later war years it seems that none of the six examining bodies, which were our central concern in Chapter 2, were active, nor did the Public Health Committee of the General Medical Council meet between 1942 and 1945 when it reconvened under the chairmanship of Sir Wilson Jameson, who in 1929 had become the first Professor of Public Health in the London School of Hygiene and Tropical Medicine. By then he was also Dean. He was more intimately concerned with teaching and examining in postgraduate public health than anyone else in the country at that time, and than any chairman of the Public Health Committee since Sir Richard Thorne Thorne who had played a critical role in the effective implementation of the original rules during the last years of the nineteenth century. Jameson was aware first hand of the difficulties involved in matching the training of his students to the needs of the service for which they were preparing themselves. During the summer of 1945, the new proposals were generally accepted and became operative on 1 January 1946. The whole process was completed within six months

[9] Ibid., 366.

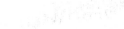

which was remarkable. The reason in part no doubt was the sense of freedom from the shackles of war.

A further attempt to extend the course achieved no more than to require candidates to commit themselves to an academic year of full-time study, or 18 months to their part-time studies. Here was a real innovation. Basic course work was to be recognized by the issuance of a Certificate in Public Health. Candidates who sought to pursue a career as a medical officer of health received their Diploma when they had satisfactorily completed their practical work, but the Certificate was intended to be a free-standing qualification for those who did not want to undertake a full apprenticeship. The idea was that men and women who wished to be appointed to specialized posts in many branches of public health, other than that of medical officer of health, would be able to acquire a knowledge of suitable standard of problems in the field of 'Preventive and Social Medicine'.[10] Certificates were not formally regis-trable by the Council, although the Public Health Committee kept a tally of the certificands and summary statistics were published in the Council Minutes. The instruction and the standards for it were, of course, monitored because they were part of the basic requirements for the DPH.

The experiment was not a success and the option was withdrawn. Almost without exception those taking the certificate went on to take the Diploma even though they had no intention of becoming medical officers of health. The reason given by the President, Sir David Camp-bell, in his address in 1953 was the introduction of the National Health Service in 1948 which, although it left the medical officer of health in the employment of the Local Authorities, reduced his responsibilities. The President also blamed another consequence of the creation of the National Health Service namely, the 'institution of a compulsory year of House Officer Service' [11] (that is to say internship). In effect, this now meant immediate employment with pay—albeit minimal pay—and board and lodging for every newly qualified doctor in the country. Heretofore most hospitals offered a pittance (indeed some of the great London teaching hospitals went so far as to charge house officers for the privilege of working with them). Other newly qualified doctors had gone straight into general practice through serving as locums or junior partners; or in many cases by putting their nameplate on the door and waiting for patients to ring the bell. Public health still had, as had been the case from Victorian times, the special attraction of providing a steady salary almost from the outset. Now, however, it faced serious

[10] Ibid. (1945). Appendix VIII, 219–35.
[11] Ibid. (1953). 5, 6.

competition in that respect. Although the revision of Rules in 1955 withdrew the provision for the award of a Certificate in Public Health, the breadth of the curriculum was further increased. It included, for instance, 'educating the public as to the promotion and maintenance of health', aftercare and rehabilitation, and International Health Organizations. The lizard was now bulging in its ageing skin; we shall see at the end of the chapter how, when it finally burst out free in 1967, it was too late for it to survive.

2. Pressures from the Empire

Thus in response to development and change in the scientific bases of public health, and in the national policy for organizing health services, our lizard did not grow because for a while after the turn of the century everything seemed to have been put right. However, new problems were developing. The skin which seemed to fit so well purported to be British, but in reality was tailored to one part of the British Isles, namely England; the public health service in Scotland was similar, but in Ireland there were considerable differences.[12] Wales, for want of political influence, was bracketed with England. As England required many more medical officers than the other countries combined, little attention was paid to the needs of the rest. Even at its best, therefore, the DPH did not fully achieve its highly specific objectives. The variations in political, economic, and cultural setting were increasingly to put the relevance of the qualification in public health, as it evolved, in question.

The British doctor abroad

The Edwardian era was a time when the territorial gains of Victoria's reign required consolidation involving the deployment of the armed forces throughout the British Empire. With this went an expansion of colonial administration and medical services. The army and the navy recruited doctors by supporting them through their medical studies and many of them were posted abroad. It was in the interests of the service and of these doctors that they should become eligible to sit the DPH, but what was the relevance of their experiences in the tropics to the purposes for which the DPH was introduced? The matter came to a head in the General Medical Council when the question arose as to whether the circumstances of their practical training could be considered outdoor work, in accordance with the Rules and Recommendations. A cautious

[12] For example, *Local Government Board (Ireland) Act* (1872). [35 & 36 Vict., Chapter 69].

start was made in 1903 by the War Office, which asked the Public Health Committee to recommend the recognition of service in Gibraltar, where, it was pointed out, a sizeable civilian population received its medical care from the forces. The request was acceded to,[13] and was soon followed by others, made on similar grounds, for doctors working under appropriate supervision in Calcutta and the Punjab. By 1911, in addition to these, outdoor work in Malta, Burma, and seven military commands in India had been approved.[14] This no doubt was a splendid experience for the public health doctor in the tropics, but it was an experience which would be of little value to an army or naval medical officer when he retired to take up the post of medical officer of health in, for example, an English shire.

The foreign doctor in Britain

Experiential unsuitability took a different form a decade or so later in the 10 years immediately following the First World War. By then, several medical schools had been founded throughout the Empire, particularly in India, and they were producing high-quality graduates recruited from among the indigenous population. A few of the best of these schools were formally recognized by the Council so that their alumni were eligible to register and sit for the DPH. However, the training experience they obtained in Britain was no more suitable for practice when they returned to their own country, than that of the discharged officer when he returned home having obtained his initial practical experience overseas. Because their degrees were not acceptable to the General Medical Council for registration, medical graduates from the majority of Empire schools were, however, automatically barred from eligibility for the diploma. Nevertheless, a British qualification, and particularly one recognized by the Council, carried with it considerable cachet. This was at a time when universities had to find all their funds from extra-governmental sources, and the examining boards were anxious to attract as many candidates as they could, regardless of residence or nationality.

It was thus in order to get around the rigidity of the law that the University of Cambridge introduced the Diploma in Hygiene which was neither more nor less than a renamed rose. Candidates need not have their names on the medical register, although they were required to have medical qualifications. They attended the same courses as the Diploma in Public Health candidates, and took the same examination. Indeed, in the last years of the Cambridge DPH examination, the two groups of

---

[13] General Medical Council (1903). *Minutes.* Appendix XIII: Report of the Public Health Committee. 29 May, p. 803.
[14] General Medical Council (1911). *Minutes.* Appendix X, p. 380.

candidates were not distinguished in the published pass lists.[15] This met the needs of those who sought, what the President of the General Medical Council was to call, 'a creditable decoration' from Cambridge University, albeit one without the imprimatur of the Council.[16] It was no more than a procedural device which no doubt swelled the coffers of the university treasury, and can be looked upon as a gesture of goodwill towards public health in the Empire. On the other hand, however, it was an expression of disdain which can have done nothing to achieve the very high standards, the attainment of which had been central to the establishment of the Special Syndicate described in the next section, nor did it support the General Medical Council in its effort to sustain national excellence. Finally, as we have just indicated, the qualification provided a highly questionable basis for tropical practice, a fact which puts the scruples of those concerned at question.

Moreover, a step had already been taken at Cambridge to meet the needs of doctors seeking training in tropical public health by the establishment shortly after the First World War of a Diploma in Tropical Medicine and Hygiene under the direction of G. H. F. Nuttall. This was available to 'any person whose name [was] on the Medical Register'. To possess it certified expertise 'in the nature, causes, prevention and treatment of Epidemic and other diseases peculiar to Tropical Countries and in the means of remedying or ameliorating those Circumstances and Conditions life therein which are known to be injurious to health'.[17] It lacked the imprimatur of the General Medical Council because it had nothing whatever to do with the work of the medical officer of health. Soon, the new School of Hygiene and Tropical Medicine would be proposing to offer its own diploma in this subject, with the backing of far stronger teaching resources than Cambridge was able to muster. In the meantime, however, the Cambridge Diploma under Nuttall proved popular and represented a serious attempt to meet the needs of those who intended to practice curative and preventive medicine in the tropics. External pressures were, nevertheless, brought to bear on the General Medical Council to broaden its definition of eligibility for admission to the examination for the DPH itself, and thereby to allow it to be used for a purpose for which it was not designed. Attempts were also made to persuade the Council to recognize the Diplomas in Tropical Hygiene and Medicine.

'But', said Sir Donald Macalastair in his presidential address in 1923,

---

[15] The *Cambridge University Reporter* lists the names of those receiving Diplomas a few days after the examinations.

[16] General Medical Council (1923). *Minutes*, pp. 8–9.

[17] University of Cambridge Archives (1922). [Min VI 53], 27 October.

'I venture to submit that the Medical Council has no Statutory Powers to control [these] studies or to recognize [these] certificates. They concern only such Medical Authorities who quite properly grant them, and they are not registrable in the Medical Register'. He continued ' . . . the course for the [DPH] must therefore not be modified and diverted from its primary and essential purpose, merely in order that the same Diploma may conveniently afford a creditable decoration for practitioners who contemplate careers other than that of the professional Medical Officer of Health'.[18] A state of siege had been declared by the outposts of the Empire on headquarters; 10 years later the walls of the fortress began to crack and after 10 further years they were breached. In a word, these new diplomas were raising searching questions about the viability of a qualification which even at a domestic level had proved to lack in flexibility what it might have gained in pragmatism. Eventually, through the Medical Act of 1950, the inevitable happened and the Council was given power to register a Diploma in Public Health acquired in a School in a Commonwealth country.[19] The first to be recognized was awarded by the University of Malaya in Kuala Lumpur[20]—hardly a suitable environment for providing training for a candidate for the post of Medical Officer of Health in England. No Diploma in Tropical Medicine and Hygiene was ever accepted as being registrable by the Council, but the Diploma in Tropical Public Health was so recognized in 1971. This was an indication of the confusion of the times, for the training it provided had little bearing on the work of a medical officer of health.

3. Standards, degrees, and economics

So much for some of the effects of the statutory law and world politics on the DPH. Another influence of equal or greater importance through the years has been that of the market. Economists are continually reminding us that we cannot spend the same dime twice; they phrase this more technically by saying that if we derive a benefit from a resource we forego all other benefits that might have been derived from that resource. It is instructive to consider the history of the DPH from

---

[18] General Medical Council (1923). *Minutes*, pp. 8 and 9; Sir Donald Macalastair was appointed to the General Medical Council in 1889 by the University of Cambridge where he was Professor of Anatomy. He became President in 1904, and four years later returned to his native Scotland to take the Chair of Anatomy in Glasgow. He finally retired after a presidency of 27 years and 42 years' service in all. Both are records. The Council has now restricted the duration of the presidency to seven years.

[19] Medical Act of 1950. [14 Geo. 6, Chapter 26].

[20] General Medical Council (1954). *Minutes*. Appendix VI, p. 241.

that standpoint because to do so gives insight to how the various examining boards had to trade off the unacceptability of high standards against the numbers of candidates they desired. In order to obtain this perspective we must turn again to events in the Edwardian era.

As the success of the national DPH programme had waxed with achievements in Cambridge, so, it would seem, the former waned with the latter. Between 1875 and the mid-1920s, Cambridge produced more diplomates than any other board and in the early days was one of the leaders in the establishment of standards, so that this is unlikely to have been a chance relationship. It so happened that Bruce Low, to whom we will return again later, had been an external examiner there from 1912 until 1915. In response to an enquiry about the maintenance of standards from the General Medical Council, he and J. E. Purvis, the lecturer in chemistry and hygiene at Cambridge who by then was responsible for the administration of the DPH there,[21] wrote separately in reply to the Council to explain that the 89 per cent pass rate in 1914 was, so far as they could tell, because the candidates were of exceptional quality.[22] The Council accepted this contention grudgingly, pointing out that there was no supportive evidence. The English Conjoint, which by then was vying closely with Cambridge for numbers of successful candidates, had similarly attracted unfavourable attention, but had answered more satisfactorily.[23] Satisfactory or not, these letters were a clear sign of deep concern in the General Medical Council.

Indications that all was not well

The numbers of examining bodies were slowly increasing, and their wares were varied. By 1918, 21 universities and boards offered a registrable qualification in Public Health; in 16 this was a DPH only, and in one, London, as we have seen in Chapter 2, it was the MD in State Medicine. Two others offered the DPH together with a variety of degrees. The Public Health Committee of the General Medical Council showed the basis of its concern about the standards by publishing tables showing considerable variation in numbers attempting the examination and in pass rates.

Some data from their analysis are given in Table 8.1. They are derived from material supplied to the Committee by the examining bodies; because very few of the candidates who failed Part I eventually proceeded to Part II, the 'number of candidates' column is taken as those presenting themselves for Part I, and the number of successes as

---

[21] Ibid. (1917). Appendix III, 288.

[22] General Medical Council (1917). *Minutes*. Appendix III, pp. 285–7.

[23] Ibid. (1917). Appendix III, 288.

Table 8.1. Candidates attempting a Diploma or Degree in Public Health, 1905–14. Ranked by numbers of candidates attempting examination[a]

	No. of candidates attempting		No. obtaining qualification	Failure rate (%)	
	Pt. I	Pt. II		of all entrants	of Pt. II entrants only
University of Cambridge (1875)	640	547	440	31.3	19.6
English Conjoint (1884)	636	469	367	42.3	21.7
Irish Conjoint (1892) (one part only)	385		261	38.2	
Scottish Conjoint (1891)	379	370	241	36.4	34.9
Victoria University, Manchester (1887)	193	178	131	32.1	26.4
University of Oxford (1876)	176	149	83	52.8	44.3

(None of the other Part II examinations for 22 qualifications offered by 12 universities were attempted by 100 or more candidates over the 10 years.)

	Statistics for the two pioneer universities				
University of Edinburgh (1875) B.Sc.	27	34[b]	25	—	26.5
D.Sc.	10	7	7	33.3	0
University of Dublin (1871)	82	72	56	31.8	22.2

[a] Report of the Public Health Committee of the General Medical Council. (*Minutes* (1917) 26 May).
[b] Some candidates who could show satisfactory evidence of appropriate previous experience were exempted Part I, and proceeded directly to Part II.

those passing Part II.[24] For instance, between 1905 and 1914, 176 candidates sat the examination in Oxford and 640 in Cambridge. Of these 56 per cent were successful in the former and 80 per cent in the latter, but the matter of special concern was that in one year, 1914, only five of 49 (10 per cent) failed in Cambridge compared with 11 of 22 (50 per cent) in Oxford. The General Medical Council therefore wrote again to the licensing

[24] Ibid. (1917). 275–83.

bodies, asking for information about the qualifications they offered, and the syllabus and examining methods for each. The final outcome was that on 31 May 1919 the Council decided that all examining bodies should again be inspected and Dr Bruce Low was appointed to undertake the work.

The doubts of the General Medical Council were not misplaced; neither the University of Cambridge nor the English Conjoint came out well from Bruce Low's visitation. He lacked George Duffey's wit but had a similarly subtle method of grading the examinations he inspected. Like Duffey, to convey his opinions, Low relied on a subtle array of nuances in the published descriptions of what he had seen.[25]

After submitting his original published reports, he was invited to discuss *in camera* his observations at a special meeting of the Council's Public Health Committee. Originally he had written of the Cambridge examination that 'it furnishes an efficient test of the competent knowledge of the candidate' and added that it was 'conducted with care and thoroughness and that the candidates who succeed in passing must possess a distinctively high proficiency, both scientific and practical'.[26] However, it seems that that was not quite the way he really saw it, for in the document which reported his talks with the Public Health Committee, and for which he was jointly responsible, the assessment of each examining body was summarized in three lines. Of the six examinations which have been our principal concern in Chapter 2, that at the University of London was considered to be of a 'very high standard' (which we may classifiy as alpha); Dublin, Edinburgh, and Oxford of a 'high standard' (beta) and in the third division, the gammas, were the Cambridge test which was considered to be 'efficient', and the London Conjoint '. . . in my opinion, quite satisfactory'. No superlatives for either, which was a turnabout from the days when Cambridge was top dog and the Public Health Medical Society was concerned about low standards in the University of London. A competitor with these two examining boards for popularity and questionable standards was Victoria University at Manchester where 'the examination requires a good standard of knowledge' (another gamma). The three of them had attracted over 50 per cent of all the candidates in the country during the decade 1905–14; there was a clear association between large numbers of candidates and high pass rates.

[25] Whether or not as a consequence of their labours, no one can say; neither man survived the experience of inspecting single-handed all the Diploma examinations in the United Kingdom for more than a year or two. Whatever the reason, subsequent rounds of inspections of the DPH were conducted by members of the Council's Public Health Committee themselves.

[26] General Medical Council (1920). *Minutes.* University of Cambridge, Public Health Examinations report and remarks by the Inspector, pp. 596–605.

Nor were low fees the explanation for the attractiveness of these Boards to candidates. Low's reports tell us that the overall fees for the two parts of the examination ranged between £10 and £12 with the single exception of the English Conjoint, which for those who were not licentiates of either of the colleges cost £21. Despite constant and conscientious monitoring it seemed that central control on behalf of the state had not been as successful as might have been hoped.

Education by examination

There was one very specific respect in which the examining bodies established by the Conjoint Boards of the Royal Colleges differed from the universities. In basic medical education, with the exception of the Royal College of Surgeons in Ireland, which prepared candidates for entry on the Medical Register,[27] none of the Royal Colleges taught, either at the undergraduate level, or for the DPH.

Successful candidates had no contact with the Colleges, nor had they privileges of any kind in them; they were simply awarded a document as an indication of their achievement, and thus were allowed to enter their names on the medical register as competent to practise public health.[28] The avoidance by the Colleges of providing instruction to candidates made no difference to the control the General Medical Council could exert over the DPH, however, because this was confined to deciding on the content of Rules determining eligibility for the examination and to conducting formal inspections to satisfy itself fully as to the nature and quality of an examination.[29] In contrast to their approach to basic medical education, they never inspected course work.

Degrees and diplomas

There were other important differences between the universities themselves. First, as we have seen, Edinburgh, from 1875 to 1915; London from 1890 to 1931; and Cambridge from 1868 and for some time thereafter, awarded degrees in public health (or state medicine) as, later, did for example Durham, Glasgow, Manchester, Birmingham, and other universities. Edinburgh, as we have also seen, required from the outset their students to prepare for the examination by taking at least one rel-

---

[27] Widdess, J.D.H. (1949). *An account of the schools of surgery: the Royal College of Surgeons, Dublin 1789–1948*. Livingstone, Edinburgh.

[28] Cooke, A.M. (1974), op. cit., Chapter 2 (note 73).

[29] General Medical Council (1893). *Minutes: Report of Education Committee*. Appendix V, Regulations of the Licensing Bodies granting Diplomas in State Medicine, pp. 8–9.

evant university course and by giving evidence of having received satis-factory instruction elsewhere; extra-mural instruction in medical sub-jects had been a tradition in Edinburgh throughout the nineteenth century and before. In the long run, students there, as elsewhere, were expected to do their course work internally.

Bruce Low was an alumnus of Edinburgh University but chose to take his DPH at Cambridge, where, as we have seen he was also an examiner.[30] This experience, when he became Inspector, must have helped to give him insight into what he found because the philosophies of those two universities were very different. There is evidence from both Low and Duffey that not only was the syllabus for university degrees probably more detailed and far-reaching than for diplomas, but that the standards of the examinations themselves tended to be higher than those for the certificates and diplomas awarded both by Conjoint Boards and by universities. This should, of course, have been the case because the status of a degree is always deemed to be higher than that of a diploma. In 1920, the year of Bruce Low's inspection, the University of Edinburgh introduced the DPH because of the fall in popularity of their science degrees (see Table 8.1). He found the examination for the new Diploma to include subjects 'not usually required by other bodies, and that candidates had to give evidence of a wide range of knowl-edge'.[31] This presumably implies that knowledge and standards for the B.Sc. which had last been held in 1915, were equally, if not even more exacting. It might therefore have been expected that the cachet of a university degree combined with more thorough training would have attracted a steady, if not large, flow of the better students. This does not seem to have been the case.

A summary is given in Table 8.1, and in Figures 2.1 and 2.2, Chapter 2, of the detailed data which the General Medical Council published about entrants, successes, and failures in the exams set by the various boards from 1890 until the end of the First World War in 1918, when the procedure was discontinued in the interest of economy.[32]

Over those 29 years, out of many more than 5000 candidates, there were only 168 entrants for the Edinburgh B.Sc. degree examination. In contrast, 1574 sat for the Cambridge DPH, and 2279 for the three Con-joint Board examinations; 1143 of them in the Royal Colleges in Lon-don, 584 in Edinburgh, and 552 in Dublin. If the B.Sc. in the University

---

[30] Biographical information in *Who's Who* and the *Medical Directory*.

[31] General Medical Council (1895). *Minutes*. Appendix XVII, pp. 625–39; ibid. (1921). 716–25.

[32] Ibid. (1917). Appendix III, loc cit., 275–90.

of Edinburgh had little appeal, the D.Sc. in public health there, with its advanced course work and research-based thesis, was even less popular. Only 34 of the 168 (20 per cent) successfully attempted it. Similar doctoral degrees were offered in Durham and Birmingham, but attracted even less interest.

The requirements for them differed considerably from those for the MD in state medicine in London. Between 1876 and 1889 London University had held an examination for the 'Certificate in Subjects relating to Public Health', of which 12 were awarded. This was then discontinued and an MD by examination and thesis succeeded it. This, in addition to the subjects laid down by the General Medical Council as necessary for registration, included a long clinical case in state medicine and a paper on mental health. The 87th, and last MD in state medicine was awarded to a candidate from the London School of Hygiene and Tropical Medicine in 1933. Its emphasis on mental health meant that by no means all its laureates took it with the intention of following a career in public health, however.[33]

Although degrees had little appeal, the number of successful diploma candidates steadily increased, so that there were 2.5 times as many in 1914 as there had been in 1895. Moreover, the proportion of these who registered their diplomas, and therefore presumably seriously contemplated a career in public health, changed from 2 of 155 (1.5 per cent) in 1890, to 132 of 238 (55 per cent) in 1914, and 49 of 62 (79 per cent) in 1918. (See Table 8.1 and Fig. 2.2, p. 75). One can only conclude that for most candidates the practical appeal of learning the application of technology greatly outweighed acquiring any kind of insight into technology itself or the sciences that underlay it. Nor, it seems, did the prestige of a university degree have any allure for those who were attracted to a career in public health.

It would appear that in England, Ireland, and Scotland alike, the most popular way for a young doctor to prepare himself for examination prior to such a career in public health was to take 'commercial courses' which may or may not have been run in universities. As late as 1896, Harvey Littlejohn, Sir Henry's son, who was to succeed him to the Edinburgh Chair, obtained from the Senatus Academicus, at a time when he had no university appointment, 'the recognition of his course of instruction in Medical Jurisprudence and Public Health and having

---

[33] Many of the statistics relating to the numbers of degrees and diplomas awarded by the various examining boards appear in the published minutes of the General Council. Almost all of the gaps have been filled from the Calendars or Minutes of the examining bodies and in a few instances from unpublished archives.

inspected Dr Littlejohn's teaching accommodation and his appliances, the Faculty recommend that Dr Littlejohn's application [to act as an extra-mural instructor] should be granted'.[34] In 1907, Henry Kenwood, who had succeeded William Corfield to the Chair of Hygiene in University College, London, records that practical instruction 'especially designed for Diploma work' was offered in the department of bacteriology and pathology, and that 13 of his own students had been successful in the Cambridge and Conjoint examinations.[35] As we have seen, by 1911 all students were required to take a course given by a university department; it was within the letter if not the spirit of the law that in 1938, six candidates who were enrolled as university students studying in the London School of Hygiene and Tropical Medicine achieved registration by taking the London Conjoint DPH.[36] This, therefore, was technical training indeed; no pandering to the wide horizon of education, or to such woolly concepts as the broadening of the mind. Health officers were practical men seeking practical instruction to do a practical job.

Issues in maintaining standards in one university

Because the pressures and problems experienced in Cambridge in the 1920s are illustrative of the national scene, there follows in some detail a description of how several closely interrelated factors, namely rigidity of curriculum, a need for revenue, the conflicts between these, and the maintenance of standards, together with a shortage of indigenous candidates seeking to pursue a career as medical officers of health, brought about the termination of the Cambridge course.

In 1922, the General Medical Council sent out copies of Low's detailed comments to all examining bodies, each of which had to reply. In Cambridge they were not at all gratified. To be described as 'quite satisfactory' by an alumnus of their own diploma course who was also one of their former examiners, must have been galling for an institution which justifiably believed that its standards were in general of the highest.

The University reacted rapidly, and in December of that year, a few

---

[34] University of Edinburgh (1897). *Senatus Academicus Minutes.* 28 October, p. 172.

[35] Watkins, Dorothy E. (1984). The English revolution in social medicine, 1889–1911. Ph.D. thesis. University of London; see also Chapter 3 for further comments on the development of academic public health in London in the late ninteenth and early twentieth centuries.

[36] London School of Hygiene and Tropical Medicine (1938). *9th Annual Report.*

days after the General Medical Council had published its new Rules, a 'special' Syndicate was established by the Council of the Senate to consider the duties of the long-established State Medicine Syndicate and the diplomas it controlled.[37] The new Syndicate faced serious problems. Were standards so low as to reflect unfavourably on the University? With a new specialist so-called 'Institute of Hygiene' to be built in London (see below), would Cambridge have any useful role to play in post graduate education in public health in the future? Were the courses which were presented in preparation for it still appropriate?[38]

The Syndicate sat half-a-dozen times, and in addition to members of the University, took evidence from the Chief Medical Officer, Sir George Newman, and Sir Walter Fletcher, Secretary of the Medical Research Council. Sir George Newman spoke of a new 'Imperial and International School of Hygiene', the general design of which would be to qualify men for diplomas in health and cognate subjects. It would be affiliated to the University of London and it was hoped that all London courses in public health would be absorbed by it. He also believed, however, that other courses outside London, at the small provincial universities, would be continued. It might, he thought, be possible for general practitioners to take the Diploma. Also, Cambridge could well adopt a higher standard—again a clear indication that things there were not all they might be. The special Syndicate, and those who gave evidence to it, were of one mind with him.

The most intriguing statement of all, however, and highly relevant to the whole issue of maintaining standards, was that made by G. H. F. Nuttall, who by then was Quick Professor of Parasitology, but previously had been Reader in Hygiene.[39] He had for many years been responsible for the teaching of bacteriology to public health students, and was very familiar both with the course and the examination. His successor as teacher of bacteriology to Diploma candidates was G. S. Graham-Smith, to whose skills as a teacher and research worker Nuttall had glowingly referred when the former had successfully supported the

---

[37] This is confusing, for the term *syndicate* has been used in Cambridge in two different contexts. One is of a standing committee with considerable fiscal independence, power, and responsibility for examinations. Such was the Syndicate in State Medicine. The term is also used for an *ad hoc* working-party established to consider matters of major importance to the University and the *Syndicate on the Duties and Responsibilities of the State Medicine Syndicate* was one such.

[38] In addition to Public Health, Tropical Medicine and Hygiene, to which we have already referred, Cambridge offered a diploma in Psychological Medicine, and another in Medical Radiology and Electrology.

[39] *Cambridge University Reporter* (1906). pp. 638–40.

candidature of the latter for a new Readership in Preventive Medicine.[40] We have already referred in Chapter 2 to the derision with which he looked upon the teaching of chemistry. C. Fraser Brockington, the public health historian who took the DPH in Cambridge in 1929, provided independent confirmation of this; he also described the teaching of Graham-Smith as magnificent and that in chemistry and physics as lamentable.[41] Nuttall went on to ask: 'Should the chemistry and physics of public health not be left to the analyst?'[42] The question of the relevance of these two subjects to the Diploma course was also being posed in London, but failed to stimulate change there either.

A further factor which kept standards of instruction down was the poor quality of some of the students in the new mixed group because combined classes were held for candidates for all three diplomas.[43] Neither in chemistry, nor in bacteriology, could it be assumed that all of the students had a sound basic knowledge of either or both subjects. The needs of the weakest had to be met, and consequently it was not possible to include advanced material, which Graham-Smith for one, considered to be appropriate to, if not essential for, the needs of the medical officer of health of the day.

Achieving any kind of excellence presented a dilemma to the special Syndicate in other ways. Despite unanimity that something should be done, it was argued that, if the course and examination became too difficult, candidates would be discouraged from applying to Cambridge. This would mean a fall in the revenue brought in by the courses and examination to such an extent that the University might have to subsidize Purvis' and Graham-Smith's salaries from its own funds.[44]

To add to their difficulties they received a visitor with gloomy news. R. J. Leiper had been Director of the Helminthology Department in the London School of Tropical Medicine, which was founded in 1905, and

---

[40] The title of Reader in a British University is broadly equivalent to that of Associate Professor elsewhere. At one time it was awarded to distinguished scholars in whose subjects there was no established Chair. Now that most universities are willing to create personal Chairs it not so commonly used, and proportionately both to professorships, and to the rest of the teaching staff, there are fewer Readers in Britain than there are Associate Professors in the United States.

[41] Brockington, C. Fraser (1978). Personal letter to Roy Acheson.

[42] Archives of the University of Cambridge [Min VI 53]. See also Chapter 2 (notes 100 and 108).

[43] In the early 1920s, Cambridge introduced, in addition to the Diploma in Tropical Medicine and Hygiene, the purpose of which was self-explanatory, a Diploma of Hygiene. This was to allow students from overseas who were not registered with the General Medical Council, and who were therefore ineligible for the award of the DPH, to gain recognition for attending the DPH course (see also note 38).

[44] Archives of the University of Cambridge (1923). *Letter from Graham-Smtih to Anderson*. 13 February [Min VI 53].

was by then Professor of his subject in the University of London. He called on some of the teachers in Cambridge because he had been involved with the Rockefeller Foundation in negotiations which were later to lead to the establishment of what was to be the new London School of Hygiene and Tropical Medicine. He discussed with Graham Smith the plans for what Newman had called a school of hygiene, referring to it as a national institute and saying that it was the intention for it 'to absorb all teaching for the DPH and perhaps give their own diploma'.[45] Although this was at variance with Newman's statement, it confirmed that the DPH at Cambridge was threatened.

The Report of the Syndicate was accepted by the University. It recommended that the DPH should be continued. In addition, it proposed an important innovation, and failed to propose another. The former was that, in keeping with other universities, 'candidates should be required to attend a course of nine months at the University'.[46] This involved residence in Cambridge for a total of 24 weeks and so was stricter than elsewhere. It almost certainly lost several potential candidates each year to the Conjoint, because there students could choose the time and place of their instruction to suit themselves; any university with a department of public health satisfied the General Medical Council. Perhaps discouragement of students was intentional, and a first step in running down a course which was to be discontinued eight years later in 1931.

The failure concerned standards. The draft report of the Special Syndicate reads: ' . . . standards . . . should be considerably raised';[47] but in its final form this had been altered to read as follows: 'standards should be carefully considered'. Not for the first time the Cambridge dons nestled back into the feathery comfort of the status quo; the University Treasurer must have been pleased that potential losses from compulsory course work might be offset but they paid the price of allowing the image of the University to become a little tarnished. The lizard's skin was therefore again subjected to stretching, but withstood it.

Not all candidates in the country sought an easy life by choosing the bodies with high pass rates, however. The Oxford examination attracted many candidates, its 45 per cent failure rate over 10 years notwithstanding.[48] Of this examination Low had to say that it was 'undoubtedly of a

[45] Ibid. (1923). *Letter from Graham-Smith to Anderson.* 1 March.

[46] *Cambridge University Reporter* (1923). Report of the Syndicate on the duties and responsibities of the Syndicate in State Medicine. 29 April.

[47] Loc. cit. (note 42).

[48] General Medical Council (1917). *Minutes.* Appendix III, Report of the Public Health Committee, p. 279.

searching quality' and that 'it appears of late to have risen . . . in popularity and the number of candidates has very materially increased '.[49]

The economic bargaining led therefore to a kind of three-way concordat between candidates seeking reasonable assurance of success in the shortest possible time; examination boards searching for a maximum income from high entrance rates; and the General Medical Council attempting to ensure that standards, if not high, were sufficient to ensure public safety. Those who believed that the open market should control education and training must have been satisfied, but others, university teachers among them, were uneasy. Not only, then, were aspirants for careers in public health practical men with practical minds, they also sought a frill-free qualification which would enable them to embark on their career as quickly and effectively as possible. They paid the piper and they called the tune.

4. Innovations in the universities

So far, we have largely concentrated on influences during the twentieth century on the Diploma in Public Health which have been outside the universities such as the General Medical Council, Empire politics, and economic forces. Between the third and fifth decades of the twentieth century, however, there were to be two innovations in the universities themselves. One of them was deliberate and the other evolutionary but both had important effects on the DPH. In 1919, Lloyd George's government established a Ministry of Health and Sir George Newman was its Chief Medical Officer. In 1922, it decided to support, in the University of London, a postgraduate institution whose sole concern was to be teaching and research in public health and tropical medicine. The second, which was more insidious, diffuse, and subtle in its origins, but at least as permanent in its longer-run influence, namely, the establishment of departments of social medicine in the medical schools of some universities and of research units under the aegis of the Medical Research Council with the same or closely related names.

The London School of Hygiene and Tropical Medicine

We saw in the first section of this chapter that during the first decade of the century, the DPH as it was originally conceived, was in its heyday and how during the war years standards fell. In 1909, a new series of events began to unfold in the University of London, which, from the

[49] Ibid. (1921), 830.

late 1920s, would radically change the picture. The University had been founded in 1839 as a body with the limited responsibility of examining candidates and awarding degrees or diplomas to those who were successful. Teaching was undertaken by affiliated but independent colleges, notably King's College and University College; such research as was done was done by them. The 12 medical schools, most of which tendered their fealty to the Royal Colleges of Physicians and Surgeons and their Conjoint Board, one by one applied for and obtained recognition as constituent parts of the University.

In 1909, preparation for the change to full status of a teaching university—which it had been proposed in government circles would take place the following year—began. The Academic Registrar canvassed the faculties for their statements of need. The Board of Studies of Hygiene in the Faculty of Medicine, which was one of some 60 similar bodies responsible for developing components of a proper academic programme, submitted a plan for the creation of a new institution within the university. This was subsequently referred to in the Senate minutes of 2 June 1913 as an Institute of Hygiene and Public Health.[50] It was to undertake postgraduate teaching, particularly for the Diploma in Public Health; it was also to employ Research Scholars, which was an important proposal because previously in Britain research in hygiene and public health had generally been conducted on an uncoordinated *ad hoc* basis. Although the Faculty of Medicine of the University approved the plan, neither University College nor King's College did, so that on 16 June 1915 the Senate of the University decided that the postgraduate teaching of Hygiene and Public Health should be 'postponed until further order'.[51]

In the meantime, Colonel Leiper, who, as has already been indicated, was subsequently to visit Cambridge, had become friendly with Dr Heiser of the Rockefeller Foundation. Their common interest was in anchlyostomiasis. On 3 August 1919, Leiper wrote to Heiser as follows:

. . . the other day . . . I had a most interesting account from [Dr Barnes] of the fieldwork in the hookworm campaigns he has personally conducted . . . Perhaps you have heard that we have secured large and excellent premises in the heart of London for a new "hospital for tropical diseases". It has been given as a war memorial for the Sailor. The Seaman's Hospital Society have decided to accomodate [*sic*] the London School of Tropical Medicine in the lower part of the building which is one of ten floors. This gives us an unrivalled position—in Euston Square—and greatly increased accomodation [*sic*] . . . the new move

[50] University of London (1913). *Minutes of the Senate.* 2 June. Report of the Board of Studies in Hygiene and Public Health, para. II.
[51] Ibid. (1915), 15 June, paras 3360 and 3361, pp. 58–61.

will strengthen our position as a school of the University and the Senate have just appointed me Professor of Helminthology in the University of London . . . The project is one which I have had at heart for several years and I am naturally highly elated at its realisation.[52]

Heiser congratulated him sincerely and added 'I hope that the next step in Great Britain will be the establishment of a great school of hygiene and public health'. The transposition of 'hygiene and public health' for 'tropical medicine ' at this early stage is interesting; the Rockefeller records show no reason for it, but of course the Rockefeller Foundation had been responsible three years previously for promoting the establishment of the School called by that name in Johns Hopkins University. In any event, the Foundation ensured that the great School was established, and although there were difficulties to be overcome, that it embraced hygiene *and* tropical medicine. Shortly after Christmas 1919, Dr Wickliffe Rose, General Director of the International Health Board, visited the new building of the London School of Tropical Medicine and wrote to Heiser describing his interest in the project.[53] There followed a complex series of negotiations between the Rockefeller Foundation, the Colonial Office, the Ministry of Health, and the University which first discussed the emphasis to be placed on tropical medicine and then went on to consider its potential as a world centre and the University's plans for an Institute of Hygiene and Public Health.[54] All of this caused rancour, and in Spring 1922, led the most distinguished member of the London School of Tropical Medicine, Sir Patrick Manson, to write to Rose expressing the view that it would 'be a calamity if . . . we would have to close our doors or become bankrupt [if the Rockefeller scheme] were to prove an opposition teaching institution'.[55] Rose assured him that this would not occur. By November, the decision had been taken to establish an organization within the University of London which combined the 1909 plan for an Institute of Hygiene together with the London School of Tropical Medicine, but which would manage its own affairs. Costs were to be

[52] Archives of the Rockefeller Foundation (1921). RG5, Series 401, Box 53, 14 March.

[53] Ibid., Series 1.1, Box 39, Folder 613.

[54] Colonial Office (1921). *Tropical diseases: summary of proceedings at a conference between the Colonial Office and representatives of the Rockefeller Foundation.* July. Colonial Office, Confidential Report, Miscellaneous No.34, Archives of the Rockefeller Foundation, RG5 (IHB/D), Series 2 (Special Report), Box 38, Folder 227; also available at Public Records Office, CO 885–27, XO 010068; see also Acheson, Roy M. and Poole, Penelope. The London School of Hygiene and Tropical Medicine: a child of many parents. *Medical History.*

[55] Archives of Rockefeller Foundation (1921). RG12.1, Series W. Rose 1916–1922, Box 53, 14 March.

divided between the Government and the Rockefeller Foundation, whose lion's share of them was in the order of $2 000 000.

Two years later, on 24 May 1924, the Board of Management of what was to be the London School of Hygiene and Tropical Medicine met for the first time at the Ministry of Health in Whitehall. W. H. Welch's idea was that his school in Johns Hopkins should be specially geared for teaching public health to medically qualified people[56] but the original plan was that the London School of Hygiene and Tropical Medicine should be exclusively medical, if not clinical, and that the sense of hygiene should broadly be taken as the science of health and its preservation.[57] Sir Walter Fletcher, with his concern for the development of medical science, and Newman whose responsibility it was to apply it particularly in the field of preventive medicine, were among the members of the Board of the new school. By September of the same year, the Board was considering an interim scheme for the introduction of a new course for the Diploma in Public Health in the London School.[58,59] Two Chairs had been included in the original establishment proposed between 1909 and 1913, but the subjects were not stipulated. In 1925, it was decided that they should be in Epidemiology and Vital Statistics and in Bacteriology and Immunology. The two foundation departments were therefore scientific and true to the name Hygiene. Major Greenwood was appointed to the former[60] and W. W. C. Topley to the latter. Of these subjects, vital statistics had been considered to merit an examination paper of its own from the time of the first examination for the Certificate in State Medicine in 1871, whereas epidemiology only received passing mention in syllabuses and examinations until 1882, when the Royal College of Physicians of Edinburgh devoted a one-hour three-question paper to epidemiology and endemiology. Thus the title

[56] Ibid. (1914). RG1.1, Series 200L, Box 185, *Conference on training for public health service*. Offfice of the General Education Board, John D. Rockefeller Fund, New York, 16 October.

[57] *Webster's new collegiate dictionary, (9th edn)* (1983). Miriam-Webster, Springfield, Massachusetts. Hygiene is defined as 'the science or art of preserving health' in the 7th edition of *Chamber's English dictionary* (1988). W. & R. Chambers and Cambridge University Press, Edinburgh and Cambridge.

[58] Archives of the London School of Hygiene and Tropical Medicine (1928). *Minutes of the Education Committee*. Vol. II. A committee was formed to work on the DPH Curriculum at the meeting on 27 December.

[59] The disparate events which led up to the foundation of the London School of Hygiene and Tropical Medicine are described elsewhere, see Acheson, Roy and Poole, Penelope, op. cit. (note 54).

[60] Major was Greenwood's given name. He held no military rank. It is interesting that Sir Austin Bradford Hill, who was Greenwood's pupil and successor, but who was not medically qualified, changed the name of the Chair to Medical Statistics and Epidemiology.

of Greenwood's professorship signified, at one and the same time, the resurgence of a science which had been the principal tool of Simon and his investigators,[61] and before them a few sanitarians such as South-wood Smith.[62] By the 1890s, when bacteriology seemed to promise solutions to all the problems of the aetiology of disease, epidemiology had been brushed to one side.

In 1928, the University of London created a third Chair in the hygiene division of the school which was in Public Health and was assumed on 1 January 1929 by Wilson Jameson. He had previously held academic appointments at University College and Guy's Hospital and had been Medical Officer of Health in Finchley and Hornsey.

By September 1930, when 22 students sat for the Diploma in Public Health in the University of London, Cambridge had already decided that its examination should be discontinued in the following year. The first part of the new London examination consisted of papers in bacter-iology, chemistry, and hygiene (which, true to tradition, and in com-pliance with the unchanging regulations of the General Medical Council with regard to meteorology, included a question on hygrometers, and on the relationship between humidity and health). Meteorology ceased finally to be required by the Council in 1937.

Fifty years after the first Certificate in State Medicine was offered, a course was planned and given, not by one or two teachers in a small university department co-ordinating the contributions of several col-leagues who devoted most of their time to other matters, but by a con-sortium of strong departments with full-time scientific staff. The potential of the new school was, as we shall see, later enhanced by the General Medical Council's imaginative recommendations of 1967. It is not surprising that the University of London through this new school began to share with the London Conjoint, dominance in the number of Diplomas awarded each year. After the Second World War, the School of Hygiene which taught the whole curriculum, became the more popu-lar of the two. Newman, when he had given evidence to the special syn-dicate at Cambridge in 1922, had said that he hoped that several small provincial schools would continue to offer the diploma; this they did, but as we shall see in the next section they had to struggle both to main-tain their standards, and to attract students. There can be little doubt

[61] Brockington, C. Fraser (1963). *Public health in the nineteenth century*. Livingstone, Edinburgh.

[62] Lewes, Caroline C. (1898). *Dr Southwood Smith: a retrospect*. Blackwood, Edin-burgh; Poynter, F.N.L. Southwood Smith—the man, 1788–1861 (1962). *Proceedings of the Royal Society of Medicine*. **55**, 381–92; Pelling, Margaret (1978). The origins of official doctrine: Chadwick and Southwood Smith. In *Cholera and English medicine 1852–1865*, Ch. 1, pp. 1–33. Oxford University Press.

that training in public health in the London School of Hygiene and Tropical Medicine was of a quality and standard which had not hitherto been reached; but the DPH as a nationally accredited qualification was long past its zenith and the school was soon to be concerned with making other contributions to training in hygiene and public health.

The examination in the London School of Hygiene and Tropical Medicine was held annually until 1968, when it was discontinued preparatory to the introduction of a new M.Sc.degree in social medicine. This was to prepare medically qualified men and women to become community physicians by teaching them the scientific basis of their work. Like all other degrees, except the baccalaureates in medicine and surgery, it was to be controlled by a university, in this case the University of London, and not by the General Medical Council. The Diploma in Public Health ceased to be statutorily controlled in 1974 when its *raison d'être*, the post of medical officer of health, was abolished. The Royal Institute of Public Health, and one or two other bodies, notably the University of Leeds, continued to offer the diploma for some years thereafter.

The social medicine movement

In the meantime, there were other changes in the world of research and education in public health in England and Wales. Among medical undergraduates, and no doubt other young people in the universities in the late 1930s, there were many who were influenced by the ideals of the time. These included the Russian Revolution, the fight to halt fascism in the Spanish Civil War, and the deprivations imposed on many in the great Depression of the late 1920s and early 1930s. They became concerned with the influence of human society on the health of its members. Some of the group, a decade later, were to develop a new kind of epidemiology. It would be misleading to suggest that John Ryle, who was of an older generation, was the leader of this group in any immediate sense, but he had a profound influence on its thinking. In particular his address to the Cambridge Medical Society in 1931[63] would appear to have made a deep impression.

Ryle was an outstanding practising physician who emphasized that all disease is a conflict between man and his environment, and that it was the physician's task to observe this interchange in its totality and to acquire an understanding of disease in man as well as of man afflicted

---

[63] Ryle, John (1931). The physician as a naturalist. *Guy's Hospital Reports*, **18**, 278.

with disease.[64] In 1947, he said 'social medicine, deriving its inspiration more from the field of clinical experience and seeking always to assist the discovery of a common purpose for the remedial and preventive services and endeavours to study [man] and in relation to his environment'. It was only at the very end of his career that he began to comprehend the methods and importance of population research.[65] His academic and professional origins were remote from public health and also from empirical research. He left at the pinnacle of his success in clinical medicine at Guy's Hospital to don first the robes of Regius Professor of Physic in Cambridge, where he spent some unhappy years. Then, in 1944, he was appointed Nuffield Professor of Social Medicine in Oxford, a Chair created for him (but he died before the 10-year tenure was complete). There he directed the Nuffield Institute of Social Medicine where Alice Stewart, a physician and epidemiologist, joined him. Shortly after Ryle's death in 1950 she was appointed to a Readership in Social Medicine which was established for her.[66,67]

Some other universities created professorial departments, most of which were called social medicine, including Birmingham (McKeown, human biologist); Edinburgh (Crewe, demographer), followed by Brotherston (public health visionary and educator); Belfast (Stevenson, population geneticist), followed by Pemberton (epidemiologist); Dundee (Mair, occupational physician); and London (Reid, epidemiologist and Schilling, occupational physician and epidemiologist). Cochrane, Doll, Charles Fletcher, and Morris were all epidemiologists, and all were employed by the Medical Research Council in units which were attached to universities. Despite their different specialties, there were two qualities in common to members of this group; one was their contribution to the development of epidemiology based on probability statistics as a method of elucidating the aetiology of non-infectious (as well as infectious) disease and the other the socialist ethos. They shared a

---

[64] Ibid.; see also Acheson, Roy (1978). Medicine, the community and the university: a century of Cambridge history. *British Medical Journal*, **2**, 1737–41.

[65] Ryle, John (1948). *Changing disciplines*, 11. London, Geoffrey Cumberlege, Oxford University Press.

[66] On Alice Stewart's retirement in 1975, the post was elevated to Professor in Social and Community Medicine, and Martin Vessey was appointed to it.

[67] Barber, C. Renate (1987). *Half a century of social medicine: an annotated bibliography of the work of Alice Stewart*. Piers Press, Billingshurst, West Sussex. This book is a kind of autobiography. The essays were chosen by Alice Stewart herself, and annotated by Dr Barber, who was a close friend of many years' standing. Most, but not all, of the material comprises research reports which she published with colleagues about her own work. Also included are some of her essays, and a report of a collateral study undertaken by David Hewitt while he was in the Department of Social Medicine at Oxford and she was the departmental head. Although she is intensely individualistic, it epitomizes as well as any single volume can, what the academic social medicine movement was all about.

concern to improve the health of mankind primarily by appropriate and effective improvements in social circumstances, and by identifying and dealing with factors which increased the risk of the development of specific diseases. The subsequent dramatic falls in frequency of some cancers, and heart and lung disease, can be attributed in great part to the application of the research of these scientists. A very few of them took the DPH of the London School of Hygiene and Tropical Medicine immediately after the war; but, that aside, few had anything to do with what was generally recognized as public health *per se*.

They developed their own instruments for presenting and discussing the fruits of their research and the problems they encountered in teaching. The first issue of the *British Journal of Social Medicine*, edited by Crewe and Lancelot Hogben, a mathematician, was published in 1946. In 1955, the Society of Social Medicine was founded; it was solely concerned at that time with research and teaching but in the 1960s took positions in medico–political matters, including the submission of evidence to the Royal Commission on Medical Education and other government enquiries. It held its first meeting in Birmingham where about 50 people attended and 20 papers were delivered.[68]

The concept of social medicine had thus attracted into some of the universities a group of brilliant scientific investigators of a quality unknown to the field in such numbers since Simon's team dispersed in 1871. The research workers in social medicine were for the most part separated from such academic workers as remained in traditional public health, not only by lack of common interests, but by strong feelings of mutual antagonism. The exponents of social medicine felt not only that the traditionalists were out of touch with the real issues of the day, but that they were apathetic about them. Naturally this was resented by those in practice.

In the meantime, the traditionalists in the academic world were

[68] Quite unlike the organizations established by the medical officers of health, of which the Society of Medical Officers of Health was the most important, the Society for Social Medicine has always included non-medically qualified members and has been strictly informal in its social affairs. It flourishes with a membership that approaches 1000. Papers then published in the *Journal* from units or departments, designated as being concerned with social medicine, covered the following topics: maternal age and birth rank in aetiology of mongolism (Birmingham), observations on 1078 peri-natal deaths (Oxford), statistical experimentation in therapeutics (Sheffield), deaf-mutism (Belfast), social and biological factors in infant mortality (The London Hospital), general practice in new housing estates (London School of Hygiene and Tropical Medicine). For more detail see *British Journal of Preventive and Social Medicine* (1955), **19** and 1956, **20**. The Journal was never the formal organ of the Society and its first name change was because sales in the United States were impeded by the mistaken view that its overriding concern was 'socialized medicine'. Subsequently, its name was to be changed a second time and is now *Journal of Epidemiology and Community Health*.

struggling to keep the DPH alive as a postgraduate qualification. They consisted chiefly of professors of public health in universities in large cities who were also serving or had served as medical officers of health or in other senior administrative positions.[69]

In 1955, the departments in six medical schools, directed by medical officers of health, were between them responsible for only 38 of the 182 diplomas awarded, an average of 6.3 each. Some of the professors of social medicine, however, such as Stevenson (Belfast), Alwyn Smith (Manchester), and Brotherston (Edinburgh), the last of whom was soon to become Chairman of the Public Health Committee of the General Medical Council, continued to offer postgraduate diplomas and degrees which satisfied the General Medical Council as being suitable for the training of medical officers of health but embraced the concepts of social medicine. A measure of consumer attitude was that the two departments of social medicine which continued to offer a DPH course despite their change in philosophy, namely, Belfast and Edinburgh, awarded 33 between them; 16.5 on average. There were 47 successful candidates who had been trained and examined by the London School of Hygiene and Tropical Medicine, where innovations such as the appointments of senior lecturers in sociology and industrial psychology were progressive, and these constituted the majority of the remainder; the Conjoint Board of England awarded 20 diplomas that year.

The reorganization of the National Health Service in 1974, together with the creation of the community physician and the establishment of the Faculty of Community Medicine of the Royal Colleges of Physicians, went a long way to closing the rift between social medicine and public health as well as to synthesizing the practical, theoretical, and professional interests of the two groups. Nevertheless, changes in the organizational structure and policy of the National Health Service, by paying stipends, albeit very small ones, to all newly qualifed doctors for the first year after qualification, and offering full salaried careers to a great majority, left public health competing on an equal basis with all the

[69] These were at: Bristol (Wofinden), Glasgow (Ferguson), Leeds (Jervis, then Bradshaw), Liverpool (Semple), and Manchester (Brockington). In the National University of Wales (Grundy) and in Aberdeen (Berry) such service was discontinued at the time of taking up the Chair. Although Grundy fits into the definition of this group he was ambivalent. He was a barrister-at-law as well as a medical man, and wrote three textbooks between 1945 and 1951 when he was Medical Officer of Health at Luton, namely, *Handbook of social medicine*, *The new public health*, and *Preventive medicine and public health*, all of which were published by Gibbs, Bamford and Co, Luton. In them he attempted to draw the two fields together, but apart from their emphasis on personal services, they differed little from other texts on public health of the time. In his prime he left his university post in Cardiff to join the World Health Organization, where he subsequently became Assistant Director General.

other specialties. Careers in public health or with the Armed Forces were attractive to young doctors who could not afford to take further specialist training, or to 'put up their plate' in practice. Now it had to face an open market.

5. Times change: The Diploma in Public Health shows the way for the faculty of community medicine

Reaction and action: 1955 and 1967

As we have seen in the foregoing section, the attempt of Jameson's Public Health Committee in the General Medical Council to broaden the applicability—although not the content—of the Diploma in Public Health proved a failure. In 1955, the Committee in its decennial revision of Recommendations and Rules discontinued the Certificate, proposed innovations which not only were wholly bereft of imagination, but left little room for flexibility. The word 'Recommendation' was removed from the title and 'Rules' for the first time stood starkly alone.[70] The rigid prescription of the number of hours which were to be allocated to each subject and course no longer appeared, however, and this was an improvement. The document was in the letter, a step back to pre-war days, but in spirit far more retrogressive than that.

A. L. Banks,[71] a member of the Public Health Committee in 1964, was concerned about this inaction in the Council against a background of continuous and rapid change in the academic world, but none in the service world. As a consequence, he challenged the Council to consider 'whether the statutory provisions regulating the registration of the Diplomas in Public Health should be continued'. A special group of enquiry was established which decided that instead of de-registration of the diploma, the Rules should be revised.[72] The outcome was that in 1967, under Brotherston's Chairmanship, the most sweeping changes of guidelines for training and education in public health were promulgated by the General Medical Council.[73]

---

[70] The name changed from time to time; originally it was 'Resolutions and Rules'.

[71] A.L. Banks was Professor of Human Ecology in the University of Cambridge, which he represented on the General Medical Council.

[72] General Medical Council (1964). *Minutes of the Executive Committee*; Ibid. (1965). Appendix VIII, Memorandum by A.L. Banks, Diplomas in Public Health.

[73] Sir John Brotherston was successively Professor of Social Medicine and Dean of the Medical Faculty in the University of Edinburgh, and then Chief Medical Officer for Scotland. As such, he sat as a Queen's nominee on the General Medical Council. There he was Chairman of the Education Committee as well as of the Public Health Committee. He was probably one of the most far-sighted medical educators of the century.

The Committee noted in its Report that although medical officers of health had become engaged in the practice of other branches of medicine beside those of local government and public health, the Council still had to ensure that the award of the diploma attested to the training and standard of knowledge appropriate to this traditional role. At the same time, the Report wished universities to experiment and to put forward proposals for new courses of study and qualifications. It added: 'Although the term "Rules" has been used on previous occasions, it does not occur in the Act'.[74] The guidelines were therefore simply titled 'Recommendations'; *inter alia* it stated that 'in future the curriculum for the Diploma in Public Health should be regarded as the academic core of a longer scheme of postgraduate training'. Moreover, before engaging on the course the aspirant should acquire 'at least one and preferably several years of experience in clinical medicine', and the training should in effect be looked upon as a common academic core for doctors seeking subsequent employment in a wide range of posts in community health practice. The biggest departure from tradition was that 'study . . . should be designed to lead candidates to the study of scientific methods'. The Council declared itself ready 'to recognize on its merits and irrespective of its title any qualification [offered by a recognized body]'.

What the Committee had to say about the content of courses was indicative and brief. A mere three or four lines expanded each of the following four headings:

(1) quantitative sciences;
(2) behavioural sciences applied to community health;
(3) genetic and environmental (including microbiological) factors in health and disease; and
(4) health services organization.

Finally the Council advised that it would recognize new qualifications as being the equivalent of the DPH and this was quickly heeded. The following year a Diploma in Social Medicine was recognized under the terms of the Medical Act of 1886 in the University of Edinburgh, followed in 1971 by the Diploma in Tropical Public Health in the London School of Hygiene and Tropical Medicine (a posthumous victory for Nuttall over Macalastair), an M.Sc. in social medicine in the same school in the same year, and one in public health in Manchester in 1973.[75] This permissive new attitude to training for statutory posts in

[74] General Medical Council (1967). *Minutes.* April, Appendix VI, pp. 215–18.
[75] General Medical Council (1971). *Minutes, Report of the Public Health Committee.* Appendix VI, p. 242; Ibid. (1972). Appendix XII, 276; Ibid. (1973). Appendix VIII, 248. The staid and proper minutes of the Council give no idea of the battle which was fought between the University of Manchester and the General Medical Council which lasted for

public health matched closely the Council's policy towards the basic medical curriculum in which schools were encouraged to experiment broadly. One can speculate that once the basic training for the task of medical officer of health had been firmly established shortly after the turn of the century, 'Recommendations' encouraging flexibility might have had a strengthening influence on the whole field of public health.

The end of the Diploma in Public Health

The late flowering came to an end in 1974, and *pari passu* the following year the post of medical officer of health[76] was discontinued. The skin had gone, and without the will or the wherewithal to grow another one, the fat old lizard had no hope of surviving. Nevertheless, he had enjoyed a full life, and had contributed much to the world around him. Perhaps he could have contributed more generously to the needs of the increasing numbers of sub-specialists who were professionally answerable to

---

three years before a final resolution was reached. Some idea of the issues can be appreciated from the fact that on the one hand the Statutes made it clear that only qualifications in public health, sanitary science or state medicine could be entered in the Medical Register, and accepted as a basis for being appointed to the post of Medical Officer of Health. On the other although BA (Econ.), or (Admin.) or (Theol.) were offered by the University, M.Sc. (Public Health) was unacceptable to the University Senate. In the fourth year of the dispute, the Assistant Registrar of the University offered 'M.Sc. (in the field of Public Health, Sanitary Science or State Medicine)'. The reply from the Council was as follows:

> I appreciate the principle which led you to suggest a wider based designation, but this would raise technical difficulties as far as the Register (which is maintained by computer) is concerned. The present computer program allocates 60 spaces (i.e. including letters, spaces, numbers and punctuation) for any doctor's qualifications. The title to which you propose for the MSc would alone exceed this allocation, and would unfortunately prove too expensive for the Council to consider.

The University yielded to this economic reality, and in November 1972 the Council acceded to their request to recognize the M.Sc. in the field of public health, which in their few remaining publications pertaining to the field, the Council abbreviated to 'M.Sc. (Public Health)' and the first degree was awarded in 1973. If there is a villain, it is not for this author to name him, but there can be little doubt that Alwyn Smith, Professor of Social Medicine, had better things to do than serve as a ping-pong ball. The relevance of the story here is that it serves as a further illustration of how easy it is for established bodies to stand in the way of the implementation of changes they themselves have approved. (*Source*: Archives of the General Medical Council, uncatalogued working papers of the Public Health Committee.)

[76] The decision to discontinue the Medical Officer of Health's Department in local government was taken on the recommendation of the Royal Commission on Medical Education (the Todd Commission) which reported in 1968 and was promulgated in the *National Health Service Act* [Chapter 32] (1973). The 'appointed day', when the medical officer of health, and all that went with him ceased to exist, was 31 March 1974.

the medical officer of health. Certainly, the earliest years aside, a varying proportion of diplomates did not register their qualification and therefore did not put their training to the purpose for which it was intended; there is no way of knowing what value it had to them. Most of them were British, but an increasing number, as we have seen, were foreigners who would be working in wholly different circumstances from those for which the qualification was designed. The contents and form of the examination, modified only by changes in the role of the medical officer of health, came to be of less and less value to doctors interested in the totality of medicine in populations, and in health promotion—and, of course, the qualification was always totally barred from people interested in public health who did not have a medical degree.

The Faculty of Community Medicine takes over

After the post of medical officer of health ceased to exist, the community physician inherited some of his duties and assumed many new ones. A new professional postgraduate training scheme was developed as the statutory responsibility of the Faculty of Community Medicine of the Royal Colleges of Physicians.[77] It too was new, but it borrowed from the past.

During 1972, the Faculty of Community Medicine started to consider its Membership examination. Partly on its own initiative, and partly in response to pressure from the professors of social and community medicine,[78] the Faculty approached the General Medical Council with two ends in view. One was to find support for retaining the DPH when it was very much on the cards that the post of medical officer of health would soon cease to exist and also to recognize the Membership of the Faculty of Community Medicine (MFCM) as a registrable qualification.

---

[77] At the time of writing, the Faculty, on the recommendation of the Government Committee on 'The public health function', has just changed its name to Faculty of Public Health Medicine. This is in part because of modifications in the responsibilities of its members and fellows for discharging 'the public health function' and partly because the title community medicine proved to be confusingly ambiguous.

[78] This informal group consists of heads of academic departments and of research units, most of the latter funded by the Medical Research Council. Originally their departments and units had titles such as social medicine and epidemiology. The group came into existence in the 1960s with a view to ensuring that the interests of members were properly represented when changes of national policy were being implemented. Among other things it gives evidence to policy making bodies concerned with changes related to their academic and professional interests. Its efforts have met with some success and it is now usual for it to be consulted when further policy changes are under consideration.

They were successful in the second endeavour. The Faculty itself held the responsibility for determining the nature of the training and the setting of the professional standards for community medicine, so that when the MFCM became registrable the event carried with it no statutory importance.

The Education and Examination Committees of the Faculty, which were responsible for preparing and conducting the new MFCM examinations and establishing a scheme for service training, leaned very heavily on the 1967 Recommendations of the Public Health Committee of the General Medical Council for their early curriculum. An important change was that there was to be a mandatory period of several years of practical experience under closely monitored supervision in contrast to the single year of what had been called 'outdoor' work which the General Medical Council had striven so hard to increase. One unfortunate difference between the Brotherston 'Recommendations' and the new syllabus was that the Faculty substituted 'social sciences' for 'behavioural sciences' and concomitantly, at a critical stage in the development of the new curriculum, failed to give due emphasis to behaviour as a fundamental factor in the origins and causes of human disease. Psychology has much to offer to the understanding of behavioural changes needed if a healthy way of life is to be adopted; but because it is not a social science, little, if any, attention has been paid to it over the first 15 years of the new training programme.

Some universities have initiated one-year Master's programmes in the field, which are academic in nature. They have formed part of the preparation of candidates for the examination for the MFCM (MFPHM), but although they substituted for the DPH they do not substitute for the MFCM. Like the British MD, they simply provide an academic qualification which is additional to what is needed for specialist accreditation.

Some differences between the United Kingdom and the United States

This educational system has developed in striking contrast to the pattern which unfolded in the United States. There apart from the Harvard–Massachussetts Institute of Technology School for Health Officers' Certificate in Public Health, at the beginning of the century, and subsequently the same qualification at the Yale School of Medicine, the standard route followed towards a career in public health has been a Master of Public Health degree awarded by university schools of public health. The vast majority of these degrees have gone to candidates without a medical qualification. Schools of public health also offer doctoral degrees, the most usual of which is a Doctorate in Public Health or in Science, which tends to be designed for people who will become senior practitioners in public health service. Some schools also offer a Ph.D. in specific fields such as epidemiology, to attract candidates whose skills are leading them to a research career. The courses lean towards providing learning in depth to the exclusion of breadth. In their nature such studies define their own boundaries, whereas the former are broader and more practical.

The very existence of the many schools of public health in the United States indicates that public health is looked upon as a discipline there. Schools do cater for medically qualified trainees, the proportion of whom in the total student body varies from one school to another, and from one specialty to another, but almost everywhere such students are in the minority. In general, however, students with and without medical backgrounds are, at least in core courses, taught side by side. It will be clear from this chapter that in Britain, such combined classes can only be held for the few in either category who are training for second degrees in a university because the DPH, to date the MFCM, and for the forseeable future the MFPHM, have only been available for registered medical practitioners. In contrast, public health, in its broader sense, has never been looked upon as a unified enterprise in Britain, but merely as a collection of specialized roles. As a consequence, most members of the public health workforce, namely those who do not have a medical degree, nor in most instances any other degree, must receive their training in other ways, and elsewhere. Until 1975, such workers were members of the department of the medical officer of health and answerable to him. Now they are no longer employed by the National Health Service, but by local government in Departments of Environmental Health. Space does not permit detailed consideration of their training, but it is relevant very briefly to describe it.

The three principal professional groups concerned have been engineers, sanitary officers—currently known in Britain as environmental health officers—and nurses, including health visitors, and in the past, midwives. Public health engineering has generally been taken as a sub-specialty of civil engineering and the training and standards of those interested in pursuing it as a career are, and always have been, controlled by the professional institutions of engineering. Sanitary officers and nurses each have to satisfy controlling bodies of their own. These are the Institution of Environmental Health Officers and the United Kingdom Central Council for Nursing, Midwifery and Health Visiting respectively and both are responsible for ensuring that those embarking on careers in their disciplines have the necessary expertise and experience, and that they maintain the professional and social standards appropriate to their practice. In each case, course work and practical experience can be pursued in a wide range of approved institutions—few if any of them universities—and the candidate sits professional examinations under the aegis of the appropriate national controlling body.[79] The Royal Institute of Public Health and Hygiene has taken an interest in developing similar standards for food handlers; technicians who work with cadavers; those concerned with community care and parentcraft and so on, but none of these endeavours is backed by statutory law.[80]

Over the past 20 years, attempts have been made to co-ordinate the education and training of people entering these major careers in public health and others like them, by the Council for National Academic Awards. As appropriate, this body enables people of suitable ability to pool experience they have obtained along the way, and to graduate to primary or advanced degrees of the Council. Subjects include engineering, health studies, and life sciences.[81]

This, potentially, is an important step along the road towards raising to the level of education, career preparation which has been little more than technical training. Moreover, the appropriateness of segregating professionals, who will eventually work together, from each other, as well as from their medical colleagues, during their formative years, is open to question. The American approach to solving this problem by way of the School of Public Health has not been an unqualified success either. In Chapter 5, Elizabeth Fee sets out some of the difficulties which were rehearsed at a famous meeting in the offices of the Rockefeller Foundation in October 1914. The issues have changed little since then. The enormously varied backgrounds in educational experience which entrants for the various specialties bring with them have made the effective management of even the most basic core courses extremely difficult. Few would question that public health is an endeavour which has yielded rich rewards but no group working within it can expect in future to achieve much single-handed. The general problem of seeking co-ordination in education and training in public health is too important to be ignored any longer.

[79] United Kingdom Central Council for Nursing, Midwifery and Health Visiting, 23 Portland Place, London W1N 3AF, *Statutory instruments, 1989, No. 109. Nurses, midwives and health visitors*; and the Institute of Environmental Health Officers, *Charter and byelaws*, Chadwick House, Rushworth Street, London SE1 OQT.

[80] Royal Institute of Public Health and Hygiene, 28 Portland Place, London W1N 4DE.

[81] The Council for National Academic Awards is to be clearly distinguished from the Open University; although the latter gives credits for suitable work undertaken elsewhere, it sets out to provide through its own staff all the instruction necessary for its degrees.

6. Is there a message?

Writers of biographies are used to telling stories with clear-cut beginnings and equally clear-cut endings, but those concerned with social institutions are not always so fortunate as we have been. For, in the case of the DPH, there was a day when it was born, another when it died, and it had a full and varied life in between. The State Medicine Committee of the General Medical Council, which carried the responsibility for its safe delivery was, with the assistance it had obtained from the chosen members of the general public, concerned to learn:

(1) what was to be taught and in what order;
(2) which subjects required practical instruction;
(3) how examinations should be conducted; and
(4) what depth of knowledge was required and what books were appropriate.[82]

In view of what transpired in the ensuing century it might be worthwhile briefly to consider these problems again.

Curriculum

As we have seen, a qualification was created—not without difficulty—and once it became established, it carried with it an enormous inertia. Even when a ponderous organization like the Council managed to form a view about change, it was not always easy to implement. Both in the late nineteenth century, when entrenched interests impeded the introduction of bacteriology, and in the mid-twentieth century, when the failure of an innovative experiment was used as an excuse to revert to a pattern established 20 years previously, the best interests of the medical officer of health and of the public he served were not always first among the motives of those who made the decisions.

In public health, where innovation must depend on a widely varied range of advances in sciences and technical developments which were previously remote from it, this is very difficult. In Britain, a century after the struggle to embrace bacteriology in the DPH curriculum took place, as a consequence of ignorance and prejudice, similar problems are being encountered with the introduction of psychology as an adjunct to sociology in the understanding of human behaviour. The basis for a fear of innovation is complex, but the comfort of the status quo is certainly

---

[82] There were other questions relating to the playing of an important role in the Courts by medical practitioners, but experience was rapidly to show these to be irrelevant to state medicine as it evolved. See General Medical Council (1869). *Minutes*, pp. 62–5; see also Chapter 2 (note 38).

innovation's enemy. The persistent retention of meteorology has been discussed above. Schools of public health might have been expected to be the ideal institutions to lead the evolutionary process. Their academic structures, however, have not kept up with the rapidly changing face of public health.

Examining

Methods of examining over the life-span of the DPH gave rise to surprisingly little contention. In the first round of inspections, Duffey, in his tour of 1894 and 1895, expressed his disapproval of a system practised, for example, in Dublin and Edinburgh, whereby a single lecturer set and marked a paper on his own course. From the outset Cambridge employed external examiners, and most distinguished ones at that, in part at least for the good reason that there was nobody in Cambridge competent to examine some aspects of the curriculum. Nevertheless, it was the General Medical Council which first established the excellent requirement of external examiners in all medical examinations, a practice which is now universal in all subjects in all British universities, and could be adopted with benefit elsewhere.

Practical instruction

The battle to ensure that candidates received sufficient practical instruction was hard fought over many years. Despite heroic efforts by the General Medical Council it was not won until after the DPH had been discontinued. Now, however, medical trainees in public health are expected to undertake a five-year apprenticeship and only then are they considered to have the maturity and competence to be accredited as practitioners to accept a responsible post. This emphasis on practical experience, which is general to all medical specialism nowadays, is by no means wholly compatible with outlooks and practices in much of conventional university education, and indeed in the past most resistance came from the universities.

Depth of learning

No lasting solution was ever found to the question about depth of learning, and we have seen how in 1922 in Cambridge, depth was quite deliberately sacrificed on the altar of economic pragmatism, and how, although the Council emphasized that its requirements were minimal, little if any attempt was made by the educational institutions to extend them. An exception perhaps was the University of London with its paper on mental health, but that was part of a course for an MD degree, not a simple Diploma in Public Health.

Adapting to change

Schools of public health might have been expected to be the ideal institutions to lead the process of change as Evans argued.[83] The present study, however, bears out a proposition made in a theoretical paper written a decade ago[84] that the fundamental problem lies not with the structure of the schools, although this unquestionably enhances it. The problem is with the men and women who staff the departments and divisions, and with the natural interest they have in how the survival of their own subjects (and indeed themselves as professionals) will be influenced by change. No longer do educators have to grapple with the statutory constraints geared to training people for a single post. Structure is after all man-made and as much a political as an administrative phenomenon which can enhance stasis. If however it is changed sensibly, stasis can be destroyed.

In 1976 Ernest Gruenberg looked optimistically ahead:

I believe that the agencies organised in the name of public health have become too preoccupied with maintaining the activities they struggled to create, have too many personal missions and have already lost such a large part of their leading role in the struggle to improve health, that we are wrong to rely exclusively upon them in the future. Just as something new was needed in 1916 [the year Hopkins School of Hygiene was founded], so something new is needed in 1976.

A social institution whose central preoccupation is protecting or preserving the peoples' health could examine every new technical discovery in social policy to weigh its potential impact on the peoples' health. It could preserve the record of past successes and failures to better the peoples' health, and continually reappraise the lessons to be learned from this accumulating experience.[85]

The straight-jacket around the DPH never allowed scope for such an approach as this. Nor, at least until the time of the First World War, with the arrival on the scene of energetic visionaries such as Newman and Rose, was there any evidence that a need to introduce radical change within training institutions weighed heavily on anyone's mind. From the 1930s, those responsible for the courses were so concerned with introducing modifications to suit the rapidly changing role of the medical officer of health, and with maintaining standards for the teaching of the

[83] Evans, John R. (1982). Measurement in management and medicine: training needs and opportunities. In *Population-based medicine* (ed. M. Lipkin Jr. and W.A. Lybrand), Ch. 1. Praeger, New York, and separately by the Rockefeller Foundation.

[84] Acheson, Roy M. (1980). Community medicine: discipline or topic? Profession or endeavour? *Community Medicine*, **2**, 2–6.

[85] Gruenberg, E.M. (1976). Personal statement. *Higher Education for public health*, p. 217. Prodist, for Milbank Memorial Fund, New York.

old pearls of wisdom in the face of economic pressures, that there was little talk of true innovation.

A school of public health may have more to offer than any other approach to improving the teaching of public health in Britain, but, among the reasons other than those given in Section 5 of this chapter, expectations of what it could do must be limited. The problem is one for which there is no single solution. A school has two quite distinct responsibilities. One is to teach and the other to research the subjects that are known to be on the growing edge of practice. Many schools do both well. What is not done by them is systematically to promote the monitoring of social and health policy implementations of new technological developments of discoveries in the physical, behavioural, and biological sciences and to weigh the potential contribution of these to public health practice.

Those who attempt such things, in practice as well as in educational establishments, may face the fighting front of professionalism. The medical officer of health, especially in a local authority with some millions of inhabitants, had great power, and of course great responsibility; he had to cope, without instruction in management science, because no such systematic instruction then existed. Yet, when the last revision of Recommendations introduced the principles of management to the curriculum—a move which five years later was to be endorsed by the Faculty of Community Medicine—many resisted because, they argued, management was no business of the medical professional. Such arguments can be extended to other fields. In the case of management this retrograde attitude played some part in the decision by politicians, probably the right one, to place the management of the National Health Service firmly in the hands of professional managers—though a few of them are medically trained.

The DPH was a child of its time. When, in the mid-nineteenth century, after 10 or 20 years of political and professional bargaining and a series of private members' Bills, the General Medical Council finally was able to control basic medical education and professional standards, it was understandable that little consideration should be given to its playing any further role in specialized medical work. Ten years later, in 1868, when Disraeli's government became aware that public health doctors also needed training, education, and standards, it was not surprising that supervising this task was placed in the lap of the Council. As we have seen, although education, training, and standards were indeed common to the two problems, that was just about as far as it went. All in all, what is perhaps surprising is that the DPH and the General Medical Council remained in wedlock as long as they did.

7. Epilogue

Of the institutions whose fortunes we have followed over the century in this chapter and chapter 2, the most important survivor from the viewpoint of the world at large, as well as from that of Britain has been the London School of Hygiene and Tropical Medicine which flies the flag of the University of London. It offers degrees in subjects other than public health but these are mainly cognate. It is in fact a school of public health, though more medically focused than any in the United States.

In a slightly different category, but in some ways more remarkable, is the University of Edinburgh which, with the exception of short breaks in war years, has continually offered a qualification, most of the time a degree, in public health and currently teaches medical and non-medical candidates side by side for an M.Sc. in community medicine. The Universities of Cambridge and Oxford teach and offer research experience for candidates for the MFPHM. The London Conjoint in Public Health went out of business in 1974 and the University of Dublin is in Ireland, which now has its own Medical Council and its own Faculty of Community Medicine.

9

Preparation for public health practice: into the twenty-first century

MARGOT JEFFERYS AND JOYCE LASHOF

1. Introduction

Earlier chapters have traced the way in which, in two industrialized nations in the last 150 years, 'the health of the public', as opposed to the curative treatment of individuals, came to be seen both as requiring public administrative action and as a subject meriting academic enquiry. They showed how the identification of specific practices, intended to improve the public's health, led to the creation of occupational roles, which, in the course of time, became formalized. In turn, institutions were designed to prepare recruits for the new tasks and roles as they developed.

What has been particularly enlightening in these historical essays is to learn that, despite the overwhelming comparabilities in public health problems in the United States and the United Kingdom as they changed during that period, there have been considerable differences in the two countries. Most noticeably, these differences are in the ways in which the public health function has been conceived and performed; in the role of the medical profession; and in the institutional provision made for training public health workers.

It is clear that there is no single or simple explanation for these differences, which have continued throughout the past century. This is despite the many factors, such as improved communication at all levels, that might have brought greater convergence in practice as well as in theory. Indeed, the value of the analyses contained in the previous chapters is to detail the historical particularities of the developments in each country in public health practice and training which, partly because they occurred at different periods, helped to give a unique national flavour to the institutional arrangements devised in each.

Several factors must be listed which helped to determine the different parts played by the medical profession in the conglomeration of occupational roles which today constitute the public health enterprise in the two countries. First is the stage of industrialization and urbanization at which a defined function was perceived and the need for trained practitioners recognized. Secondly, the extent to which the fortunes enjoyed by medical practitioners in their traditional clinical fee-for-service activities influenced their willingness to enter salaried positions. Thirdly, the strength of collectivist as opposed to individualistic popular ideologies affected public activities as well as private behaviour. Finally, the degree to which other occupational interests and the public challenged professional claims to disinterested conduct and to monopolistic practices. There have been considerable differences in all such factors as well as in others in the United Kingdom and in the United States. Nor can the weight of tradition itself be discounted, especially in the case of the United Kingdom. Origins imply roots, and unless there is some overwhelming ground swell to disturb them, they are deeply embedded enough to continue to ensure the particular shape of all subsequent developments, even when the verdict of history may be to show them as obsolete, if not bankrupt.

Three questions must be addressed which concern the present and the future of public health and of its training institutions. These are prompted by the analysis of the recent past as presented in previous chapters. The first is whether it is possible to discern changes which are likely to affect the whole mode of public health practice and hence of educational preparation for it in the near or more distant future. The second is whether predictable changes are likely to lead to more or to less international comparability between the public health roles and the institutions which prepare people for them. A third, over-arching question is whether the training institutions themselves influence the shape of public health practice, or whether they are merely responsive to the demands made on them by the practitioners of public health and by their paymasters—the latter most commonly the organs of state at a local, national, or international level.

In seeking to answer these questions, we consider first how far the two countries will have problems of public health in common in the next few decades. Then we ask whether those who will determine future public health policy in both countries—and this includes politicians of different persuasions and the employees of state bureaucracies, as well as those currently engaged in public health practice, teaching, or

research—are at present contemplating similar operational and educational objectives, or whether they assume that their options are
limited by the legacies of their national pasts. We end the chapter, not by
coming to hard and fast conclusions ourselves, but by asking readers of
the book, whose concern for an improvement in public health can be
taken for granted, themselves to enlist in the ongoing debates about
how this vital collective function, and preparation for it, can best be
conducted in the future.

2. Challenges to the public's health

As the twentieth century nears its end, it is clear that the challenges to
public health today are as serious, if not more so, than those at the end of
the nineteenth century. Nor can they be contained within the boundaries of single nation states. Those problems sanitary reformers a century
and a half ago thought that they were confronting—poor, unhygienic
environments, malignant miasmas, and a level of poverty which pre-
cluded a healthy, adequate diet for the majority—are still there for many
if not for most of the inhabitants of Third World countries. Even industrialized nations like the United States and the United Kingdom have
not been able totally to eliminate such environmental or social structural
causes of avoidable illness, disability, and premature death. Some medical interventions have successfully reduced infant deaths in impoverished countries. What are now required are equally urgent measures to
reduce fertility levels in these countries and to secure a better social distribution of scarce economic resources.

   This is not the place to debate the question of how much the decline in
death rates and increase in life expectancy which characterized both the
United States and the United Kingdom as well as virtually every other
industrialized country were due respectively to the successful control of
some lethal environmental hazards, to the often compulsory implementation of specific prophylactic procedures, to a fairer distribution of
income, or to the wider dissemination of health knowledge leading to
better health practices on the part of more and more people. Clearly, all
were responsible to some extent. Nor is it appropriate to consider here
the various explanations which have been given for the changes in state
policies which initiated or encouraged these changes. It is more important in the context to point out that these undoubted success stories did
not lead automatically to the health millenium, to a universal lived-
happily-ever-after syndrome. As a result, the United States and the United
Kingdom, and to a greater or lesser extent all advanced industrialized

countries, face other public health challenges which are either specific to the late twentieth century or remarkable now because in earlier epochs they were not so visible or were swamped by other, more pressing concerns.

One of the most insidious yet important effects of the public health successes in mortality reduction at early ages which have taken place in the twentieth century is to put on the agenda the need to consider seriously the health and living conditions of the increasing numbers in each successive cohort who survive into extreme old age, which so often brings with it multiple handicap and a loss of personal independence in activities of daily living. Neither the United Kingdom nor the United States has yet evolved services which, at one and the same time, are adequate to meet the needs of most of the survivors and gain the willing agreement of younger generations that it is in their own best interests—in the present as well as in their own ageing future—to invest in measures designed to improve health in old age.

In the late twentieth century, mankind is increasingly hoist by its own petard. That is to say, the technical advances which have enabled us to increase exponentially our productivity, that is our capacity to produce goods and services, not merely to prolong and sustain life but to enrich the variety and quality of choices which individuals can exercise during their lifetimes, have been found to have unexpected and unwanted side effects. In turn, these have become the public health problems of our day. Our economic and technological successes, accompanied, however, by military and economic struggles for the control of resources, have engendered a vast range of problems, including some which, in contemplation, seem likely, if not tackled in the near future at the technical, economic and political levels, to have a devastating effect on the sustainability of our environment.

Public health practitioners, because their brief includes attempting to control those factors in the environment which affect adversely the health, broadly defined, of the populations whose representatives employ them, cannot ignore the current and future threats which emanate from the use or abuse of nuclear power, the production of 'greenhouse gases' and resultant global warming, and the release of toxic chemicals into the environment. Nor can they dismiss the threats to whole population groups of the production, distribution, and consumption of natural and man-made addictive products on a massive scale. They are forced to consider the potential public health effects—beneficial as well as sinister—of recent developments in genetic engineering, if they were to be applied to human beings. Further, as if to keep the guardians of the public health on their toes, the appearance in the last decades of the twentieth century of a previously unknown but now recognized as a lethal retrovirus, HIV, leading, it seems inexorably to AIDS, challenges them to find ways of preventing an epidemic which threatens to engulf and destroy people, usually in the prime of their lives.

The present speed of scientific discovery and of technological innovation means that issues which only 20 years ago seemed to belong to the world of science fiction are now on the current social and political agenda of national states throughout the world. Scientists, including those involved in understanding and promoting health, have a fearsome responsibility to comprehend these changes and to instruct their politicians and their populations of the health implications, including those which, at first sight, seem to have little to do with human health.

There was a period—the years following the Second World War in particular—which was marked by an extreme optimism concerning prospects for health among other aspects of human existence. That is no longer the mood today. Yet it is important that we do not succumb to the predominant pessimism which the size and complexity of present-day threats seem to warrant. There is a danger that defeatism can act as a self-fulfilling prophecy and paralyse the effort needed to find solutions.

3. The challenge to public health institutions and practitioners

Before considering the specific issues facing the institutions which prepare individuals for various aspects of public health practice, it is necessary briefly to sketch the main characteristics, at the end of the twentieth century, of the statutory organizations which, in both countries, are charged with the protection and promotion of the public health. Earlier chapters have traced broadly the development of these organizations and so attempted to account for their present form.

In the United States, responsibility for the control of public health practice is shared by federal, state, and local government. The federal government provides overall direction, establishes national priorities, and sets standards which may reflect both consensus and party political policies. Federal agencies encourage research and practice development by financing research institutions and by promoting communication among researchers, and between them and the practitioners.

Federal agencies also have significant regulatory power to control production and distribution practices which may impose a threat to public health throughout the nation; these include toxic chemicals, food, drugs, both licit and illicit, and environmental pollutants. Some of these dangerous substances are fairly well regulated; but there are contradictory policies concerning some drugs, such as alcohol and tobacco, and very ineffective controls over others, for example, cocaine and heroin. Moreover, the fragmentation of control among the different federal agencies responsible for different aspects of public health is conducive to inefficiency.

By and large, however, the practice of public health, whether preventive or promotive or coercive, is carried out at a state, city, or county level. It is the staff employed at this level who form the bulk of public health practitioners. Senior management staff may have initial qualifications in a variety of academic disciplines or applied subjects, including technology and business management. Whatever their preliminary training, it is likely to have been at university level and broadly based. Moreover, they are likely to have been prepared for their posts by obtaining a master's degree or even a doctorate in public health, granted by a school of public health, after a period of full- or part-time training. Some of them may be physicians. The majority will have been drawn from other professions and disciplines.

In the United Kingdom, the departments of central government set standards, and, theoretically at least, monitor performance where public health functions are mandatory rather than permissive. (The constituent parts of the United Kingdom, namely England and Wales, Scotland and Northern Ireland, have separate but generally comparable legislation governing their public health provision.) Since 1974, at the local level (except in Northern Ireland), public health functions are shared by two statutory agencies—Local Authorities and the District Health Authorities of the National Health Service. Local government has had its public health activities restricted, except in so far as it also has responsibility for the social support and care as well as the housing of chronically ill and disabled people and the frail elderly. The National Health Service is responsible for promoting measures designed to maintain and improve maternal and child health, and for the prevention of chronic disease in middle and late adult life. A newly established Health Education Authority is particularly concerned with helping to improve standards of health behaviour relating to such matters as diet, exercise, addiction, and sexual activities.

Within the National Health Service, managerial responsibility for public health is, *de facto* if no longer *de jure*, in the hands of medical practitioners who have also obtained the postgraduate qualification in community medicine (since 1989, renamed public health medicine), standards for which are set by the Faculty of that name of the Royal Colleges of Physicians of the United Kingdom. They have the status of consultant in the National Health Service, comparable to that enjoyed by clinicians in medical specialties. They are supported by registrars who are medically qualified junior doctors in training posts, as are consultants in other branches of hospital-based medicine. Non-medically qualified members of the National Health Service departments of public health are employed only in a technical capacity (for example, to give statistical or technical advice) and are not eligible for consultant and hence managerial posts in the specialty.

In local government, medically qualified staff are notable by their absence. Responsibility for health as it relates to the control of the environment is in the hands either of environmental health officers, whose training has been to technical diploma rather than university degree level, or of engineers who, after their initial degree or diploma have specialized in water, sewage, industrial pollution, and other aspects of environmental control. Acheson describes training programmes in these fields in more detail in Chapter 8.

Given the differences in the organizational structure of public health institutions in the two countries and in their personnel, it is not surprising to find substantial national differences in the ways in which the educational and research establishments regard their responsibilities for preparing practitioners for their work, despite the comparability of the major public health challenges. In the following two sections, we examine the educational and research strategies being pursued or advocated first in the United States and then in the United Kingdom. In our concluding remarks we cast a critical eye on the two national scenes and ask whether the proposals are sufficient to meet the public health challenges of the near and more distant future.

4. The United States: future obligations of schools of public health

As earlier chapters have shown, there has been a longstanding assumption in the United States that the basis of public health knowledge is multidisciplinary, and that the contributory disciplines need to be brought together within schools of public health. It follows that the United States' profession of public health is not homogeneous, and that its practitioners, as well as those who teach them, are drawn from several basic disciplines. Factors which give the profession coherence are first, the focus on community rather than individual health; and second, the principle of commitment to the public good, to social justice, and to the egalitarian ethos. In turn, this focus and these commitments dictate the underlying objectives behind educational programmes.

Given that public health is a field of activity devoted to the protection of health and the prevention of disease, the academic preparation of its practitioners is increasingly designed to make them aware, not only of the nature of the many environmental threats to health and the technical means of overcoming them, but also of what constitutes effective public health action. This, in turn, depends on social, economic, scientific, and political forces in society at large. To educate public health professionals to function in the complexities of the real world, to carry out the basic and applied research required to expand knowledge and secure its application, and to train researchers to address the general and specific issues of public health, are recognized by the schools of public health as the challenges which they will face in the twenty-first century.

In March 1987, a conference on education, training, and the future of public health brought together the deans of the United States' schools of public health and leading public health practitioners to examine the relationship of education to practice.[1] Not surprisingly, identifying the problems proved easier than providing the solutions. Among the issues discussed, relevant to our concerns with the comparison between the United States and the United Kingdom, were the tension between clinical medicine and public health, the collaborative efforts of schools of public health and public health agencies, and the relationship between professional and academic education.

The tension between clinical medicine and public health.

As earlier chapters have shown, the tension between clinical medicine and public health has pervaded the history of public health education and practice in both Britain and the United States. In the United States, one of the manifestations has been the comparatively low status of the medical officer or public health physician *vis-à-vis* the clinician. Although the role of many ancillary public health workers has been accepted as conferring considerable status on the non-physicians who enter the profession by that route, the status of the physician in the field has been persistently debased, especially by fellow physicians.

There is, however, a real potential for change as the century nears its end, and as the part played by physicians trained in public health alters. The reasons stem from the changing requirements of the medical care system. It is now struggling to cope with the maintenance of a system of

---

[1] *Proceedings of the conference on education, training and the future of public health, 1987.* (In press).

ambulatory care of patients with chronic disease and the increasingly ageing population at a time when hospitals are becoming more and more concerned with the high-technology management of short-stay patients.

These developments demand more closely integrated systems of care, and increased community-based resources for the chronically ill. They also demand more sophisticated means of making decisions regarding the allocation of scarce health care resources. This last requirement calls for the recruitment of physicians with additional training in epidemiology, economics, methods of evaluation, and administrative skills. In the last few years more physicians have shown themselves interested in obtaining such knowledge in order to play leadership roles not only in government agencies at the federal and state level, but also in Health Maintenance Organizations and hospital systems at local levels. Schools of public health are setting out to attract more physicians in order to prepare them to assume these new responsibilities and are enlarging the scope of their curriculum, often joining with schools of business administration and public policy to achieve this purpose. As this new group of physicians takes on these responsibilities, be it in the public or the private sector, it is probable if not certain that their status, if not their popularity, will improve.

In addition, medical schools are showing renewed interest in improving the preparatory education for those involved in ambulatory and primary care, including preventive medicine, and this has resulted in an expansion of departments of community medicine. The Kellogg Foundation has recently announced a new initiative designed to establish centres of excellence for the teaching of primary care. These centres are to bring together for education and practice the primary care disciplines of medicine, nursing, and dentistry with public health. Such a development should also help to break down the barriers between public health and clinical practice.

Collaborative efforts of schools and agencies.

Much public health effort during the past decades has been directed towards changing those aspects of the life-styles of individuals identified as the major determinants in the prevalence of cardiovascular disease, cancer, chronic pulmonary disease, and unintentional injuries. Little attention has been directed to the influence of the environment, both social and physical, on life-styles. There is, however, a growing realization that the time has come for schools of public health to reassert the importance of a population or community-based approach, not only in the identification of risk factors, but in their control as well. For example, although change in the behaviour of individuals remains the goal of anti-smoking, low-fat, high-fibre diet, and exercise campaigns, if the efforts to bring about change are to be successful, they will have to take into consideration the social and economic environments which induce high-risk-bearing activities in the first place.

Schools of public health need to take the lead in understanding how tax policies, advertising practices, and regulatory measures, for example, affect the use of tobacco and alcohol. They also need to examine why health status is inferior and all risk factors more prevalent among the poor, and how an individual's sense of self esteem and of control over his or her own life influences his or her health behaviour. The schools themselves are increasingly prepared to explore these issues and bring a multidisciplinary approach to the development of programmes aimed at defined populations and executed by the communities themselves. Their objective is to educate their students to implement appropriate programmes and play a role in policy development. Although clinical medicine increasingly must incorporate preventive advice, including health education, into its repertoire, it is more likely that future advances in primary prevention of chronic diseases will come from the population-based public health field, as have past successes in conquering many of the infectious diseases.

If these efforts are to be successful, however, education in public health will have to re-focus its attention on providing its professionals with the means to make a community diagnosis, to identify community health needs, and to develop interventions and strategies for their implementation, as well as with the competence to evaluate them. The basic knowledge and skills required to perform these functions are now part of the curriculum of all schools; they include epidemiology, biostatistics, survey research methods, programme planning, techniques for mobilizing community resources, and the evaluation of interventions. Added to these must be more systematic consideration at both the academic and the practical level of the political process at all levels of society and how to function effectively in it.

While it is clear that all students of public health should recognize and have a basic knowledge of the disciplines and skills which underpin the public health enterprise seen as a whole, it is clear that no one person can be skilled in everything. The multidisciplinary character of the faculty and students of the schools of public health must serve as a model for the public health agency, where there is an equal need for a team approach and for the cross-fertilization of the expertise of the epidemiologist, the sociologist, the political scientist, the economist, and the health educator, among others.

The challenge is even greater than this, however, because it is now becoming clear that there is a need to integrate the existing type of public health approach into the delivery of primary care.[2] This is well exemplified by the World Health Organization's Alma Ata declaration on Primary Care[3] and their 'Health for all in the year 2000' campaign among nation states at every level of technological sophistication as well as their 'Healthy cities' initiative in the developed world.[4] Community oriented primary care, a concept developed in particular by Sidney Kark in South Africa and Israel,[5] has recently received renewed attention in the American context. Following a report by the Institute of Medicine in the United States in 1984,[6] the Public Health Service at the federal level sponsored studies and encouraged further development of the community oriented primary care model by community health centres; by Health Maintenance Organizations (where the enrolled population constitutes the community); by county health agencies which have assumed responsibility for the delivery of primary care services to indigent populations; and by rural area private practitioners in collaboration with their rural hospital and their health department.

Under the terms of this federal initiative, the School of Public Health in the University of California at Berkeley, for example, began to work with community health centres supported by the United States Public Health Service in order to identify opportunities for and obstacles to the implementation of the various elements of the community oriented primary care model. It also developed a training manual to assist health centre staff in implementing these principles.[7] It is now co-operating with a California county health agency to explore the potential for developing the model for county-wide use. If it can be shown that community health is best served by the collaborative effort of public health and clinical medicine, then progress will have been made in overcoming the historic tensions between the two.

[2] Ibid.

[3] World Health Organization (1978). *Declaration of Alma Ata. Report on the International Conference on Primary Health Care.* Alma Ata, Union of Soviet Socialist Republics, 6–12 September. World Health Organization, Geneva. (*Health for all series, No. 1*)

[4] World Health Organization (1981). *Global strategy for health for all in the year 2000.* World Health Organization, Geneva. (*Health for all series, No. 3*)

[5] Kark, S. L. (1981). *The practice of community oriented primary health care.* Appleton-Century-Crofts, New York.

[6] *Community oriented primary care, a practical assessment* (1984). National Academy Press, Washington DC.

[7] University of California at Berkeley, School of Public Health (1988). *Community oriented primary care in action: a practice manual for primary care settings.* United States Department of Health and Human Services, Public Health Service Health Resources and Services Administration Contract, No. 240–84–0124, Washington, DC.

The dual responsibility of schools of public health

A related but broader issue is that of the dual responsibility of schools of public health as both professional and academic educational institutions. It is clear that, although the schools primarily developed as a result of the need to train practical workers, in recent years they have become increasingly oriented to research and hence have expanded their academic M.Sc and Ph.D. degree programmes in addition to the MPH and Dr.P.H. degrees.

Given the complexity and diversity of the field of public health and the increased scientific expertise required to address the great variety of public health problems, this expansion is not surprising and, indeed, is highly desirable. The faculty of the schools today is therefore drawn from an even wider range of disciplines than ever before. What characterizes the research effort of this diverse faculty is the application of their various disciplines to current public health issues. For example, in the field of environmental health there is a need for toxicologists to identify toxic agents and their mechanisms of action; for engineers to determine how to decrease the output of hazardous wastes; for industrial hygienists to explore methods of protecting workers; for epidemiologists to identify environmental hazards; for health educators to work with communities; and for social and political scientists to devise and develop governmental policies relating to control and regulation.

In health administration, economists are needed to study how resources can best be related to access to and the use of care; clinicians and systems analysts together should study the effect of organization and financing on the quality of care; and ethicists and social and political scientists to address issues of burden, equity, and justice in the determination of priorities. Assertive measures directed to health promotion as well as disease prevention are rightly receiving increased attention and have also to be viewed from a broad perspective. The researcher in the behavioural sciences must address the interplay of societal and individual influences, and of genetic and environmental factors which affect behaviour and endanger or promote health.

If the overall objective is to create a society that maximizes health, then the combined efforts of all these disciplines are required to develop and test theories. Theory-testing, in particular, cannot be done without close communication with both the field of practice and colleagues in various academic departments. The range of knowledge and related skills required will rarely be within the resources available to any one school. Hence, the development of joint degrees must continue, most commonly awarded in collaboration with schools of business management, public policy, and law. Joint teaching between such institutions has already led to collaborative research which bridges internal university divisions as well as disciplinary boundaries.

Individual status within the faculty is highly prized but highly dependent on the quality of a member's research output. Schools thus accord priority to research, in preference to community service. As a result, some public health practitioners consider that the schools are divorcing themselves from practice and consequently lacking in the ability adequately to train practitioners. However, this need not be the case.

If field practice is an integral part of the MPH curriculum, as it undoubtedly should be, it will ensure that students gain experience in applying their classroom knowledge to the solution of real problems. Training in field work, moreover, can be effectively used as a mechanism for involving practitioners in the educational process, not merely as preceptors but as adjunct faculty. In addition, if members of the faculty are more actively involved through consultation and seminars around the problems students find they are addressing in their field experience, the requirement itself can play an important role in bridging the gap between the university and the service worlds. Of course, a certain degree of tension between the academic and the practical is inevitable and, indeed, even healthy; but the relationship should and can be complementary rather than divisive.

5. The United Kingdom: through community medicine and back to public health

Not surprisingly, much of what we have said about the present and future challenges facing the United States institutions charged with preparing public health practitioners for their work and advancing their knowledge base applies with equal or greater force in the United Kingdom. The masters degrees of the university schools and departments now offered to those entering the field of public health, as well as the examinations for the Membership of the Faculty of Public Health Medicine[8] place the same degree of emphasis on epidemiology, biostatistics, health economics, and the social and behavioural sciences, as do the American MPH and Dr.P.H. courses.

Intra-professional tensions in the United Kingdom

There have also been tensions, still by no means resolved, between clinical practitioners and teachers on the one hand, and, on the other, those

[8] See Chapter 8 (note 77).

whose practice, teaching, or research concern not so much the individual as the collectivity at national, district, or local level. In the medical
fraternity, some clinical specialists, to coin a phrase, have been more
equal than others; as a consequence, hospital-based clinicians have been
able to exercise greater influence on the distribution of health care
resources, (including those who teach medical students), than have
those whose post-qualification training in public health or community
medicine is deliberately intended to equip them to give informed advice
and guidance to policy makers and managers on such matters.

It was hoped that the formation in 1972 of a Faculty of Community
Medicine within the Royal Colleges of Physicians of the United Kingdom would provide a more prestigious and satisfying career for those
doctors who chose to work in non-clinical posts. It was also intended at
one and the same time that this would be combined with providing a
special place for the community physician in the administrative structures at all levels of the National Health Service, and with persuading
clinicians of the value to them of having someone with medical qualifications on decision-making bodies affecting their work.

In Chapter 6, Lewis has considered why these aspirations for a better
deployment of medically qualified doctors, who chose to practice at the
population or group rather than the individual clinical level, were
largely frustrated in the 1970s, and why the subsequent changes in
National Health Service management structures in the 1980s appeared
to place in further jeopardy the roles which the Faculty of Community
Medicine had designed for its members.[9] Furthermore, it was feared
that the changes would be to the detriment of preventive medicine as
well as primary care to which community medicine had sought to give
priority. Suffice it to say here that the specialty now mainly sees a threat
from non-medically qualified managers rather than from clinicians, and
is gravely concerned about the way in which environmental health
issues have been handled.

The Report of the Committee on the Public Health Function,[10] which
sat under the chairmanship of Sir Donald Acheson in 1987 and 1988,
underscored the need for revitalized professional groups responsible for
promoting and monitoring the public health in its widest sense, and
intended to influence how professionals in those groups should be

---

[9] Department of Health and Social Security (1983). *Report of the National Health Service
management inquiry* (The Griffiths Report). Her Majesty's Stationery Office, London.
[10] See Chapter 6, Section 6; Chapter 8, Section 5 and note 77.

prepared for their future roles.[11] The name of the specialty has already been changed to Public Health Medicine and the Report and its major recommendations were accepted by the government and enthusiastically endorsed by the Faculty of Community Medicine, which represents practitioners, academic teachers, and research workers.

For other reasons, however, it is as yet too early to assess whether past rifts between public health practitioners and clinicians are likely to be perpetuated or to diminish as we enter the last decade of the twentieth century. As we write, the government proposes to create an 'internal market' in the National Health Service and to permit, indeed encourage, hospitals to become self-governing and large general practice units to hold their own budgets and make contracts with hospitals for the care of their patients.[12] The organizations representing different branches of the medical profession, while accepting the need for greater efficiency and acknowledging the need to provide general practitioners with incentives to improve still further their disease prevention and health promotion activities, have joined together in general opposition to the plan. If, as is probable, the government's proposal is implemented, it could lead in either direction, that is, to a closing of the ranks within the medical profession to resist the managerial controls to which they object, or to a regrowth of internal professional dissension based on differences in perceptions of the effects of such managerial decisions on resource allocation or monitoring.

Collaboration between academics and practitioners

In one respect, however, namely that of collaboration between the academics and the practitioners of public health, greater progress may have taken place in the United Kingdom than in the United States in recent years. As previous chapters have indicated, before the formation of the Faculty of Community Medicine in 1972, there had been an ongoing cold war between on the one hand, the practitioners, represented by the medical officers of health, and on the other, the members of academic departments of social medicine who were mostly research epidemiologists; see also Chapter 6, Section 4 and Chapter 8, Section 4.

During the late 1960s there was a growing recognition of the damage done to the promotion of the public's health by the continued rift between the universities and the world of service in public health. The

---

[11] Department of Health and Social Security (1988). *Public health in England: The Report of the Committee of Enquiry into the Future Development of the Public Health Function* [Chairman Sir Donald Acheson], Cmnd. 289. Her Majesty's Stationery Office, London.

[12] Department of Health and Social Security (1989). *Working for patients: the health service caring for the 1990s*. Her Majesty's Stationery Office, London.

academics took the initiative in trying to heal the breach by proposing common membership for practitioners and academics of a newly created Faculty of the three prestigious Royal Colleges of Physicians,[13] and the medical officers agreed to accept the contemporaneous, if not synchronized, proposal that, henceforth, their roles in prevention, promotion, and administration should be carried out within the bureaucratic structures of the National Health Service rather than within those of local government.

With hindsight, it is easy to see that the job descriptions for community physicians in the management structure of the National Health Service in 1974 bore little resemblance to the positions they actually occupied. They were often powerless to fulfil their role as guardians or promoters of the public health. Many felt that they had been relegated to subordinate positions in hospital management rather than being allowed to act as policy makers concerned with the equitable distribution of scarce health care resources. As a consequence, morale fell and recruits for this specialty were insufficient to fill the vacant posts. The prospects were further undermined by new National Health Service management proposals in the 1980s, which, as they were implemented, appeared further to erode the public health function.[14]

On the other hand, perhaps paradoxically, the trials and tribulations which the National Health Service and the teaching and research institutions were undergoing in the changing socio-political atmosphere, which came with Margaret Thatcher's government, brought a radical new view of the way in which public sector enterprises should be run. By holding public health practitioners and teachers to account, they brought them closer together in a number of significant ways.

In particular, the new proposals for an internal market in the National Health Service, which broke down the previous political consensus regarding the inviolability of this post-Second World War pillar of the Welfare State, require that all those concerned with the public's health consider afresh and together their professional goals and the means of attaining them. They require that, together, they redefine their objectives first for public health in the very widest sense of that term, and second for the educational means of producing competent public health practitioners. The Committee of Inquiry on the Future Development of the Public Health Function's recommendation for even closer relationships between academics and practitioners—incidentally, much along

---

[13] These are the Royal College of Physicians of London and of Edinburgh and the Royal College of Physicians and Surgeons of Glasgow.

[14] See Chapter 6, Section 6.

the lines proposed by the Deans of the American Schools of Public Health—was, to some extent, pushing at an already open door.

6. Unresolved issues

There is no doubt that the re-affirmation of the worth of the public health function, implicit in the British Government's acceptance in principle of the main recommendations of the 1988 Report[15] helped to improve morale and hopes for their own future among practitioners and academics. Any euphoria, however, was destined to be short-lived. In the early months of 1989, government proposals for radical changes in the management of the acute medical services[16] seemed largely to ignore the specialty and its concerns.

As we write, the rapidity of change which the Conservative Government requires from health service managers and practitioners and the small amount of time allowed for consultation with professionals add to the difficulty we would in any case have faced in predicting the likely future, immediate or long term, for education in public health in the United Kingdom. As the role which public health practitioners can perform in the revamped National Health Service becomes clearer, the structural changes may well require still further shifts in the educational policies which the specialty was beginning to formulate before being confronted with further immediate and critical problems.

At the considerable risk of being shown with the passage of time to have been unnecessarily Cassandra-like, we feel that it is worth setting out in brief some of the issues concerning the future of public health educational establishments in the United Kingdom, which, despite the recommendations of the Committee on the Public Health Function, are either unresolved or remain problematic as the century nears its end.

The first question is whether the United Kingdom's schools of public health and the variously named departments of medical faculties, which at present alone or in collaboration with one another prepare the medically qualified for community medicine practice, can become, as envisaged by Sir Donald Acheson's committee, the institutions responsible for preparing recruits from assorted backgrounds for a much wider gamut of public health posts. In short, are British universities now ready for developments which have much in common with the United States' schools of public health?

The obstacles in the way of transforming what have hitherto been

---

[15] Department of Health and Social Security, op. cit. (note 11).
[16] Department of Health and Social Security, op. cit. (note 12).

largely uni-disciplinary institutions, concentrating on converting doctors with a set of clinical, diagnostic, and therapeutic skills into practitioners capable of diagnosing community-based health problems and taking appropriate action, are formidable. It is true that some of these institutions have for some decades recognized the need for help in their present task from biostatisticians who do not necessarily possess medical qualifications. More recently, too, they have spasmodically called upon medical sociologists and social anthropologists, and more consistently upon health economists.

It has to be said, however, that those without medical qualifications have commonly felt themselves to be confined to 'non-commissioned' positions in institutions where the 'officer class' is exclusively medical. In other words, the former are often on short-term contracts associated with research projects, or members of other university departments and as such usually unpaid for their service teaching, or postgraduates writing theses and paid by the hour or session. Whatever their position they have hitherto had little or no say in the construction of the courses in which they participate. If they do obtain a tenured, faculty position in a community medicine department or school, their chances of promotion to full professorial status are markedly less favourable than those of their medically qualified colleagues. The equality of disciplinary status which marks a genuinely multidisciplinary establishment is still lacking. In addition, the special economic status afforded the medically qualified in the universities in the United Kingdom, which is justified on the grounds of maintaining comparability between salaries paid to clinicians in the universities and the National Health Service, even though it is given to those no longer engaged in clinical medicine, has always rankled with other academics. As a consequence, medical faculties may not be able to expect help from other university departments, especially at a time when resources generally are severely limited and pressure is being placed upon them to become more 'efficient' with their more thinly spread manpower.

The single national school of public health—the London School of Hygiene and Tropical Medicine—and a few medical departments with various titles in some universities have, in the last three decades, offered courses in a limited range of subjects within the general field of public health which are open to non-medically qualified as well as to medically qualified students. For example, the London School of Hygiene and Tropical Medicine has developed masters and/or diploma courses in medical statistics, medical demography, health economics, nutrition, tropical hygiene, parasitology, and so on. The medical faculties of the Universities of Manchester, Nottingham, Glasgow, and Edinburgh all have postgraduate specialist courses in one or other aspect of public health which are open to non-medical as well as to medical graduates. The University of Liverpool's School of Tropical Medicine has a variety of courses designed solely for students preparing to work in general or specific aspects of public health in the developing world. These have all been positive developments which, albeit to only a limited extent, have brought medically qualified faculty and students of public health medicine together with non-medically qualified staff and students who intend working on matters of public health interest.

There is the strong probability that the Department of Health will give active encouragement, including financial support, to some universities to create full-blown schools of public health to replace the more modest educational provisions of the existing departments of community medicine and/or epidemiology. As we write, it is not yet clear how far these schools will be charged, more generally, with the educational preparation of National Health Service managers. Some fear that the emphasis in the schools will be more on business efficiency than on the promotion of public health *per se*.

The success of this new initiative for the public health function will also depend on whether non-medically qualified recruits to the field of public health will enjoy comparable career prospects to those whose names appear on the General Medical Council's Register. If this is not the case, able non-medically qualified graduates may be deterred from entering the public health field, if not health service management in the acute sector.

The proposed new schools will also depend on the relationships they establish with other educational institutions involved in specialized training for health professionals and researchers. Since 1988, the polytechnic colleges, a sector of higher education, which, in Britain, parallels the universities, have been freed financially from what had become for many of them the shackles of local government control and finance. Encouraged by new forms of central government funding, they have been developing innovative courses at various educational levels, especially for occupational groups who work in health and welfare fields, including environmental health and health service management. They are essentially multidisciplinary institutions which, like the technology institutes in the United States, deliberately set out to combine the academic with the practical, the scientific and technological with the counselling and the caring, and the efficient management of resources with ideas of equity and social justice. They may well make offers to prepare health service personnel for their future roles, offers that the employing authorities would find it difficult to refuse and which may compete favourably, at least in economic terms, with anything the new schools of public health can provide.

The major issue facing the institutions involved in public health education now and in the future is how to resolve the continued ambiguities which still surround the role of those medically qualified doctors who enter the field. The Committee on the Public Health Function categorically asserted the need for a medical specialty in public health; this understandably was enthusiastically welcomed by the Faculty of Community Medicine in 1988, but the changes which its report recommends appear more cosmetic than fundamental. The change in nomenclature— from 'community medicine' to 'public health medicine'—was a symbolic gesture which, although vociferously opposed by a minority, had a strong, initial placebo effect on the morale of the majority in the specialty. By attaching the word 'medicine' to the term 'Public Health', members of the Faculty were reassured that medical people still had a special role, and non-medical members of the public health labour force may not feel excluded as they might have done had the faculty labelled itself 'public health'.[17]

As the Faculty itself recognized, however, the Committee of Enquiry placed less emphasis on 'the way in which community physicians now and in the future contribute to the decision-making processes in the National Health Service', that is, on their role in management.[18] The Faculty nevertheless interpreted the Committee's recommendations as 'giving ample scope for the development of the planning and management function, for which, it is known, community physicians are now valued by Health Authorities'.

The Faculty went on to claim, but not to demonstrate convincingly, that surveillance, policies, priorities, and evaluation are tasks particularly appropriate to the medically qualified, while other, unspecified, aspects of management are not. The implicit assumptions, rather than explicit rationale, behind its position appears to be that a knowledge of epidemiology is the essential ingredient required for these tasks and that this, in turn, cannot be effectively acquired except by those with a previous training in clinical medicine.

Once again, it is not easy to predict whether the Faculty of Public Health Medicine and the schools which expect in the future to train con-

---

[17] The Faculty has recognized another need which was highlighted by the Report, namely that public health medicine should accept once more a dominant role in the control of infectious diseases. The recognition of the importance to public health of the control of chronic disease had brought with it a relative neglect in specialty training programmes in the principles of infectious disease control.

[18] A Statement made by the Faculty of Community Medicine, London, 9 May, 1988.

sultants in public health medicine will be successful in clarifying their educational objectives, given that governmental proposals for the future of the National Health Service are dominated by concern for the financing of the acute sector and of care in the community for elderly and chronically disabled people.[19] As, however, they seek to carry out their functions as directors of public health, or consultants in public health medicine, they may well continue to find themselves in conflict with general managers who, because they hold the purse strings, are bound to be the winners.

7. Into the twenty-first century

As the present century draws to a close, the problems faced by both United States and United Kingdom educational establishments, of preparing a cadre of individuals able to plan policies for the public health and secure their adoption and application, are indeed formidable.

Recent proposals for educational development in the United Kingdom suggest that the new schools there may, in future, come to resemble more closely the schools of public health in North America. These have been largely prompted by the need to defend public health perspectives against narrower concerns for the provision of facilities for the treatment of the acutely ill and the care of the chronically sick and disabled in the community. In the United States, the emphasis, at least in rhetoric, on health promotion and disease prevention provides a basis, which has been lacking in the past, for establishing a broad constituency in support of increasing resources devoted to public health and to the education of public health practitioners. In addition, the growing recognition of the need to determine the effectiveness and opportunity costs of therapeutic measures offers an opportunity to direct attention to their general effect on the health of communities as well as on the experience of individuals. Unless those responsible for public health keep their mission in high profile, the danger remains that, in both countries, the politicians' and the publics' crude perceptions of societal needs, combined with unfettered commercial interests, will continue to thwart the measures which could lead to a substantial improvement in the health of populations at local, national, and global levels.

[19] The government proposes that local government social workers rather than National Health Service public health workers should manage care in the community; see Department of Health and Social Security (1989). *Caring for People*. Her Majesty's Stationery Office, London.

It is salutary to remind ourselves that the state of the public health is dependent not primarily on the knowledge and skills of experts, whether or not they are trained in clinical medicine, but on the complex economic, social, cultural, legal, and political influences which govern the ways we produce, distribute, and consume resources, on the character of health risks and on the means of purposeful intervention. Nevertheless, unless there are experts with knowledge and dedication to the promotion of the public health perspective, the outlook for the year 2000 and beyond will be bleak indeed.

INDEX

DATE DUE

DEMCO 38-296